UNDERSTANDING SURGERY

A Comprehensive Guide for Every Family

by

JOEL A. BERMAN
M.D., F.A.C.S.

BRANDEN BOOKS
Boston

Library of Congress Cataloging-in-Publication Data

Berman, Joel A.
  Understanding surgery: a comprehensive guide for every family
  / by Joel A. Berman.
    p.cm.
  Includes bibliographical references and index.
  ISBN 0-8283-2061-6
  1. Surgery--Popular works.
  2. Surgery--History--Popular works.
  I. Title.

RD31.3.B47 2001
617--dc21
                2001018500

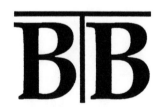

BRANDEN BOOKS
Division of Branden Publishing Co.
PO Box 812094
Wellesley, MA 02482

To My Wife Andrea

and

To The Memory of My Father

Leon G. Berman M.D., F.A.C.S.

A Skillful Surgeon, Compassionate Physician,
Teacher, Writer, Scholar,
and,
Eternal Student

ACKNOWLEDGMENTS

I deeply appreciate the efforts of Adolfo Caso of Branden Books for his belief in my ability to write this book as well as my first book, *Comprehensive Breast Care and Surviving Breast Cancer*; in today's publishing world, "It Ain't Easy To Get A Book Into Print!"

Although the writing of this book has been solely my effort, I have valued the comments and reviews of the following chapters by their respective specialists:

"Orthopedics" by Dr. Kenneth Kengla,
"Urology" by Dr. Melvin Novegrod,
"Gynecology" by Dr. Charles Moniak,
"Neurosurgery" by Dr. Abraham Rayhaun,
"Thoracic Surgery" by Dr. Santosh Mohanty,
"Cardiac Surgery" by Dr. Himmet Dajee,
"Plastic Surgery" by Dr. Malcolm Paul,
"Ophthalmic Surgery" by Dr. Mark Bronstein,
"Ear, Nose and Throat Surgery" by Dr. Douglas Tran,
"Pediatric Surgery" by Dr. Ali Kaviani.

The illustrations have been masterfully done by Faith and Adrian Van DeRee and I am indebted to them for their comments and reading of the manuscript. The cover design was done by Danny Berman.

Wanda Atkinson and Lena Bodnar have extended themselves in the secretarial work needed for this project. I also would like to express my appreciation to Marissa Saplala for typing and proofing the manuscript, and Quan M. Nguyen for providing computer expertise.

And finally, to my wife Andrea Berman, RN, OCN for her constant support and encouragement during the many months of writing this book, I am again eternally grateful.

Joel A. Berman
M.D., F.A.C.S.

The purpose of human life is to serve and
to show compassion and the will to help others.

Albert Schweitzer

CONTENTS

If you are curious about this book and want to know the facts,
But can't be bothered by information or reading between the cracks,
I've gotten together the subjects all arranged from A to Zed,
Which you can easily master even sleeping in your bed.
So if you think you'd like to know about this fable of nonsense,
You can open to this page and just peruse the table of contents.

PART I

PART II

A. **GENERAL SURGERY**

B. **VASCULAR SURGERY**

C. UROLOGIC SURGERY

D. ORTHOPEDIC SURGERY

E. GYNECOLOGICAL SURGERY

F. NEUROSURGERY (BRAIN AND SPINAL CORD)

G. THORACIC (CHEST) SURGERY

H. CARDIAC (HEART) SURGERY

I. PLASTIC AND RECONSTRUCTIVE SURGERY

J. OPHTHALMIC SURGERY (EYES)

K. OTO-RHINO-LARYNGOLOGY (EAR, NOSE AND THROAT)

L. PEDIATRIC SURGERY

DIAGRAMS

PART I

Chapter 1
INTRODUCTION

I sat one day in the library and looked at a surgical text,
It weighed too much, had rarely been used, and left me quite
perplexed.
Now why in heaven would anyone want to wade through all those
pages?
It seemed so dull, though I must admit, it was written by dozens of
sages.
So I said to myself, I know what I'll do, I'll write a book just plain
and simple
Explaining to every man, woman and child the art of removing a
pimple.
Surely a book about cutting and sewing would be to the layman's
liking,
As long as the words were quite simple, and the subject and writing
were striking.
So here is the tome that I've written for you, it's been more than a
minuscule chore.
And if when you're through, you don't like it, don't tell me, or I will
be hurt to the core.

The major texts of surgery, written for students and physicians, are usually upwards of two thousand pages and filled with complex medical vocabulary, and this makes it all but impossible for the layman to understand the procedures and the bases for surgical practice. It is my intent to give a simplified but comprehensive presentation of surgery for the general populace.

The objectives will be to offer information and guidance to patients and family about the most common surgical procedures, which physicians have often failed to make sufficiently clear to those they are treating.

This is not a textbook for surgeons or students, but a guide for all individuals who want to understand the basics of surgery. While the focus will be primarily on what is called general surgery, I will also include sections on the most common sub-specialties such as Vascular (dealing with blood vessels), Cardiac (heart surgery), Pediatrics, Orthopedics, Neurosurgery (Brain and spinal cord) and several others.

I am not interested in giving you only a reference text, but in presenting you with a pleasant read about the past, present and future of surgery, and hopefully in such a way that it is not just filed away on a shelf as a book only to be used when one has a surgical problem or question. A study of the human body, its function, failings and surgical correction can be fascinating, even exciting when set forth in the appropriate way. I hope this book will let you marvel at the beauty, the complexity and the ability of the human body to be repaired in the hands of the trained physician, and perhaps when you finish you may glean some of the fascination and excitement which I have found in my day in and day out experience as a practicing surgeon.

Chapter 2
HISTORY OF
SURGICAL PROCEDURES

When Will and Ariel Durant wrote their Story of Civilization
In thousands of pages and eleven large books, 'twas a massive publi-
cation
But using my art of brevity, I'll write this medical history, as I should,
And only use eight pages...cause, damn I'm really good!

L et us look through a mythical telescope back to the earliest days of creation and see what we can conjure up about the ability of primordial creatures to take care of themselves. Imagine some slimy thing crawling across the ocean floor, getting bitten by another slimy thing or somehow becoming injured. Our little creature had two outlooks, dying or somehow repairing the damage and surviving, albeit probably for a shorter period of time. Now we can postulate on how that repair took place, most assuredly without conscious understanding by Mr. Slime, either by secretion of some internal healing substance or by an instinctual reaction by the organism which caused it to repair the injury. Sound far-fetched? Well maybe, but this same process is going on millions and millions of years later throughout the animal kingdom of today. Creatures have some inherent ability to heal themselves without conscious awareness and this type of healing has led to the eventual development of present day medicine and surgery. Big step in reasoning, you may say. Possibly, but it leads us to that day millions of years ago when man first became able to reason even at the most fundamental level.

When a "lower" species was cut or injured, it depended on the body to heal itself. Blood flowed from a wound until the blood vessel went into spasm and allowed the coagulation system to form a clot. And one day a primordial humanoid found that he could stem the flow of blood by applying pressure to the bleeding site...and surgery was born! He then showed his discovery to his cohabitants who showed it to their offspring and so on through the ages.

The beast of the forest that injured itself and developed an abscess, somehow knew through instinct to chew upon the area until it opened and drained. Drainage even today is the treatment of an abscess or locked-in infection. But it took the conscious intellectual human mind to look at the abscess on a limb and know that it must be poked with a sharp stick in order to drain and allow him to survive.

And because man could not understand the reasoning behind his sickness he probably attributed it to spirits, spells (put upon him by other people, animals or demons), or the unknown and thereby began to perform incantations along with his early surgical and medical exploits. So, now let us put away this mythical scope and jump to the dawn of civilization. We know that in ancient Peru, France, and Britain, human skulls have been discovered which showed that trephining or trepanning was done, which consisted of making a one to three inch hole in the skull. This apparently allowed evil humors to get out and scientists examining the skulls say that the "patient" often lived long after the procedure! This practice may still exist among some primitive peoples of the world. So we can look at aboriginal or South American tribal cultures and possibly see what the prehistoric or primitive man used for healing. This included vegetable drugs, binding wounds and removing foreign objects (such as sticks or arrows!), and also included charms, talismans and incantations. A great deal of early medicine was done by the "medicine men" and witch doctors with much of the result being the effect of fear or belief, such as we see in placebo effects even today.

Now, in reviewing medical and surgical history, there are great gaps highlighted by the masters of each age, usually individuals who collected the history of medicine to that date and wrote it down as their own treatise. The progression of surgical care was very slow over the early millennia and over the last several centuries. To give you a brief background of historical highlights is to give you the names of the individuals who made these compilations in the early periods and to note the innovators and geniuses of the last five hundred years who made the sentinel achievements whereby medicine and surgery took giant steps forward.

Let us start with the invention of writing and the information found on clay tablets which we call the Code of Hammurabi, apparently written by a Babylonian king 3800 years ago. One such pillar tablet is preserved in the Louvre Museum in Paris and gives rules about treatment and also the punishment of physicians whose patients die in the course of treatment

- they would have their hands cut off! (Fortunately our rules are somewhat less severe today.) And in ancient Babylon, the sick were placed in the street for anyone to offer help or information about treatment (the first curbside consultations!). Sacrifice and incantation was a major part of medicine.

Moving on to ancient Egypt we find the name Imhotep, a chief minister of King Zoser, who not only designed the pyramid but was an early "healer" and became immortalized as the Egyptian God of Healing. The Edwin Smith and Ebers Papyri discovered in the eighteen hundreds, in Egypt, gave voluminous information about treatment, incantations, and notably a long treatise on the care of wounds and battle injuries.

In India we find ancient writings, two to four thousand years old, about a medical system called Ayurveda, mostly spiritual; this was followed from 800 B.C. through the first millennium A.D. by the more advanced ideas of two individuals, Caraka (an internist) and Susruta (a surgeon) with writings about wounds, tumors, and abscesses as well as medical diseases. The early Hindu surgeons drained abscesses, removed simple tumors and did crude treatment of fractures and sewing up of wounds.

In China, the culture extends back several thousand years with traditional Chinese Medicine and its dualistic theory of the Yin (female, dark and passive - the earth) and the Yang (male, light and active - the heavens) principles. The human body was made up of five elements (fire, water, earth, metal and wood) and these, with balances between yin and yang, determined health or illness. The Chinese described tying off (ligation) of arteries, the presence and importance of the pulse and said the body consisted of five organs: heart, lungs, liver, kidney and spleen. We all have heard about acupuncture; the Chinese also used hydrotherapy (i.e. cold baths for fever) and had a great pharmacopoeia of herbal medicines, many of which are still used today such as castor oil, camphor and iron for anemia.

Western Medicine progressed slowly over several thousand years from Early Greece with Asculapius slowly drifting away from the supernatural. By the fourth century B.C., Hippocrates, often called the father of medicine, had written his "Aphorisms" (the best known being the first: "Ars Longa, Vita Brevis - Art is long and life short") with many descriptions of observations and diagnosis, with only but the most basic in the way of surgical intervention. He left us the famous Hippocratic Oath, which has been stated by graduating medical students for many years. I include it for you to peruse since it is universally known about, but rarely seen.

"I swear by Apollo the Physician, and Asclepius, and Health and All-heal, and all the gods and goddesses...to reckon him who taught me this Art equally dear to me as my parents, to share my substance with him, and to relieve his necessities if required; to look upon his offspring in the same footing as my own brothers, and to teach them this art, if they shall wish to learn it, without fee or stipulation, and that by precept, lecture, and every other mode of instruction, I will impart a knowledge of the Art to my own sons, and to those of my teachers, and to disciples bound by a stipulation and oath according to the law of medicine, but to none others. I will follow that system of regimen which, according to my ability and judgment, I consider for the benefit of my patients, and abstain from whatever is deleterious and mischievous. I will give no deadly medicine to anyone if asked, nor suggest any such counsel; and in like manner I will not give to a woman a pessary to produce abortion... Into whatever houses I enter, I will go into them for the benefit of the sick, and will abstain from every voluntary act of mischief and corruption; and, further from the seduction of females and males, of freemen and slaves. Whatever, in connection with my professional practice or not in connection with it, I see or hear, in the life of men which ought not to be spoken of abroad, I will not divulge, as reckoning that all should be kept secret."

Another Greek, Galen, in the first century A.D. postulated an entire body of medicine, much of it false, which was to be followed, essentially unchallenged, for fifteen hundred years. He stressed the importance of anatomy but since dissection was forbidden, the anatomy of the day was often poorly conceived or completely in error.

The Muslim empire produced the genius of the Persian Rhazes, who wrote many texts and actually distinguished between measles and smallpox. He was later followed by another Persian, Avicenna, who wrote the "Canon of Medicine". But as much as these tomes expounded on diagnosis and medications, there was a surprising paucity of knowledge in the area of surgery.

You may ask "Why?" and the answer is actually quite simple. A good basis for surgery depends on a firm knowledge of accurate human anatomy, and up to this point dissections were carried out on animals or on parts of humans, and the anatomical knowledge was often based on centuries-old texts which were often incorrect or flights of fancy of the author. During the late fourteenth and fifteenth centuries new anatomy texts appeared and were much more complete than those we had seen for two thousand years. In 1543 Andreas Vesalius published his "De Humani Corporis Fabrica" (On The Structure of the Human Body) which was based on careful human dissection and the diagrams are for the most part as accurate as anatomical treatises of today. His work was followed by a host of books on anatomy and physiology and this may well be considered the beginning of modern surgery. Within the next one hundred years there was an explosion of scientific and cultural advancement with the likes of the genius of philosopher Rene Descartes ("I think, therefore I am."), Isaac Newton (Laws of Physics - remember the apple falling on his head?), Galileo (the telescope), Robert Hooke and Anton Leeuwen-hoek (the discovery and use of the microscope) and the great discovery and publication of "De Motu Cordis" on the circulation of blood and the function of the heart by William Harvey (1628).

Surgery then took great strides forward when the physician could understand the anatomy and some physiology, and attempt to correct its problems. Likewise, there were advances in the parallel field of medicine such as Edward Jenner's description of Smallpox inoculation in 1796, Johannes Muller's description of physiology or how things work in the 1830s, and the description of the bacterial cause of disease by Semmel-weiss (child bed fever - women dying of infection after being examined by physicians with dirty hands) and Robert Koch (who discovered the organism that causes tuberculosis).

The most famous contribution to surgery and its advancement came with the discovery of anesthesia by several individuals, Crawford Long and Horace Wells, and by William Morton who first demonstrated a painless operation at the Massachusetts General Hospital in 1846. Nitrous oxide, ether and chloroform became the drugs of choice and led to the advancement of more complex surgery. In the end of the nineteenth century, Conrad Roentgen's discovery of X-rays led to the opening of new horizons in the field of diagnostics.

With the twentieth century came the development of chemotherapy for syphilis, by Paul Ehrlich, followed soon by the discovery of Sulfonamide and the discovery and use of Penicillin, by Alexander Fleming in 1928, and its purification and widespread use at Oxford by Howard Florey and Ernest Chain, ten years later.

Liberated from the time-warped problems of pain, infection, and armed with a host of new techniques, surgery came of age in the twentieth century. I won't go into much detail about the advances, but suffice it to say that because of the two World Wars, medicine and surgery were "forced" to make great strides including immunological advances, and a whole host of support technologies including the invention of plastics and inert metals which could be used in surgery. Advances in technique which had been started during the last decade of the nineteenth century by such surgical giants as the Viennese Theodor Billroth (abdominal surgery, including ulcer surgery on the stomach), and William Halsted (the radical mastectomy), propelled surgery into the twentieth century and the development of neurosurgery by Harvey Cushing, and thoracic surgery (removal of part or all of a lung) by Harold Brunn, Rudolph Nissen and Evarts Graham. By 1944, John Garlock in New York City was able to successfully remove an entire esophagus for cancer using part of the colon as an interposition "graft". In the early 1920s and 30s surgeons began operating on the heart but successes were rare and true cardiac surgery didn't start until the 1940s, with the early development of extra-corporeal circulation, first in animals, then in humans by John Gibbon Jr. Soon it was possible to put the heart completely at rest, stopping the "beating", and allowing surgeons to remove and replace damaged heart valves and bypass blocked coronary arteries. Alexis Carrel had perfected the suturing of blood vessels back in 1905 and vascular surgery has made great strides since that time. This led to experimentation with organ transplantation and the victories over rejection with greater understanding of immunology and immunosuppression. In 1967 the world was made aware of the first heart transplant by Christian Barnard in South Africa, a procedure which has now become routine and standard at medical centers throughout the world.

This has been a very brief outline of four thousand years of medical and surgical history, and we should be happy that we live at a time when most of the pain and suffering of surgical intervention has been all but relieved. Let us move on now to understand more about the training that these physicians have in preparation for taking the patient into consultation and the scalpel in hand.

Chapter 3
EDUCATING THE SURGEON

In thirteen hundred and forty two
To become a doctor, there was little to do.
Climb a hill, raise your arms in a humble position
Yell once and dance and...you're a physician.

The training today is much more intense,
The course work is hard and it just makes no sense
To work all those years with no compensation,
And wondering when you will bring home the bacon.

The days are so long and rewards long in coming,
The work is quite hard and the hours are numbing.
The MD degree is just too hard to reach,
I think I'll just go be a bum on the beach.

Now I can imagine that most people don't give two hoots and a holler about the education of a surgeon, but I want to spend a little time on this subject so you know what the surgeon has gone through for the privilege of taking out your gall bladder, repairing your heart or removing your cancer. I have mentioned that the first doctors or "medicine men" were more connected with the "spiritual", using chants, incantations and "witchcraft", with folklore passing down from one individual to the next, the art of repairing fractures and treating wounds.

The education of the healer was through observation and a type of apprenticeship which lasted for centuries up until the development of great schools of learning. The first of these appeared in Salerno, Italy in the early 1200's, with the support of Holy Roman Emperor Frederick II. At the Salerno school, the physicians were taught how to fix hernias and fractures and performed amputations. For the most part, they were taught diagnosis for diseases, which they could do little about, and often prescribed rest, bathing or diet, or gave emetics (drugs to make people vomit), and frequently "bled" patients to remove evil humors. Their knowledge of narcotics allowed them to give opium for pain relief along with near toxic doses of alcohol.

In the Middle Ages great hospitals were established throughout Europe, usually affiliated with religious institutions such as abbeys, convents and monasteries and most of the physicians were religious personnel since they usually represented the major portion of the educated populace who could read during that period. Books were all hand written, making them rare and expensive and information about medicine and surgery if not passed down from person to person, could only be read by those who understood Latin (in which most books were written). The literate few during this period were the monks and other ecclesiastics, and healing was a combination of physical and spiritual modalities. Throughout this period childbirth and what we know as obstetrics today was practiced only by the midwives.

With the invention of the printing press and moveable type by Johannes Gutenberg and the first printing of the Bible in 1455, books became more available. The first forty-five years saw a tremendous upsurge in the writing and printing of books, called incunabulae (the first of anything is called an incunable) and these books often were printed to look like hand written manuscripts. With the massive increase in relatively cheap books, the populace became more literate and the universities and medical schools grew rapidly and were inviting, not just to the clergy, but to the many upper class individuals who, prior to this time had, for the most part, been unable to read. Great medical schools arose in Europe with major centers in Pisa, Leiden, Oxford, London and Edinburgh to name a few. By the seventeenth and eighteenth centuries regular curriculae for anatomy, physiology, pathology and pharmacology (the study of drugs) were established and the remaining specialties found their way into the medical schools over the subsequent two centuries.

In the United States a sentinel occurrence was the Flexner report in 1910, supported by the Carnegie Foundation for the advancement of Teaching. Flexner essentially took medical education out of the closet of mystery and outlined the need for trained full-time academic teachers in medical schools and emphasized the need for libraries, laboratories for anatomy and science, lecture rooms and access to a hospital where students could learn by being in contact with physicians treating "real" patients.

Now I won't bore you with more details about the history of the schools because I want to outline for you briefly the education of a physician and surgeon at the beginning of the twenty-first century. It is important to recognize that until that last quarter of the twentieth century, most medical students were male whereas now there is a significant percentage of women graduating with M.D. degrees.

The requirements for entering medical school vary slightly from college to college, but the basics are pretty much the same. Except for the rare program that combines undergraduate and medical school in a single facility for only six years to the M.D. degree, most undergraduate college students will be required to achieve a Bachelor of Arts or Science degree (B.A. or B.S.) and usually a good grade point average (A's and B's) and in the top ten percent of their graduating class or higher. This does not take into account the many programs established throughout the United States to help minorities get into medical school, and for many years special emphasis has been placed on recruiting African American, Native American and other minority groups to fill a noticeable cultural and ethnic gap in the physician force of today. Although the premedical courses may stress the inclusion of biology, physics, inorganic and organic chemistry, and zoology, the medical schools are also seeking well-rounded individuals with an additional knowledge of literature, history, English and philosophy. In addition to the grades of an applicant, the medical schools usually require recommendations from teachers and community leaders and a personal interview as well as the scores from the Medical College Admission Test. To all this I must add that many Medical Schools only accept 5% of the applicants and students may have to take further postgraduate studies or work in laboratories or hospitals to make their application "look better" before reapplying again. Getting into a medical school is only the first hurdle!

Most medical colleges have a four-year curriculum divided into two sections, the first two years being pre-clinical, namely the studying of the science of medicine, the last two years being the clinical years where the student learns by being in contact with patients and practicing physicians.

The first year the student is bombarded with a massive amount of information in embryology (about the development and formation of embryos), Gross Anatomy (which usually involves dissecting a human cadaver under the careful instruction and guidance of the professor, while memorizing all the parts!), Microscopic Anatomy (seeing what the tissue looks like under a microscope - i.e. brain cells, kidney cells, skin, bone),

Physiology (functions of the parts of the body - i.e. how a muscle works, why kidneys can excrete waste, how the stomach functions and produces acid), and Biochemistry (the study of the chemistry of life processes, i.e. how cortisone is produced, sex hormone production, thyroid function). And that's not all; the first year student also studies Cellular and Molecular Biology (how things work at the cellular level and even smaller, the molecular level), Neuroscience (the study of brain and spinal cord, and nerve anatomy and physiology), Genetics (the study of genes, heredity and variation) and then a broad introduction to medicine and society.

The students that complete the first year, (and who don't throw in their marbles and go into some other business) can look forward to the interesting second year and a whole new set of courses. These include Microbiology (the study of microorganisms like Staphylococcus and the germs that cause TB, or syphilis or a sore throat), Immunology (your body's defense system to help fight off disease), Nutrition, Pathology (the study of abnormal anatomy - i.e. cancer, pneumonia, diabetes mellitus) and Pharmacology (the study of all the drugs used today like digitalis, pain medicines and hormone replacements). Then there's Epidemiology (the study of the causes of disease), Introduction to Clinical Medicine (such as how to use a stethoscope to listen to the heart or lungs and how to use an otoscope to look into ears), Family Practice Introduction, and a course of behavioral sciences. Some programs also have lectures in Alternative and Complementary medicine (modalities including psychosocial interactions and the more unusual non-Western medical practices like acupuncture, diet therapy, meditation, etc.).

So, you've survived the first two years, somehow, and are then ready to see your first live patient. Quite a frightening experience for most young physicians-to-be! The last two years of medical school introduce you to the various specialties of medicine, (the surgical ones which we shall discuss in the next chapter). They are Medicine, General Surgery, Pediatrics, Obstetrics and Gynecology, Neurology and Neurosurgery, Ophthalmology (eyes), Psychiatry, Radiology, Orthopedics, Ear, Nose and Throat (Otorhinolaryngology), Anesthesia, Preventive Medicine, and Urology. Additional studies for the fourth year may include Prenatal Obstetrics, Ambulatory Surgery, Emergency Room Medicine, Geriatrics, and Primary Care.

And, you graduate and get your M.D. degrees to the sounds of "gaudeamus igitur" and all that stuff and usually someone reads the

Hippocratic Oath and now you're a doctor. Unfortunately, that's just the very basics and doesn't really prepare you for much because you haven't had enough clinical experience. Most United States medical students take the National Board Examinations before they get their degree and this helps them to get licenses in states other than where they went to medical school. But in most cases the new doctors go on to get further training in a specialty of their choice such as Family Practice, Emergency Room Medicine, Radiology, or a host of other interesting areas. We will discuss the surgical specialties in Chapter IV.

Oh! You might reflect on the fact that while you are sweating away in medical school, most of your college buddies are well established in some business, making a living and raising a family. (Some medical students are married, but it creates a great stress on the family and the husband or wife usually needs to support the student for many years.) It's a difficult period to go through and yet for the individual fascinated by medicine and intent on helping others, it never becomes tedious or boring. After these four years, the new physician may opt for additional training so that many doctors don't even start their own practices until they are almost thirty years old!

Chapter 4
INTRODUCTION
TO SURGICAL SPECIALTIES

When I was young in college, to feel good I had to lie,
To other guys who often seemed much cleverer than I
So I went off to med school, and determined I would find
A specialty that I could use to give me peace of mind.

And after four hard years I found my niche in general surgery
Where I could talk to patients and not be accused of perjury.
And when I meet old college pals (on benches in the park)
I can truly say I always have the final cutting remark.

When the physician has completed his studies for an M.D. degree, he may decide that he wants to go on into a surgical specialty. This will require him to enter into a postgraduate training program called a residency (sometimes including a first year called an internship) and may spend as many as six to eight more years expanding his knowledge and experience. He is generally taken on as a special resident physician at a university hospital, clinic, or private hospital and paid a meager salary during this period of time. Depending on the specialty, he may be on duty thirty six hours and off twelve hours including weekends or may just have an eight-hour day and be available for emergencies.

In Part II of this book, we will discuss the various specialties and each major procedure in more detail. At this time I just want to familiarize you with the main fields of surgery and outline for you the types of procedures they do.

First, and my own specialty, is general surgery. At one time about a hundred years ago, this encompassed all the areas of surgery and the general surgeon could handle all surgical procedures including the chest, heart, orthopedics and pediatrics. Over the years each specialty has advanced to the point where one individual cannot have an expertise in all areas and young surgeons have learned to choose which area is most interesting for them.

General Surgery encompasses Abdominal Surgery (stomach, intestines, colon, appendix and rectum, pancreas, liver, spleen, gallbladder and adhesions), skin, breast, thyroid, parathyroid, hemorrhoids, pilonidal disease, esophagus, hernias in the abdomen, abscesses, "Lumps and Bumps" and a diverse selection of cancers throughout the body. Although this is not a complete list, it includes most of the procedures which the practicing general surgeon does today. For this he is usually required to take an internship for one year and four to six years of residency training. In some programs, such as the one I went through, the resident does research in an area of his interest and may write a thesis and get a Masters of Science in Surgery Degree.

The second area I want to address is Peripheral Vascular Surgery. This usually requires a surgeon to take an additional one to two years of training after the general surgical residency although some comprehensive programs combine the general and vascular surgery in one training program. Vascular surgery includes suturing, repairing or replacing the major blood vessels of the body such as the Aorta in the chest and abdomen down to the smallest one millimeter vessels in the hands and feet which can be approached surgically. In the arms and legs, the arteries are considered medium sized and are much more amenable to repair than the tiny vessels of the hands and feet. Vascular surgeons are the ones who sew arteries and veins together for use during dialysis for kidney failure, and place all kinds of artificial shunts and bypasses, either to get around blocked vessels or for dialysis access as we will explain in a later chapter. This specialty also corrects problems of the carotid artery (which supplies blood to the brain - narrowing may cause a stroke), renal (kidney) arteries (narrowing of which may cause hypertension (high blood pressure), and vein problems (varicose veins and venous ulcers). The most recent advances in vascular procedures are in the field of endovascular surgery, where a trained specialist can repair an artery using balloons and special devices placed in the damaged arteries through tiny incisions, obviating the need for major vascular surgery.

Urology is the surgical sub-specialty which includes Kidney, Ureters, Bladder, Prostate, Testicles and internal and external Genitalia. In this field we have the kidney, ureteral and bladder stones, prostate enlargement and various types of cancers specific to this area.

Orthopedics (which literally means "straighten the child"), is the medical and surgical treatment of bones and joints including the spine (which is shared with the neurosurgeons) and all types of trauma involving the bones and joints. They handle back pain and joint pain, amputations and endoscopic surgery on the joints. Some orthopedists go on to further specialize in complex back and spinal surgery or hand surgery including procedures which require microsurgery (using special magnifying lenses to repair tiny vessels in the hand). A whole field of reimplantation surgery has developed for severed limbs which requires further expertise and training.

Gynecological surgery centers on the female reproductive organs, the vagina, cervix, uterus, tubes and ovaries, including hysterectomy (removal of the uterus), salpingectomy (removal of the fallopian tubes) and oophorectomy (removal of the ovary). These surgeons also may do diagnostic or therapeutic laparoscopy (using small incision and placing a small camera in the abdomen to avoid large incisions) such as tubal ligation, or identification of pelvic infections or other problems. A whole advanced field of Gynecologic Oncology has developed requiring two to four additional years of training to learn how to remove all cancers involving female organs.

Next we move on to Neurosurgery, which is the specialty focusing on diseases involving the brain, spinal cord and nerves. It requires two years of additional training after the general surgery residency and the neurosurgeon must be well versed in the diagnostic abilities of a neurologist to identify the problems in brain function. We will go much more into detail about neurosurgery in later chapters.

Thoracic surgeons, not surprisingly, operate on the thorax or chest cavity which includes the esophagus, lungs, ribs and chest wall. They remove lung cancer and other tumors, benign and malignant, and do surgical procedures for infections in the chest called empyemas and lung collapse secondary to trauma or emphysema (a disease where the lungs contain abnormal air pockets that may rupture).

The Cardiac surgeons operate on the heart, replacing heart valves that are diseased and bypassing coronary arteries (the blood vessels that supply the heart itself). They also may surgically correct congenital deformities, although pediatric (children) heart surgery is a sub-specialty all its own. Cardiac surgeons usually require a two year fellowship in addition to the regular surgery residency.

Plastic and Reconstructive surgeons take several years training in their specialty to do cosmetic surgical procedures such as breast augmentation and reduction, facial plastic procedures (face lift, brow lifts, rhinoplasty [nose job], and acid and laser skin peels), liposuction, and abdominoplasty. They also do reconstructive surgery after trauma, congenital defects, breast reconstruction after mastectomy, and complex skin grafts and "flap" procedures which I will explain later and which include Tram flaps, Pedicle flaps and Rotation flaps.

The Ophthalmologists, in addition to the medical management and examination of the eyes, also perform the delicate and often complex procedures including cataracts, retinal and eye muscle surgery, trauma and the new laser and LASIK procedures.

The Otorhinolaryngologists must learn to pronounce their specialty first and then learn how to take care of problems involving the ears, nose and throat including sinuses, parotid gland, tongue, tonsils and adenoids, and facial nerve, and have special training in removing cancers in this area.

Pediatric surgery emphasizes that children are not just little adults and have special problems all their own. They have a host of congenital deformities as well as the usual problems of hernia and appendicitis, and these specialists are specially trained to handle the delicate management of tiny infants.

In Part II of this book we will discuss these surgical specialties and their procedures including the diagnostics, anatomy, techniques and complications.

Chapter 5
THE SURGEON'S OFFICE

My surgeon has an office on the ocean in a barge.
The place is kinda dirty, the reception room is large.
He doesn't have a license, but he has a lot of saline,
He says it's from the ocean, he collects it when he whaling.
He's not too highly skilled, and his hands are quite a fright,
But hey, you can't have everything, and wow...his price is right!

When I asked my office manager to list what she considered most important about an office, she gave the following comments. First she stressed location and that included parking. If you're sick and not feeling well or if you've had surgery, you don't want to have to travel a long way to see your doctor and then not be able to find parking. Simple but important!

Next, when you walk into someone's home, one glance will give you a good idea as to whether the person is well organized or not. Similarly, when you walk into an office you should get a feeling of professional organization, with decent lighting, seating and tasteful decorations. If the doctor and his staff don't care enough to take an interest in the details of his office, it may reflect on how he will take care of you! The office should be clean and orderly. Now this doesn't mean it has to be expensively decorated and super-high tech; many physicians can't afford this. But it should reflect a care and concern about presenting a good face to the public.

Another point brought up was that this office should have personnel who appear pleasant and happy with their jobs and surroundings. Disgruntled staff may reflect poorly on the "boss" and in a setting where tests are ordered and surgeries are scheduled, job dissatisfaction can lead to mistakes and unpleasantness. The patient is usually not ecstatic about going to see the doctor, and to have to put up with moody or cheerless staff is unacceptable. The staff should be polite, helpful, efficient and knowledgeable. Though it sounds banal, YOU are the customer and should be treated well whether you are the CEO of a major corporation, an unemployed day worker, or a single mom with kids in tow.

The last point my office manager stated was that the office personnel should know their business. They should know about disability and health insurance and be able to answer questions to make you feel "okay" about your upcoming surgery arrangements or about problems you are having after a procedure. The office staff are the doctor's up-front representatives and their failure to be polite on the phone or in person is unacceptable.

I have seen some doctors who routinely keep patients waiting several hours for appointments and I don't understand why patients tolerate this. Of course there will be times when unscheduled surgeries or emergencies arise, and I always call my office to let the patients know. They can wait or reschedule as may be the case. When I return to the office, I always personally apologize to any waiting patients and give a brief explanation for my tardiness. Common courtesy is often forgotten by busy physicians and is not excusable!

Now, I wanted to present this chapter for two reasons. First, to let you know what goes on in the doctor's office (what you see and don't see) and second, to give you my own ideas as to what should be the rule of thumb in taking care of the needs of patients.

Most surgeons' offices are located near a hospital complex so that if any problems or emergencies arise with patients, the doctor will be immediately available and can call for assistance if needed. Different surgeons have different types of facilities in their own office, in some instances complete operating suites, or maybe just the ability to remove small lumps and bumps. This necessitates either disposable instruments or a sterilization unit. Many physicians find it easier to take their work to a nearby emergency room, outpatient surgical center or hospital and not have to concern themselves with the problems of maintaining a sterile operating facility. Nevertheless, all surgeons have the equipment and instruments needed to remove sutures and skin staples, remove drains and change dressings. Most also have needles and syringes to do local biopsies, give injections and aspirate fluids or blood samples. They will have appropriate facilities for disposing toxic waste materials and the offices are checked by OSHA which is a governmental agency inspecting for cleanliness and safety provisions. In today's world of serious infections and AIDS, patients deserve to know that the office they are in is safe as well as comfortable.

I think it is important for any physician to have some type of reference library, either consisting of books, journals or computer access to information in dealing with day to day problems and to keep up to date with advances. Many hospitals have excellent medical libraries with librarians available to do searches for physicians on any topics. Affiliation with regional medical centers or university centers and teaching hospitals will assure the interested physician a place for continuing medical education as well as additional consultation.

Now why do I mention these things? Merely because medicine is a never-ending educational experience and if your physician is not on the "cutting edge" of the newest advances, he's soon relegated to the "glue factory" because you shouldn't and won't seek out his opinion and care. When you look for a surgeon, keep these factors in mind and don't be shy about asking questions about the office if you are interested. Proximity to a hospital and a source for continuing education is important.

The doctor's consultation room should be comfortable and private and the patient should be able to sit and talk if he or she wishes. Understandably, in some high volume clinic situations this may not be possible, but at any time you should be able to say that you want to talk about the proposed test and procedure, and have your questions answered to your satisfaction. You're not buying a car or a house; it's your body we're talking about!

We will talk more about the physician-patient interaction in Chapter 10.

Chapter 6
THE OPERATING ROOM

Somewhere between joy and doom,
Lies the operating room.
Many people daily work there,
And some nurses go berserk there.

And in this place of fact and fable,
Stands the operating table,
Where the surgeons work their wiles
With sharpened blades and sneaky smiles.

So if you've made the big decision,
(Watching shows on television)
To have your hernia fixed tomorrow
Go to the hospital without a sorrow.

But be sure to know that factor:
That your surgeon ain't an actor!

I n my book *Comprehensive Breast Care*, there is an excellent chapter by one of the operating room nurses called "The Masked Strangers", in which she artfully describes the various people you will meet and the functions they provide. Suffice it to say that you will encounter a number of "masked strangers" in the surgical suite. From the attendant who will transport you to the surgical department dressed in his "scrub suit", you will be introduced to the "holding room" nurse who will answer any questions you may have. She will make sure your laboratory work, chest x-ray and electrocardiogram are in order, and will assemble all the paperwork including the history and physical examination, and make sure the consent is properly written and signed. We don't want to take off the wrong leg or fix the wrong cataract! You will also meet the anesthesiologist who will be giving you the anesthetic agent that you--your surgeon and he, have decided upon. He usually starts your I.V.

(intravenous lines) for giving fluids and medicines and will reassure you about any questions you may have, especially if you are going to sleep. We will talk more about the anesthesiologist in Chapter 21.

You will then meet another nurse who will work with the holding area nurse and accompany you with the anesthesiologist to the operating suite (or room if it's not fancy!) where you will meet a scrub nurse or technician. During the procedure, the scrub nurse, in sterile gown and gloves, will be handing the instruments to the surgeon and the other nurse, the circulating nurse, will be available to get any needed supplies in or outside the room while you are asleep. The nurse and the anesthesiologist will attach blood pressure and cardiac monitors to you before you are put to sleep and once you are sleeping may do other procedures to monitor your vital functions. These might include placing a tube in your stomach (an NG or nasogastric tube), your bladder (a Foley catheter) or a central venous or arterial line (placed in a vein or artery, respectively). Often these tubes are removed before you wake up, but usually your doctor will tell you if he plans on leaving any in place after you have awakened so it won't be a total surprise.

After the surgery is completed, you will be brought to the recovery room where a specialist nurse will take care of you for about an hour until you are stable enough to go back to your room. Again, I would recommend your reading Carol Metcalfe's chapter on the "Operating Room Nurse" for her comprehensive and often amusing insights.

But let us consider when and why we use a hospital based operating room as opposed to office surgery, an outpatient surgical center, or the emergency room. The hospital may be the only fully equipped facility in your community or it may be the only one fully accredited for use by your insurance company. But aside from these issues, the acuity and severity of the surgery will often determine where it should be done. Whereas small procedures such as removing moles and simple biopsies may be done in a well-equipped emergency room with a local anesthetic, hernias will need more anesthesia and a larger number of instruments and will need a regular operating room such as in a hospital or surgical center. Understandably, there may be some cases such as hernias which can be done in either facility and this may be done according to surgeon, insurance or patient preference. The hospital operating room is the place for major surgeries where the patient may be staying overnight or where there is the potential need for services only available in the hospital. Should any problems or unforeseen complications arise, it's important to have a full staff of trained experts to take care of the problem. Obviously brain and heart surgery and complex intestinal surgery must be done in a hospital setting. There are also some procedures, as we will see later in this book, which require very expensive, high-tech equipment that are only found in hospitals.

All operating rooms are subject to strict quality controls and must have constant checks on sterility and equipment, and the quality control is often a point for competitiveness among the hospital suppliers. If suture material is breaking or stapling machines for intestines are not working well, a competitor will immediately fill in the void with a better instrument or suture. Competition often breeds better quality. Hospitals and surgical centers have committees overseeing every aspect of medical care to bring the possibility of error or malfunction as close to zero as possible. True, mistakes are occasionally made, but most of the time they are very minor and do not impact patient health or safety. In choosing your site for surgery, you can check out its safety record and its relative scoring with an agency called The Joint Commission on the Accreditation of Hospitals. If the facility to which you have been recommended has scored poorly or has a problem with accreditation...go elsewhere. There are many fine institutions. Go where you feel safe and comfortable!

Chapter 7
OUTPATIENT SURGICAL CENTER

Hey, you need a surgery and want it done real quick
Like takin out a bullet or a knife that made ya sick?
Well come on over to my place, behind Gilhooly's bar
My private surgicenter is a souped up ragtop car.

I wantcha to be paying for the service with small bills
And I can get ya any kind a mainline stuff or pills
I use a knife that's pretty clean, I cut you while I drive,
And I can vouch, some of my patients, dey is still alive.

Over the past decade surgical centers have been popping up all over the United States. They are the alternative to in-hospital operating rooms when a patient needs more than a minor procedure and will require general anesthesia or anesthesia standby. The operating rooms are much the same as those found in hospitals, offering full nursing facilities and pre operative, intra operative and post operative care. The patients usually stay for only a few hours and then have a relative or friend take them home since they will have been sedated to some degree. Some Surgical Centers actually have facilities to keep patients overnight for observation. Frequently the outpatient surgical center is near a hospital so that patients who have problems during surgery or the recovery phase, can be transferred to the hospital for overnight observation or more specialized care.

In today's world of cost control, many insurance companies prefer to have less serious surgeries done in the outpatient center because the cost is less and the greater requirements for hospitalization do not have to be met or are less stringent. Still, history and physical exams are required and sometimes basic laboratory work, chest x-rays and EKGs may be needed. Most surgical centers can arrange for a pathologist to be on hand for doing frozen sections (quick stains for evaluating tissue) when a surgeon wants to remove a skin cancer and needs pathological confirmation that all the margins are clear of tumor!

The typical outpatient center has a waiting room for family, a dressing room and a preoperative area where a nurse takes a brief history, an intravenous line is started and you have a consultation with the anesthesiologist. (He may call you at home the night before and answer your questions and remind you not to eat anything after midnight). You are then taken to the operating room, your procedure is done and then you go to a recovery area where you remain at least an hour or until you are stable enough to go home. A nurse will usually help you into the vehicle and give care instructions to your family or friends who are driving.

All in all, the Outpatient surgical center is often more convenient for patients because there are not as many patients in the admitting area as in a hospital and you probably receive more individual attention, purely on the basis of numbers; fewer patients allow the nurses to spend more time with you both before and after surgery. Also, because the acuity and seriousness of the procedures are often much less than in a hospital, the atmosphere is usually more relaxed and thereby more comfortable.

If you are in need of minor surgery such as hernia repair, breast biopsy, removal of small skin problems or minor orthopedic or podiatric (foot surgery) procedures, you may want to consider an outpatient surgical center.

Chapter 8
THE EMERGENCY ROOM

If you have a touch of plague or meet up with a missile,
Or if your two year old has swallowed his brand new plastic whistle,
There is a place that's waiting for your rendezvous with doom...
It's your friendly, local, understaffed... Emergency Room.

The physicians are all dedicated to serve and save humanity
With nurses who are unafraid of squalor and profanity.
And if you have a mother-in-law who's getting on your nerves,
Give her a dose of poison and then call up the reserves.

As long as you can show the world you cared to send for aid,
No one will even ask you why the old bag swallowed Raid.
Just tell the friendly E.R. Doc, old mum was suicidal,
Give him one hundred bucks and he won't call it homicidal!

As recently as twenty years ago anyone with an M.D. degree could apply for and usually get a job working in an emergency room. It was generally a low paying thankless job that few physicians wanted and it was often manned by licensed physicians who were in the residency training and needed the extra money. Now, most of these physicians were adequate but there was also a whole host of physicians and "new M.D." graduates who worked in the Emergency Room to augment their income and sometimes these physicians were not well enough trained to manage the more severe problems that presented themselves at the E.R. doors.

Today we are in a new century and Emergency Rooms have kept pace with all other areas of medicine. For the most part, physicians working there are highly trained specialists who have taken an accredited three or four year residency in emergency medicine and most of the programs have trauma center experience. When you arrive at a major emergency room you can be assured that the staff can expertly handle all types of medical problems, including pediatric emergencies, heart attacks, trauma, lacerations and gunshot wounds as well as colds, asthma, flu, back aches and broken bones. It's a whole different world today and the quality of care has taken a giant step forward.

All major emergency rooms are required to have an on-call panel of specialists who can take over in their specialty after the patient has been seen, evaluated and at least temporarily stabilized by the E.R. physician. These usually include primary care physicians, pediatricians, general and vascular surgeons, cardiologists and cardiac surgeons, neurologists and neurosurgeons, psychiatrists, ear, nose and throat specialists, eye doctors and orthopedists. These physicians usually have to be available to arrive at the hospital within thirty minutes of being called. Frequently the emergency patient may be uninsured or minimally insured, and the physicians who take "all comers" are usually donating a significant amount of their time and service "gratis" to the indigent and needy, and should be commended for this.

It is important for the public to realize that the emergency room is not a clinic to be used because it is convenient. If patients have minor problems, they should contact their own physicians during the day rather than crowd an already overused system with common colds and minor problems in the middle of the night, that could wait till morning and be seen by a family physician or general practitioner.

Frequently, when the place is very busy, the nurse in the waiting room will use a triage selection system to bring the sickest patients in first. This sometimes leaves those bypassed very angry and complaining because they often do not see the urgency of the patient who is taken before them. Obviously a patient with a heart attack in progress or a stroke needs to be seen immediately as a life saving measure, and similarly patients who are bleeding or having difficulty breathing, as with severe asthma, must be attended to as soon as possible. So the E.R. physician pleads for understanding and patience from the public.

The emergency room is also the "dumping ground" for the obstreperous, obnoxious and sometimes dangerous patient who has overdosed on illegal or legal drugs and the alcoholic with one of the many complicating problems of acute alcoholism. These patients are often very difficult to manage and try the most patient, considerate nurses and doctors.

Another use for some emergency rooms is as a minor surgery site. Many physicians, especially those who work in the hospital all day, find it more convenient to meet their patients in the emergency room for giving injections, taking blood, doing spinal taps, removing small skin lesions or checking on problems with surgical wounds. Frequently I will ask a patient with a problem to meet me in the emergency room so I can evaluate the condition and have the option to run more tests, admit the patient or send the patient home.

So, if you need to visit your local emergency room, be aware that these doctors and nurses are highly trained and able to help you, but they also have a job which can at times be stressful, difficult and tiring and they need your understanding too!

Chapter 9
THE PREOPERATIVE WORKUP

I've fallen in love with Betty, the gorgeous pre-op nurse,
I keep on having surgeries, so we can just converse.
I've had three hundred blood tests and forty EKGs,
And had 600 x-rays from my tonsils to my knees.

I think that Betty knows me now, but how shall I explain
The reason I keep coming back, perhaps she'll think I'm vain.
I think I'll have a heart transplant, and then I'll have a chance.
If I give her my own heart, she'll know it's true romance.

Surgery is obviously a stress on the human system. Not only the emotional anxiety of going through a procedure or worrying about whether you have some severe problem that's correctable, but also the physical impact. This type of stress from the anesthesia to the actual surgery itself can be anticipated by your doctor, and to evaluate the situation, he will perform certain tests in the days before you go for your surgery.

The first preoperative workup is the history and physical exam. Sometimes most of the workup has been done by your primary care doctor and this has been relayed to the surgeon. Nevertheless, between the two of them a complete history and physical must be done. Briefly this consists of a description of the present illness ("I have a pain, or a lump or a hernia"), the length of duration and/or how it happened. There must be a past history including allergies, medications you are taking, previous surgeries such as breast biopsies, hernias, hysterectomy, heart transplants and complications or drug reactions, and a list of all your medical problems, such as heart disease, diabetes mellitus, high blood pressure, and AIDS. Note must be made of your social history (married, single, divorced, widow, children, significant other), whether you smoke and how much alcohol you drink. A review of systems is included which consists of questions about general health, cardio-respiratory system (heart and lungs - i.e. shortness of breath, chest pains, palpitations, coughing up blood), gastrointestinal system (such as nausea, vomiting, constipation, diarrhea, vomiting up blood, black or bloody stools, ulcer history) and genitourinary system (problems with the kidneys, ureters, bladder or other genitalia). This review also includes a gynecological history for women including age at first menarche (menstrual period), age at first pregnancy, whether you're still having periods and their regularity, age of menopause (when you stopped having periods), and whether you're taking birth control or hormones. Then there are questions about neurological (nerve problems) and psychiatric history, as well as any orthopedic and skin problems.

By then your physician should have a pretty good history about your risks and this will be followed by a complete physical examination. Naturally, a specialist such as a heart doctor, urologist or gynecologist will tend to focus more on his/her area of expertise, but a brief physical exam is always needed. This will include a general description of you (young, elderly, weak, in pain, thin, obese, etc.) followed by an exam of the head, eyes, ears, nose, mouth and throat. Then the neck exam is done, looking for stiffness, lymph nodes, thyroid gland enlargement and abnormal sounds from your carotid arteries which supply the brain. General examinations of the chest, breasts of both men and women, lungs, and heart sounds are done, followed by abdominal and flank exams for tenderness, masses, and hernias, to name a few.

A woman should have a regular gynecological exam every year after age 21 and males should have a testicular and rectal exam by their family doctor every year. A limited exam of the arteries and veins in the arms and legs, and a neurological evaluation is recommended. The examining physician will also want to give his impression of the patient from an emotional and psychiatric point of view, to help in alleviating fears and misunderstandings. The physician must be sure that the patient comprehends what is being said and the nature of the surgery that is going to be performed.

This is a brief list of what is expected in a history and physical examination, and it should be completed to some degree before a patient has any major surgery.

Obviously if someone is going to have a minor procedure such as a lymph node biopsy or removal of a skin tumor under local anesthesia, the physical may not need to be as comprehensive at the time of the surgery. But everyone needs a good, complete H&P (History and Physical) on a regular basis (every 1-3 years).

Okay. So now that's done. Next, the doctor will need to order some special studies to help in assessing your physical condition and risk for surgery and to further evaluate a condition which he has already diagnosed. I will list a few of the more common studies: Chest x-ray, electrocardiogram (EKG = heart evaluation), and a series of blood tests among which may be CBC which means a complete blood count including hematocrit and hemoglobin, to determine how much blood you have and whether you have been secretly bleeding. There are the electrolytes, Na (Sodium), K (Potassium), Cl (Chloride) and CO_2 (carbon dioxide), these are measures of the chemistry of the blood and can tell a lot about the status of your health. Blood sugar is measured to determine if you have diabetes mellitus, BUN or blood urea nitrogen and Creatinine to evaluate kidney function, and the clotting factors PT or protime, PTT, partial thromboplastin time and platelet count, a measure of how well your blood clots. Another study is the urinalysis checking for problems with the kidneys and infections in the urine. These are the basics, but there are a myriad of other blood and urine tests your doctor may order. You can ask him about these and how they apply to your specific problem.

The pre-op tests may cause the surgeon to delay your surgery until certain things have been corrected or rechecked. I always say that when a blood test comes back very abnormal and doesn't make sense...repeat the test! If your EKG is abnormal, you may be referred to a cardiologist for further studies including a stress test where you walk on a moving platform while your heart function is monitored to evaluate for coronary artery problems. This, in turn, may lead to the need for coronary angiography which is an x-ray with dye of the arteries to your heart.

An abnormal chest x-ray may lead to getting a CAT scan, or computerized axial tomography of your chest to rule out cancer, tuberculosis or other problems.

Be aware that as we increase in age, the chance for abnormalities in the preoperative workup also increases and your physician may need further studies to get you cleared for surgery.

This brings up one further issue. If the surgery is an emergency, then obviously it cannot be delayed by laboratory values, but these values will help the doctor to correct problems just prior to or during the surgery itself. If the surgery is elective (does not have to be done NOW!), then the patient should be made as healthy as possible before being brought to the operating room. This means that your surgeon must use common medical sense and never rush anyone into elective surgery without a proper workup.

Sometimes the patient is such a poor surgical risk, that alternative and second best options for treatment must be considered. The adage "The operation was a success but the patient died" is a hard one to explain to a family and for the surgeon to explain to himself.

That is the preoperative workup in a nutshell. Arranging for these studies, getting them done, evaluating them and getting surgery scheduled appropriately takes time and usually involves multiple phone calls by an office staff person. And this doesn't include the ins and outs of getting permission from an insurance company or a managed care group. Multiply this situation by ten or twenty in a surgeon's office, and you will understand why getting a surgery scheduled may not be as easy as it seems. Be patient and understanding...eventually everything will get done safely and completely.

Chapter 10
TALKING TO YOUR SURGEON
Second Opinions, Credentials and Qualifications

You can bet your britches, and I can bet mine too,
That if you become a surgeon, you may rue the day you do.
'Cause every time you do a case someone will go inspect
The whole shebang to see if you have done the thing correct.

I mean, does every workman and contractor have to prove
That every corner done has just a perfect tongue in groove.
So what if you forget to tie a vessel off or two?
Why should everyone come out and point a thumb at you?

In what other profession do we ask for 100 percent?
Why can't these stringent rules, just a little bit, be bent.
Then I could advertise in public and the daily press.
I'm a real surgeon and guarantee 80% success.

Now if you were in school an 80% would be a solid B
Enough to get you by with some respectability.
Unfortunately with surgeons, it doesn't work that way,
Everyone expects you, to always have an A.

Your kindly family doctor, Dr. Noodledorf, examines you and tells you that you have a hernia and recommends that you have it repaired. He refers you to Dr. McGillicutty who is in the suite next door so you make an appointment to see him and discuss the situation. Now, if you have been a patient of Dr. Noodledorf's for twenty years and have a high regard for him professionally, you may say to yourself: "Hmm. If my doctor recommends this guy, he must be good", and you may well be right in assuming so. But let me advise you about surgeons so that you can make your own informed decision.

Although not trained specifically in surgery, every physician who graduates from medical school has a license which lists him as a physician and surgeon. In other words, anyone is potentially able to do surgery legally. Of course one wouldn't be able to get privileges in any reputable hospital or surgical center without proper credentials, but anyone can do just about anything in his own office. So, beware and look for the training and credentials and be sure your surgeon is indeed a trained surgeon. He should have gone through an accredited residency program in that type of surgery in which he specializes and this usually means completing the senior residency or chief residency. Then he should be eligible for or have passed the specialty boards in his specialty such as general surgery, orthopedics, neurosurgery, etc. Board Certification is something all physicians are proud of and they usually have "board certified" on their business cards and the certificate is usually displayed in their office. Look for it or ask the secretary about board certification if you want to be sure. It's your one guarantee that the individual has met a least the minimal requirements of the National Specialty Board for practicing his profession.

Next, you should get a general impression from others who may know the community and ask about this surgeon. But be aware that this can be dangerous in both directions. I know a very poorly trained surgeon who has a very good bedside manner. He has more complications than most of his colleagues, but the problems are overlooked by the patients because his personality is so charming. Conversely, I also know another surgeon who is well-trained and highly competent who is very abrupt with patients and has a poor bedside manner. These are obviously the extremes, but I bid you take caution that you get a well trained, competent surgeon; comments from former patients may not give you the entire story. Do your homework, ask nurses or other doctors and you may get a better idea with whom you're dealing. And remember, almost every doctor has lawsuits. The number may reflect how busy he is, the type of surgery he does or the location in which he is working. Sometimes doctors are sued for nonsense reasons and yet it's cheaper for their malpractice insurance carrier to settle the case for twenty or thirty thousand dollars rather then put up a defense which may cost twice that amount. And I have known excellent surgeons who have been sued and lost cases when nothing was done outside the standard of practice. The legal system sometimes fails, as we have seen in a recent well publicized murder trial. No one can predict the behavior of a jury, especially when someone has suffered pain or severe illness, whether or not the surgeon is responsible for doing something wrong. The general impression is that the suffering patient needs to be compensated and a scapegoat is sought. There are many cases where the physician has done grievous harm and yet the case is thrown out for some nonsensical legal reason. It works both ways.

You might want to look at what a surgeon does in the way of education, lecturing, and what positions he holds in the medical community. How is he regarded by his colleagues? Has he been a chief of surgery or given lectures on some area of his specialty? Most specialties have a highly respected College of that specialty; in general surgery, it is the American College of Surgeons. The Surgeon who has been evaluated by this college and accepted into its ranks has the right to use F.A.C.S after his name (Fellow of the American College of Surgeons). There are colleges in several countries and many foreign physicians have several credentials you should look at. Conversely, there are several initials which can essentially be "bought" and placed after your name just by receiving an application and sending in your membership fee. Be careful what you accept as legitimate credentials!

You should always ask your surgeon what his qualifications are and how often he has done the proposed procedure. There are some cases which I do every week such as gall bladder or appendectomy surgeries, and then there are some that I may only do once a month such as thyroid or stomach. And yet I have been well trained to handle these procedures. I have probably done five hundred to a thousand gall bladder procedures over thirty years, and far fewer thyroids. And yet I feel equally qualified to handle each one. If I only did one thyroid a year and only two gallbladders a year, I would probably be less qualified, but depending on my training, my ability and my overall competence, I may be very able to do each of those procedures well. So choosing a surgeon is not an easy matter and a number of factors must be weighed carefully.

In summary, the strongest basic recommendations I would make are: (1) A completed residency program, (2) Board Certification by the American Board of that Specialty, (3) Fellowship in the American College of that specialty, and then take into consideration all the other factors I have mentioned.

To get onto another topic, I want to talk briefly about Second Opinions. In today's world with patients much more informed, especially with the Internet availability, the surgeon will be asked more questions and the patients will demand more information and answers. Remember that the Internet information is not screened and edited by experts and a lot of what you see may not be "the truth and nothing but the truth". Don't believe everything you read. Often it takes a physician to clarify medical situations to you and you shouldn't be afraid to ask about conflicting information. Some patients always want a second opinion and that too is a double-edged sword. First, a patient may ask around until he or she receives the answer that is wanted, whether it is the best medicine or not. I have seen some surgeons undermine the opinion of another just to get the business of a patient (sounds bad and is bad - people are sometimes greedy and unethical).

When seeking a second opinion, if the recommendation is very different, maybe you need a third opinion to straighten out the confusion. I always tell my patients to seek out second opinions if they wish but I also give them some guidance as to where to go. I select a few prominent surgeons in the community and then also offer the names of large teaching hospitals and medical centers, which may be in your area - names like City of Hope, The Mayo Clinic, Scripps Clinic, Norris Cancer Center at USC, etc. This will protect the surgeon as well as the patient, and if your patient comes back, he/she will be more comfortable with the surgeon's recommendations in the future.

In conclusion, I recognize that there are many confusing areas in this presentation. Suffice it to say that it is important to do your homework, follow the guidelines I have given, and then you will have the best chance of being satisfied with the surgeon and with the surgical outcome.

Chapter 11
POSTOPERATIVE CARE

You've had your operation; now please get up and go.
This ain't a never-ending cheerful horse and pony show.
I've done my job, you've got your pills, so will you please be fair,
Get dressed, and say goodby, good luck; just get out of my hair.

When you go shopping for a car, you take your car and drive,
That's just the kind of action that a patient should derive.
Take your body, leave the body parts that I excised.
And scram, be happy you got out in one piece and alive.

Does that sound like your surgeon? (I'll clue you - you've got the wrong guy!) There is an expression we use in the profession called "the itinerant surgeon". Basically he is the guy who "cuts" and runs. It probably evolved at the time when the surgeon was the only trained guy for many miles around and would go from town to town plying his craft, and then leaving the patients in the care of a primary physician or a skilled nurse. If problems or complications arose, the follow-up personnel would have to handle them, sometimes with disastrous or even fatal outcomes!

Today's surgeon is expected to follow up on each of his cases himself or else sign out to a qualified partner or colleague who can handle any problem that might arise, and do it with about the same skill as the operating surgeon. In most cases this holds true, but there are some surgeons who are only interested in the "surgical case" and disappear after it is completed. I know a heart surgeon who is very busy and after he finishes each case, he leaves the follow-up care to any other doctor on the case. Now he is responsible enough to have a skilled backup person available, but the ethics of the situation are strange because he does not treat the patient as a whole, he just treats the heart. Nevertheless, he is a skillful surgeon and generally his patients do very well.

In one sense, he is doing his job as a technician, but in another, to my eyes, he is failing miserably as a physician. This, of course, is my own view, but I like to think of the physician, whether he be a heart surgeon, family practitioner, general surgeon or other specialist, as a person who reflects a long tradition of concern and caring for the patient as a human being. And to this end, he should be available and concerned for his patients, except when he is out of town or in some way incapacitated. Is that a big responsibility? Yes. But, that is the responsibility that each physician, in my humble opinion, takes when he completes his education and takes on the caring for the sick or injured.

So what does postoperative care mean? Of course it means writing the appropriate postoperative orders for the patient, which includes some type of diet, or if the patient cannot eat, then intravenous fluids. It also includes pain management such as intravenous or intramuscular Morphine, Demerol and Dilaudid, and oral Vicodin, Percocet, or Tylenol. There may be need for anti-nausea medications such as Compazine, or Zofran and the physician may want to check for bleeding or treat infection with one of the hundreds of available antibiotics such as Penicillin, Cephalosporin, and Erythromycin. There are also many appropriate blood tests to follow the patient's progress (*see* Chapter 25). The orders after major surgery usually include a plan for activity which may include being out of bed or bathroom privileges. The surgeon should take precautions to prevent pneumonia with breathing exercises, and pulmonary embolism (*see* Chapter 19) and to assure that emotional needs are met. The doctor should discuss the patient's surgery and the orders with the recovery room nurse who will convey the information to the "floor" nurse. In the case of outpatient surgeries, the surgeon will usually discuss his findings with the patient and the family, and give written postoperative instructions and prescriptions for pain medications, antibiotics, and other medicines.

We will talk more about the postoperative care for specific surgeries in Part II of the book. The surgeon will need to follow the patient in his office for varying lengths of time in the recovery and postoperative period, and deal with any minor or major complications which may occur. This part of surgery is often the most pleasant for me and sometimes the most difficult if I am dealing with incurable cancer or complex problems. But that, to my understanding, is a major part of my being a physician. It is sad to see so many modern "itinerant surgeons" who have given up their role as comprehensive "healers" and have become mere skilled technicians. It reflects poorly on the profession and perhaps is one of the reasons physicians are not regarded with the high public esteem they had seventy five years ago.

Postoperative care, like others aspects of surgery, is an art which unfortunately has been given less attention in our hurried world with crowded clinics, HMO's, and volume oriented specialists, rather than individual patient-oriented physicians. Don't feel uncomfortable about asking your surgeon how often he will be visiting you after surgery or if he will be visiting at all, and for how many weeks or months you can rely upon him for any problems, after the surgery is completed. After all, when you build a house or have plumbing work done, you expect your contractor or plumber to be around after the job in case problems arise. Expect at least this much from the person who is operating on your body!

Chapter 12
COMPLICATIONS

Though an earthling, made from sod,
The surgeon thinks he's just a god.
So if you mention complication,
He may ask what drugs you're takin.

Crazy as it all may seem,
This perfect person cannot dream,
That in some way his operation,
Caused some major aberration.

Now I can tell he shouldn't oughter,
Think that he can walk on water.
But you see the facts remain
He walks on water in his brain.

Okay. I hate to burst your bubble. But your surgeon is not a god, does not walk on water and unfortunately makes mistakes and has complications. Now we should say at the outset that there are many causes of surgical complications and actually very few are directly caused by surgeon error or incompetence. They are, of course, usually in direct proportion to the patient's overall health, the type, length and severity of the surgery and a host of pre, intra and post operative factors that we will discuss as briefly as possible. The ever troubling question of the patient to the surgeon: "Why did I have that problem or complication?" should be answered by your surgeon as completely and simply as possible. Once a problem or complication arises, the patient may begin to lose faith in his doctor, and this can be prevented by careful and timely explanation.

First, I should emphasize that the surgeon must plan his surgery and outline to the patient and his family the potential adverse events that can occur. I do not mean to frighten a patient who is already concerned about a procedure, but it is important that he have a realistic understanding of the possibility of problems such as anesthetic problems, wound infection, or less-than-perfect surgical results.

The surgeon, of course, must plan carefully, have experience, be meticulous about procedural items and have minimal blood loss and a timely surgery. I have seen some surgeons who take three to four times as long as the average surgeon for a simple procedure, claiming that they are taking care not to let any complications occur, and yet the longer a patient is asleep, the greater the risk for anesthetic problems and the longer the exposure to microorganisms that could cause infection. Surgery should be done carefully, artfully and swiftly for the best results! In the postoperative period, he should anticipate the potential problems as we have outlined in Chapter 11.

Now, let us go down the list of complications and problems with which the patient and the surgeon must contend. I emphasize the physician also because we surgeons do lose sleep worrying about problems and complications; it's not like changing a muffler on a car and then going on to the next repair!

The only true surgical emergency is hemorrhage. Of course, I am not minimizing all the medical problems such as cardiac arrest, respiratory arrest or other acute medical emergencies. I am just stating that the purely surgical emergency is hemorrhage, and every surgeon is aware of this potential problem, and knows he must handle it swiftly. When an artery is cut, the natural response is for it to constrict. Evolution has graciously given us a method for our bodies to stop minor bleeding by having the muscles in the artery wall cause the vessel to retract and constrict. During the short period of time that this occurs, the body's coagulation (clotting) system works to plug the open end of the artery so that when the artery muscle relaxes in a few minutes or hours, no more bleeding occurs.

Unfortunately, the clotting system is sometimes not good enough to clog a cut artery and when the muscles in the artery relax, bleeding may start again and result in life-threatening hemorrhage. Now, no surgeon is going to knowingly leave a surgical sight with bleeding still occurring, so when he leaves a dry field, why does bleeding occur one or two hours later, sometimes necessitating taking the patient back to surgery. It may be caused by a clip or tie coming off a vessel but it may also be from inadequate clotting in vessels that the surgeon cauterized during surgery. Sometimes bleeding is minimal and can be observed, but if the patient shows signs of falling blood pressure, increasing pulse and falling blood count such as hematocrit and hemoglobin (*see* Chapter 25), the surgeon must take the patient back to surgery and stop the bleeding.

Aside from the problem of bleeding or hemorrhage, the first thing commonly seen after surgery is an elevated temperature or fever. Many experts claim that a mild fever is a natural response to surgery for the first twenty-four to forty-eight hours but it is always important for your doctor to evaluate the cause of the fever. The most common cause during the first two days after surgery is usually due to a pulmonary or lung problem. During surgery or in the period directly afterward, the lungs may not be completely expanded and this condition, called atelectasis, can cause fever. It is corrected by deep breathing or a procedure known as incentive spirometry, where a patient breathes against a resistance to fully expand the lungs. Inspiring or breathing in through a tube, has this effect and will clear the atelectasis and prevent the development of pneumonia. As you can imagine, in some children, debilitated and older people, this can be a major problem.

The next most common cause of postoperative fever is urinary tract infection, which may be due to catheterization or preexisting problems and is treatable with antibiotics.

Wound infection problems come next. First, let's consider minor phlebitis which may be as simple as an infected site where an IV has been placed, to a more extensive involvement of the veins in the arms or legs. The problem at the IV site is usually managed by changing the site of the IV and applying warm compresses, but antibiotics may also be indicated. Other wound problems may be infections in the surgical site skin, and leakage at a connection in the intestine. These kinds of infection usually occur after three or four days and may lead to actual separation of the wound called dehiscence or a more serious condition called evisceration, where the whole wound closure breaks down and the abdomen opens up.

Other less common but serious postoperative causes of fever are pancreatitis and parotitis.

The next problem the surgeon must watch for is major phlebitis in the large veins in the legs or pelvis. More common in obese patients, this problem can occur in anyone, especially if they are in bed for prolonged periods. That is why many surgeons use special compression stockings and foot pumps which keep the blood circulating in the legs and prevent blood clots in the veins which may cause blood clots to go to the lungs, pulmonary embolism. In Chapter 19, we will discuss this potentially lethal complication in more detail along with another similar problem called fat embolism.

After surgery other complications may be related to heart function such as arrhythmias, abnormal heart rates where it beats too fast, too slow or irregularly, heart attack (myocardial infarction), or an acute problem called "shock". Now the word "shock" is bandied about by everyone and yet to a physician it has a more specific meaning, namely a failure of the blood circulation with poor blood flow into the tissues. Obviously this leads to failure of many organs such as the heart itself, the kidneys, lungs, liver and brain and can cause death rapidly. We won't go into the complex management of shock except to say that we try to prevent it by anticipating problems that may lead to it. These include heart failure, severe infection throughout the body called sepsis, and hypovolemic shock, due to rapid loss of large volumes of blood or severe dehydration by loss of fluids from the blood into the tissues.

Another group of postoperative complications is psychiatric in nature. I have seen many patients, especially those who have to be in the intensive care unit for any period of time, develop what we call postoperative psychosis. They become disoriented and act "crazy". Frequently they are individuals who are normally in very good control of their emotions and also in control of their own lives. When placed in a situation where they are totally dependent on doctors and nurses for their every need, something inside them "clicks" and they develop this psychosis which often requires help from a psychiatrist, and special medications and sedatives may be needed. The condition almost always clears when the patient recovers fully from the operation.

We will talk more about the specific problems and complications of surgeries in Part II of the book under each heading rather than discuss them here. Additional general problems, however, can include kidney failure, gastric distention or failure of the stomach to empty (it enlarges and causes you to vomit), acid-base imbalance, a complex problem with the fluids and chemicals in your blood, liver failure and abdominal abscesses. Anesthetic problems will be covered completely in Chapter 21.

So I admonish you to be aware of the fact that surgery is an art and a skill, that the human body is not like a machine, and it may not always react to the stress of surgery as we expect. Be realistic and understanding and know that the well-trained surgeon may have complications with a patient even under the best of conditions.

Chapter 13
INFECTIONS AND ANTIBIOTICS

"On the Antiseptic Principle in the Practice of Surgery"
Written in 1867 by Lister became a sort of liturgy,
When physicians learned about nasty small "bugs"
And then learned how to treat 'em with drugs.

This was the third of the three great discoveries
That opened the door for surgical recoveries.
The first, you recall, was the tying of vessels.
Number two, anesthesia, by Morton and Wells.

So now we will challenge the worst of infections,
With drugs we have made with some complex confections,
And E. Coli, Staph and Strep can be driven,
When antibiotics correctly are given.

In the mid-eighteen hundreds some remarkable research was done by Louis Pasteur in the study of bacteria which led eventually to the publishing by Joseph Lister of his book "On the Antiseptic Principle in the Practice of Surgery". We have to imagine back one hundred and fifty years when it was considered normal for physicians to go from patient to patient without washing hands and to perform surgery with the very minimum of cleanliness. Ignasz Semmelweiss noticed that the wealthy women patients in the obstetrical ward where babies were delivered had a much higher incidence of puerperal sepsis or infections during childbirth, than the poor women, and he discovered that the reason was that doctors were frequently examining the wealthy women in labor without gloves or washing hands, and carrying bacteria from one patient to the next. The poor women were rarely examined and surprisingly had almost no puerperal sepsis. He tried to convince his colleagues to wash their hands between exams but they scoffed at him, and he was ridiculed to the point where he eventually went crazy! In retrospect we owe him a great deal of gratitude and credit for his pioneering work in antisepsis.

Penicillin was discovered in 1929 by Alexander Fleming and began to be clinically used by the 1940's. Since then there has been an explosion of drug development so that today we have a very large armamentarium of drugs to use in the treatment of infections. There is even a specialty in medicine called Infectious Disease and I frequently use these physicians to help me in managing particularly difficult infectious disease cases.

Now, I don't propose to give you a course in the use of antibiotics, but rather to give you some understanding of the types of microorganisms that are found, how they work and some factors that influence whether patients develop infections and what influences their recovery or demise.

In general, bacteria are divided into two groups that are called Gram Positive and Gram Negative depending whether they stain red or blue when prepared on a slide with a Gram's stain.

Bacteria produce substances called toxins, which are poisonous compounds, and these toxins act in the body to make you very sick. Living Gram positive bacteria often produce exotoxins and dead bacteria produce endotoxins. These toxins may alter your body's ability to fight off or destroy bacteria or may cause bacteria which normally inhabit your body to become pathogenic and cause disease. Still other toxins may cause tissue to die and become liquefied, may cause blood vessels to clot off, or may cause swellings, bleeding and shock.

What happens when you get an infection? We will call an early infection cellulitis, -itis being a suffix that means "infection of" or infection of the cells. The old Latin words associated with infection are tumor meaning swelling, dolor meaning pain, calor meaning heat, and rubor meaning redness. If you take a moment, you can think of many English words which come from these basic Latin words such as tumor, dolorous, rubious, and caloric. When a physician sees any of these signs, he must determine whether there is an infection and treat it appropriately. If the infection is allowed to progress, pus will form; an enclosed space with pus is called an abscess. The treatment of abscess today is much the same as it has been for thousands of years - open it and drain it.

When an infection spreads from one area it may travel by way of a system called the lymphatic which is just another type of vessel to carry waste from any area of the body, and this brings us to local collections of lymph in structures called lymph nodes. When you have a sore throat and it is red and painful, the infection may spread to the lymph nodes in your neck and we say you have swollen glands.

When pus and bacteria get into the blood stream, this is called sepsis and can cause high fever and rapid and severe progression of illness leading to death if not controlled.

Well, what things lead to infection? From the point of view of the surgeon, he must be careful in his handling of the tissue, avoid injuring the blood supply to an area and do his utmost to avoid getting a buildup of blood called a hematoma in the operative site. In certain patients there may be an increased risk for infection, and these will include underlying diseases such as Diabetes Mellitus, Cancer, Anemia, Chronic diseases, certain medications such as steroids, and radiation therapy.

First, we should think of a situation where bacteria can get into the body. This is called contamination such as may occur when you get a cut and the skin protection is breached, during an operation or when someone suffers a knife or gunshot wound which injures the intestine and contaminates the surrounding body.

Several things will influence whether you develop a severe infection. First, how strong or dangerous are the bacteria which have entered the system? Next we need to understand that the amount of bacteria is also important, as well as the length of time of the contamination. The method of contamination is important, i.e. was the patient stuck with a dirty nail, or splinter of wood which is still in the body? We will talk about different parts of the body in Part II of this book and will touch briefly on the types of infection that can occur there. The general health of the individual and the part involved will make a big difference. When there is good blood supply to an area, then the body's own defense system can get to the involved area and fight off infection. If the area has poor blood supply because of arteriosclerosis or hardening of the arteries, tissue damage, diabetes mellitus which effects small blood vessels or just general debility in very old or chronically ill people, then the bacteria may have an easier time growing and cause severe disease.

The physician will evaluate his patient for the presence of infection daily by looking for any of the four Latin word symptoms we have mentioned and if they are present, he will perform certain laboratory tests to help him in the diagnosis and treatment. These may include chest x-rays for signs of pneumonia, CAT scans, special radioactive injection studies called nuclear scans such as Indium or Gallium, or a whole host of other radiological studies. In addition, he will do certain laboratory tests which we will discuss in Chapter 25. Suffice it to say that a blood count, urinalysis, and cultures of any pus or wounds are very important in determining what type of antibiotic should be used.

Sometimes the organism causing a disease is not a bacteria but a fungus such as in athlete's foot or "yeast" infections or a virus as in AIDS, and these need different tests and different medicines for treatment.

This has been a lot of information to digest, but I do want to touch on some other points. First of all some individuals are very allergic to certain drugs. They may have a bad reaction which can be mild with a rash, to itching, breathing trouble and sudden death. Physicians always ask a patient about any side effects from taking a medicine, and this is always highlighted on a medical chart. In the case of severe reactions, many patients have "Medic Alert" bracelets to inform anyone treating them of the danger.

When you have an infection, your doctor wants to treat you with the best drug which has the least toxicity or side effects. You don't use a cannon to kill a fly and conversely a peashooter will not kill an elephant. Physicians learn what types and amounts of drugs are best for each situation and when it involves stronger drugs which are much more dangerous to use but may be the last resort. They have to watch for hearing loss, kidney and liver and other problems. The field of infectious disease has become so complex that when I have a patient with a ruptured appendicitis or ruptured colon I often get consultation from the infectious disease specialist.

Just for your interest, I'm going to name some of the bacteria we see in a surgical practice. Gram-Positive organisms are Staphylococcus aureus, Pneumococcus and Streptococcus. Gram-Negative organisms include Meningococcus, Escherichia Coli, Salmonella, Klebsiella, Haemophilus influenzae, Proteus, Clostridium, Pseudomonas and Aerobacter. And these are only a few of the many, many organisms we find in human infections.

Some of the antibiotics used are Penicillin, Ampicillin, Flagyl, Erythromycin, Cephalosporin, Gentamicin, and Floxin, just to name a few. Take a look at the "Physician's Desk Reference" which lists all the drugs we commonly use and you will find hundreds of antibiotics. You will also see a listing of the dosages and side effects, which can sometimes be very scary.

Treating infections can sometimes be very simple, but other times it may involve intravenous medications and frequently multiple combinations of medications.

Sometimes a surgeon will give you what we call prophylactic antibiotics in anticipation of contamination or possible infection to prevent or lessen the impact of the bacterial contamination. Examples are gall bladder and intestinal surgery and certain orthopedic procedures.

This has been an overview of infection and antibiotics and I hope it helps you to understand some of the problems which a physician will encounter in dealing with this situation.

Chapter 14
KNIVES, LASERS AND CAUTERY

Knives, scimitars, dirks and cleavers
Daggers, shivs and snickersneevers,
Jackknives, rapiers, spears and krisses
Tomahawks, swords, stylets, cutlisses.

These all are very fine for fighting,
And if you slay enough, for knighting,
The saber cuts from guzzle to zatch,
But I thinks it's finally found its match.

For all the above are good for killing,
But I've got one that's used, God willing,
Instead of for wounding or taking of life,
It's used to cure - the scalpel knife.
Why on earth write a chapter on knives, lasers and cautery?
Just cause I oughtery!

I can vaguely recall the first time I held a scalpel in my hand and drew it across human skin to make an incision. I was an intern at a prestigious hospital in New York City and was doing my first appendectomy with the guidance of a gray-haired surgeon who couldn't keep his hands out of the wound. I cut his hand! Just a tiny nick but it was enough to make me the laughing stock among my colleagues. That was the last time I did that, but to me it seemed like an inauspicious start to my surgical career. Reminiscing brings back many good and bad moments during my training program, I digress. We're talking about knives, lasers and cautery.

The first two are methods of cutting, the first of these is time worn, used since man first made stone tools and the second is a child of the late twentieth century. Many of my patients inquire whether I can do their surgery with lasers and are somewhat disheartened when I tell them that a laser is just another method for cutting. Laser is an abbreviation of the first letters of Light Amplification by Stimulated Emission of Radiation, and its use in general surgery is actually very limited. It was early on used for cutting and coagulating during certain laparoscopic procedures, but the side effects and complications made it fall into minimal usage. However, in certain procedures such as hemorrhoidectomy, eye surgery and certain brain operations, it has become an important tool for the surgeon. Lasers can cut, coagulate, vaporize tissue and selectively destroy tissue. There are several different types of lasers including CO_2 - carbon dioxide, Nd:YAG - neodymium (yttrium-aluminum-garnet), Ho:YAG - holmium, Er:YAG - erbium, and the KTP - potassium-titanyl-phosphate. Anyway, the word laser sounds good and many surgeons who advertise use the word laser in their "ads" because it sounds high-tech, modern and has a catchy patient appealing sound to it. "Hey doc, I want my surgery done with lasers."

I feel like saying, "We'll bring in Dr. McCoy from Star Trek and use ultra-gamma-neutrino-lasers for your surgery, sir! Beam me out."

But to get back to real cutting, scalpels, some completely disposable and the handles of some are often reusable, are very fine, ultra sharp instruments and can become dull cutting through tough tissue and frequently have to be replaced several times during a surgery. They also come in several sizes and types, some broad, some tiny, some with round or pointed tips and others adapted to certain special operating conditions. Another modality used in the surgical operation is electrocautery; this can either be monopolar or bipolar. Cautery is used for cutting in place of a scalpel or for cauterizing or sealing off bleeding vessels with heat, a modern adaptation of the middle ages technique of using boiling oil or fire to stop bleeding, but they didn't have much for anesthesia! It has become an irreplaceable modality for many surgeons to cut, and then dry the operative field using this tool, whereas many years ago the surgeon had to tie off each bleeding vessel with a suture, requiring much more time and prolonging the surgical procedure. Another relatively new device is the argon beam coagulator which uses the gas argon and electrons to seal off bleeding areas and has a very minimal tissue depth penetration and can be used on the surface of vital organs without damaging the organ, as may occur with standard electrocautery.

I am sure in the years to come new and even more efficient tools for cutting and stopping bleeding will be discovered and used in surgical operations, but somehow, I think the scalpel will still hold sway in the hands and minds of the surgeons.

Chapter 15
LAPAROSCOPY

They say that Isaac Newton was sitting under a tree,
When an apple fell upon his head, and he found gravity.
And likewise, after centuries had passed, to please society,
Someone sat under that very tree and found laparoscopy.

It's just the product of a brilliant and inquiring mind,
That finds a new idea and leaves the old ones far behind.
With laparoscopic surgery we have turned a brand new page,
And ushered in a new and different type of surgical age.

We put a camera in a joint or abdomen to see,
What was causing all that person's symptomatology,
And without making big incisions we can take out many organs,
With such success that we'll be known as surgical J.P. Morgans.

When I first heard about laparoscopic cholecystectomy, taking out the gall bladder using four tiny holes, a camera, and some strange instruments, I said "It'll never fly. Too risky. Not me!" Now I do two or three every week and rarely do the old type of procedure using a large oblique incision under the right rib margin. My patients are done as outpatients, coming to the hospital and going home the same day, and have minimal pain and almost no incisional scarring. They are usually back to work in a few days and eat normal food. It's the closest thing to the invention of the wheel I have ever seen.

The first laparoscopic cholecystectomy was performed in Germany in 1985 and though pooh-poohed by surgeons like me for years, by 1993 nearly half a million procedures were done that year alone. Laparoscopy is a method of operating which uses only a few small openings into the abdomen. A special needle is inserted into the abdomen and carbon dioxide gas is insufflated into the peritoneal cavity inside of the abdomen, allowing an interface between organs and the abdominal wall. Then a ten millimeter camera attached to a television screen is inserted through this port and a general exam of the intra-abdominal contents can be done. Under direct vision, at least three more ports are placed and using special clamps, scissors and cautery the gall bladder can be dissected out, the veins, arteries and bile ducts sealed with staples, and the gall bladder can be dissected out of its location under the liver and brought out through one of the ports. Then most of the CO_2 gas is removed. Any remaining CO_2 may sometimes get caught temporarily under the diaphragm and this may cause some patients to have an annoying aching pain in the right shoulder after abdominal laparoscopic procedures. The gas gets absorbed by the body in about six to twelve hours and the pain goes away. I have known some patients to get very worried about this, and knowing its cause and that it will soon go away is usually all they need to hear!

Abdominal laparoscopy is not without complications and I will mention a few of the general considerations now and more specific ones under the particular types of surgery later in the book. The trocars that are placed in the abdomen can be very dangerous in untrained and uncareful hands and may result in severe injuries to the intestines and more seriously injury to major blood vessels such as the aorta, the vena cava, the iliac arteries or their accompanying veins, or may just cause nonspecific bleeding. These injuries usually require making a large incision in the abdomen and repairing the damage. However, sometimes the damage is not immediately apparent. As an example, a surgeon made a hole in an artery during what should have been a routine laparoscopic appendectomy. Because the blood vessel had a lot of peritoneum and fat around it, the bleeding stopped temporarily when the vessel contracted and closed off. The procedure was completed without any warning signs and in the recovery room the patient went into shock from sudden loss of blood when the vessel began bleeding again. Only an emergency surgery saved the young man's life. It should not have happened!

In general, laparoscopic surgery saves the patient a big incision, the dividing of abdominal wall muscles and affords a much more rapid recovery, much less pain and less tissue damage. The patients are often only in the hospital for the day and are back to work in a few days. We will discuss other laparoscopic procedures under their appropriate specialty in Part II along with diagrams showing where the holes in the skin are made. Laparoscopy is relatively simple and much less invasive with less tissue morbidity than the older methods, but does require expertise and special training.

Once laparoscopic cholecystectomy became popular, several other procedures were tried and several specialties began using the same basic method for their procedures. We will go into specifics under each specialty in Part II. As of now the laparoscopic procedures that have been accepted by surgeons are: cholecystectomy, diagnostic laparoscopy--which means just looking around inside--including those for cancer diagnosis, appendectomy, hernia repair, liver biopsies, and hiatus hernia repairs. There are also small and large intestine resections, taking away adhesions and lymph node biopsies.

Surgeons have also done the following procedures but to a limited degree and their acceptability will be increased in the coming years. These include: cancer operations on the colon, stomach operations, ulcer operations and certain bypass operations. Gynecologists are now using the procedure to make diagnosis of gynecologic pathology, both benign and malignant and can frequently remove lymph nodes and small tumors laparoscopically. Of course tubal ligations have been done this way for a long time. The chest surgeons use scopes to examine the lungs in a procedure called thoracoscopy and can do some biopsies and other procedures in this manner.

Orthopedic surgeons are now looking into joints with arthroscopes to repair ligaments and clean out disreputable joints.

Laparoscopy and its cousin procedures have made a strong impact on several different kinds of surgery and we shall discuss this more with each specific subspecialty as indicated, including an overview of the types of complications which may ensue using this modality.

Chapter 16
PERITONITIS

Before the time of Lister and Pasteur,
Opening the belly would cause a disaster.
If one allowed germs to get inside us
We patients would die of a peritonitis.

Before we can talk about peritonitis or inflammation of the peritoneum, we better clarify to the non-medical person what the peritoneum is. Imagine a room filled with chairs, tables, dishes and other objects. Then take an imaginary plastic spray gun and cover everything with a thick plastic coating. This coating would essentially make a contiguous connecting sheet around everything and leave the center of the room as being inside the plastic coating or balloon. That is essentially what the peritoneum does. It covers all structures in the abdomen as if we had blown up a balloon inside.

The peritoneum is a real structure with blood supply and nerves and can be important to a physician when something causes it to be disrupted or get infected. Inflammation of the peritoneum, or peritonitis, has many causes. The more common causes of peritonitis are ruptured appendicitis, perforated diverticulitis or hole in the colon secondary to infected diverticulae (*see* the chapter on Colon), perforated ulcer of the stomach or duodenum, problems of infection in the abdomen secondary to injury as by local "knife and gun club activity" and breakdown of connections called anastomosis made by a surgeon.

The symptoms of peritonitis are abdominal pain, fever with chills and sometimes diarrhea, nausea and vomiting. The abdomen will often be distended and very tender and when the physician listens to the belly with his stethoscope, he may not hear any sounds. Normally we can hear bowel sounds indicating the normal back and forth movement of the intestines. A silent abdomen is often indicative of something wrong.

Why, then, have a chapter on peritonitis? Mainly because it can act to warn the patient and his doctor that something is going on inside and somebody better do some studies and find out what it is! Although most people recover from peritonitis when the underlying cause is treated, as with removing the diseased appendix or colon, it remains the greatest cause of death following abdominal surgery. When a patient comes to the physician with abdominal pain, one of the first things the doctor will do will be to determine if the patient has peritonitis, looking for peritoneal irritation signs of pain, tenderness, fever, or silent abdomen. He will look for something called rebound tenderness which means that when he pushes in on the abdomen and lets go suddenly, there is a sudden severe pain due to sudden movement of an inflamed or infected peritoneum.

If the doctor determines that there is peritonitis, then he needs to do x-ray and laboratory studies to pinpoint the cause and make plans to correct the problem. He will generally want to start an intravenous line since the patient is often dehydrated from vomiting and not eating, and will give pain medication and some broad spectrum antibiotics.

**Peritonitis means something is wrong
Insideus!**

Chapter 17
REHABILITATION

Habilitate means to make one suitable,
Especially those who haven't a cluetable.
So to re habilitate,
Assumes you were once in a suitable state.

Now most people I know are downright strange,
With behaviors and actions that they oughta change.
They wouldn't do well with rehabilitation,
For that would only cause more frustration.

Instead of re anything I would suggest,
Buying a large metal-lined chest,
And take all the people you want to rehabilitate,
And ship them all off to a totally different state.

There's an old expression that has become overused: "Let nature takes its course". When surgeons in days past completed their handiwork, the patient was sent home to heal and more often than not, nature took its course - right to the grave. In the twentieth century we developed the concept of rehabilitation which focuses on the individual as a functional member of society. It was not enough just to have a successful surgery; it was the responsibility of the physician to bring the patient as close as possible back to his prior normal physical and emotional status.

Over one hundred years ago it was shown that early ambulation of patients reduced complications and yet it took another fifty years for physicians and patients to believe this line of thinking. It's almost as if when you treat the patient as being sick, he will continue to be sick; if you try to get him functioning again, he will recover more rapidly.

In situations where patients have been critically ill with tremendous weight loss and thereby muscle loss, the program of rehabilitation may take months, whereas after simple surgeries it may take several days or weeks.

We need to understand that rehabilitation nowadays is a comprehensive program involving the patient, but also with direct or indirect assistance from nurses, psychologists, physicians, physical therapists, occupational therapists, speech therapists and sometimes prosthetists, the people who make and apply artificial limbs or other replacement parts. The sooner these individuals are involved in a case, the sooner the patient will get the optimal amount of improvement. I was surprised to find that several of the major surgical texts included almost no information on this important aspect of total care for the surgical patient. And yet, it is perhaps the one aspect of the case that interests the patient most. "So you're gonna remove my zingwatch and my dohickey, Doc? When can I resume my golf game, go back to work and resume sexual relations?"

Any surgical program in a major hospital prides itself on the quality of its rehabilitation program. I will give you a brief outline of some of the things you should look for as you are recovering from surgery.

First, and most well known and utilized is physical therapy. The objectives are to use exercise to bring back as much function as possible. Obviously this may be more apparent with orthopedic cases, but it applies even to the patient who's had an appendectomy or a gall bladder removed. The objectives include exercises for strength, coordination, range of motion and endurance, just to name a few. The therapist will work with the patient in an active or passive way. From the simple activity of getting out of bed and walking, to a complex set of active exercises where the patient moves himself, to passive ones where someone else moves the patient or his limb, and everything in between!

Physical therapists use massage, heat therapy, which can include many different types - hotpacks, whirlpool, infrared and water therapy, electric currents stimulating nerves called electrotherapy, cold therapy with ice compresses and just plain encouragement.

Occupational therapy helps get the patient back to doing things that will be worthwhile for him as a functional member of society and the work force, or just to be able to get along in daily life, whether it's managing a colostomy, a wheelchair or at home activities. This is very important for recovery and the surgeon must be aware of all the modalities available to help his patient in the postoperative period.

Psychiatric and social work rehabilitation is also an area where we as physicians often fail in our care. With our focus on the surgical problem, we may ignore major emotional or psychosocial problems which leave the surgically-healed patient effectively incapacitated.

If you or a loved one is anticipating major surgery, be sure you ask about the rehabilitation services in your hospital; frequently it's better to arrange for help before the surgery rather than afterwards. I will talk about amputations and prosthesis in the orthopedics chapter, about paralysis and dealing with the problems of the paraplegic and quadriplegic patient in the chapter on neurosurgery, and problems with urination in the urology section.

Patients with new colostomies and ileostomies, where for medical reasons the large or small bowel is brought out to the skin level where a bag is applied, need tremendous support from nurses who will tell them about the care of the opening at the skin called a stoma, and may need psychosocial support and also may benefit from talking with other individuals who are living with the same situations. I personally know many famous celebrities, always in the public eye, who function well with their postoperative disabilities including colostomies and prostheses without having it effect their lifestyles or public image to a great degree, if at all. In my book on "Comprehensive Breast Care", I talk extensively about the problems encountered by women who have had mastectomies or axillary dissections. Similarly, patients who have a disfigurement secondary to cancer surgery or temporary problems such as hair loss during chemotherapy have someone to turn to in a comprehensive program to help them get through the problems of daily living.

In conclusion, be sure that your surgeon and his hospital are sensitive to these important issues and can outline a rehabilitation program prior to and after a surgery.

Chapter 18
HEMORRHAGE, COAGULATION AND TRANSFUSIONS

Whenever you are angry, you speak of "seeing red".
To a surgeon this expression causes sirens in his head.
And though the right wing zealots spoke of "Better dead than Red",
We know that surgically speaking, too much red and you'll be dead.

Ho hum, you say, if blood comes out, then put a little in.
It should be just as simple as to close a safety pin.
And so it is with surgeons, as we ply our nasty trade.
If blood emerges while we work, we get a blood bandaid.

Lose a little, get a little, sounds so simple now,
Yet hemorrhage is a problem, much more complex than the Dow.
For blood is not just colored water, to be put in later,
Much the way you pour the water in your radiator.

Blood is really an organ, with complex, and diffuse conjunctions.
We need the volume, but we also must have all the other functions.
There's red cells carrying oxygen, electrolytes, and serum,
Platelets that form blood clots, immune proteins, and right near um...

Are white blood cells that help us fight off some obscure infections
And water and some lipid fats, and Rh fact connections.
So when the blood is gushing out upon an OR table,
Try remember all the parts, that is, if you are able.

I want to present a simplified chapter on blood, hemorrhage and transfusions. You should understand that this is a very complex subject which has been covered in large volumes and about which hematologists or blood specialists spend years learning. I will divide it into several sections and give some basic information about each one.

First the components of blood. As in the poem, blood is a complex of red blood cells or corpuscles which compose about 45% of the blood and carry iron and oxygen to your cells; the white blood cells scavenge debris and fight off infection and contain immunological substances, and platelets or thrombocytes help form blood clots. It also contains many different clotting factors, which I will describe soon, which help the formation of blood clots with the platelets. The blood also contains many chemicals needed by your body to function properly, including what are called electrolytes: Na - sodium, K - potassium, Cl - Chloride, as well as Ca - Calcium, Mg - Magnesium and glucose all suspended in a 90% watery substance called plasma. When a physician orders an intravenous solution, he must be sure to order the right components, the right amount of glucose and remember that diabetics have too much sugar in their blood and electrolytes depending on the results of blood tests he has taken. Similarly, if a patient has been bleeding, we must not only replace blood volume, but also specific blood clotting factors and calcium which is used up in clotting.

If a patient loses a small amount of blood, say one pint, there may not be a need to replace anything, since the body continually produces new blood. However, when massive bleeding occurs such as in gunshot wound trauma, ruptured aneurysms which are large ballooned out blood vessels or during surgery, then transfusions may be needed, and attention must be paid to all the parameters of the blood components. If the patient has a low platelet count and you give him blood, he may continue to bleed and not form blood clots. So hematologists are often called in to help us restore normal blood homeostasis.

Now to some other basics. The average adult has about 10 pints of blood and this varies with weight, age, sex, body build, etc. and can lose about a pint without much problem. When you donate a unit of blood that is about a pint. The volume you lose with the donation is made up rapidly with transfer of fluids from one part of your body to the blood stream so that the total volume remains the same. It takes about two weeks for your body to produce and replace the red blood cells.

The blood circulates through your body in a continuous circular pattern, driven by the contractions of the heart. It goes from the heart through the arteries to the tissues such as brain, stomach, kidneys, skin, etc., where it gives off oxygen and other nutrients to the cells, and then returns to the heart by the veins. It is pumped into the lungs where it picks up more oxygen, returns back to the heart and then starts the trip again. Simply put, the flow of blood, with a certain volume present, gives us our blood pressure. If the amount of fluid in the system falls, as with bleeding, then the blood pressure falls and the heart beats faster to keep the total amount of blood circulating at a constant number. So when there is hemorrhage, a patient's blood pressure usually goes down and his heart rate or pulse goes up. Those signs, together with measurements of the blood, will let the surgeon know how much a patient is bleeding and how much to replace. We'll talk more about the actual numbers in Chapter 25 when we will also discuss the white blood cell count (WBC) and other blood factors.

When a patient's blood count, amount of blood or red blood cells falls too low, he may need a blood transfusion. We generally say that 9 grams of hemoglobin is the cutoff level with normal being between 13 and 15 grams for most healthy people. But for many reasons, including religious (Jehovah Witnesses refuse any blood transfusion), the choice of no blood or of, under certain circumstances, blood be given. Frequently, when a patient knows he will be needing blood, he will give his own blood in advance or have friends or relatives donate for him.

As far as coagulation is concerned, I am going to show you a schematic version of the clotting pathway which includes factors I-V and VII through XIII. I never remember all the specifics myself and always have to refer to specialists or books to understand all the pathways, but I thought you might be interested to see how much is involved in forming a blood clot and stopping bleeding when you get a scratch or cut. The factors and their synonyms are:

   I = Fibrinogen
   II = Prothrombin
   III = Tissue Factor
   IV = Calcium Ion
   V = Proaccelerin (labile factor)
   VII = Serum Prothrombin Conversion Accelerator Factor
        (stable factor)
   VIII = Anti-hemophilic Factor
   IX = Christmas Factor
   X = Stuart-Prower Factor
   XI = Plasma Thromboplastin Antecedent
   XII = Hageman Factor
   XIII = Fibrin Stabilizing Factor and then there are platelets.

We sometimes refer to the expression consumption coagulopathy which means that because of continued bleeding and the body's attempt at stopping the bleeding by forming blood clots, many clotting factors are used up or consumed and this must be managed by physicians with in-depth knowledge of the clotting pathways and their replacements.

In certain situations like hemophilia, kidney disease, and Von Willebrand's disease, special factors are needed and must be supplied by the hematologists. Another problem called disseminated intravascular coagulation or DIC is the name for a number of conditions which cause severe problems with coagulation and can lead to death if not rapidly and appropriately corrected. Some of the things that can cause DIC are massive bleeding, problems with labor and delivery, severe infections, burns, liver disease, crush injuries and malignancies. DIC is a difficult problem to counteract and sometimes results in death even in the most experienced hands.

Now let us turn to the whole area of transfusions. Blood contains substances which are called antigens, and without being more specific, we have to receive a blood transfusion with blood containing pretty much the same antigens as our own. Otherwise severe "allergic" reactions and even death can occur. The first blood group discovery was made in 1901 with the determination of A, B, and O types. Later on many other subgroups such as Rh, Kell, Lewis, and Duffy were discovered making it much safer to receive blood transfusions. In the early 1980's with the beginning of the AIDS epidemic, we were unable to identify contaminated blood. Now we can determine contaminated HIV positive or AIDS blood making the blood supply safe and dependable.

In conclusion, let me review briefly the hemostatic process, or how bleeding stops without our external help. After a minor injury causes an opening in a vein, or an artery or small artery called an arteriole, the vessel contracts and partially closes off. Then a mass of platelets join together to form a plug, like a finger in a dike, stopping the bleeding and allowing the hole to heal with a collagen scar (*see* Chapter 21). So, the next time you have a cut and are bleeding, think about all these considerations I have mentioned and by the time you have reread this chapter the bleeding had better have stopped; if not - see a doctor!

Chapter 19
PULMONARY EMBOLISM

Blood clots in veins where they shouldn't be found,
Can be a great problem if they should abound.
And if they break loose and go to the lung,
A patient may die with the reason unsung.

More than half a million will get this bad disease,
With blood clots from their pelvis, or their ankles to their knees.
And ten percent will die within an hour, sad to say.
So one must make the diagnosis soon, with no delay.

And of the 90% who live beyond the very first hour,
About a third will die in spite of all the medical power.
So face it, blood clots in your veins, are a very serious matter,
And shouldn't be taken lightly or be treated by a Mad Hatter.

If you are diagnosed and treated with the proper drugs
The doctor can dissolve the most pernicious of the clogs.
And using anticoagulants, blood thinners to the public,
You'll probably survive to next New Year's and be able to
drink some bubblic!

In reviewing the literature for this chapter, I was surprised to find that so many people have pulmonary emboli and that a large proportion of them die of the disease. When a large clot breaks loose in a vein and travels through the venous system to the heart and through the right side of the heart into the lungs, death may be instantaneous when the body is unable to get oxygen. There are other factors involved which we don't need to consider, but it's important to note that almost 50% of patients dying in the hospital have some degree of pulmonary emboli. If the diagnosis is made, then ninety percent will survive; if the diagnosis is not made, only seventy percent will survive, so it is important to know the signs and symptoms and be sure that your physician knows about them and starts appropriate therapy rapidly.

But let's go back a few steps. Who develops these blood clots and why do they develop? Normally, blood flows continuously from the legs into the large vein in the abdomen and chest, the vena cava. But under certain circumstances, blood flow is diminished and sets up a background for coagulation or clotting to occur. As long ago as the 1880s the famous German physician Rudolf Virchow determined that three factors were responsible for blood clots or thrombosis to occur. They are known today as Virchow's triad and consist of (1) stasis or slowing down of blood flow in the vein, (2) injury to the vein, and (3) an increased tendency for the blood to clot called hypercoagulability.

The causes of this triad are many but the main ones that concern us here are those related to surgery. When a patient has an operation he often is lying down for a prolonged period with no muscle activity; the patient is often paralyzed by the anesthesiologist so that the surgeon can operate in a motionless field. This operative inactivity and the postoperative bed rest are highly conducive to stasis in the veins and thrombosis or formation of clots can occur more readily. This problem may be more common as we get older and it takes longer to recover and ambulate.

When a patient gets dehydrated or if there is a decrease in blood thinning factors then there will be an increased tendency for clots in the vein. Because of the increased pressure in arteries, blood clots are less common and any clots that occur don't ever go to the lung - it's the wrong direction; as you recall arteries take blood away from the lungs and heart to the tissue; veins take blood from the tissue to the heart and lungs!

What exactly is an embolism? It is a blood clot carried in the blood vessel. A pulmonary embolism is a blood clot that has gone to the lungs. The risk for pulmonary embolism, PE, is high in patients over 40 years old who have a history of vein problems called phlebitis, a surgery lasting longer than an hour, and with orthopedic procedures on the hips and knees. There is a also high risk after trauma, especially if veins or surrounding tissue have been badly injured.

What should your doctor do to prevent this problem? First of all is the awareness of the problem. Second is an anticipatory treatment of the patient before it occurs. This means applying special stockings or compression apparatus during many surgical procedures. In the very obese or high risk patient, the physician may want to give the patient prophylactic anticoagulant treatment.

The most common anticoagulant is heparin or a similar drug, and getting repeated blood tests (*see* Chapter 25) to make sure that the blood is "thin" enough. The patient may be changed over to a pill, coumadin, which can be taken daily at home. The physician must carefully monitor even this drug, for if the blood gets too thin, the patient can bleed massively from the slightest injury, from the intestinal tract or the urinary tract.

What are the symptoms of formation of clots in the larger veins deep in the leg? There may be no warning signs and that is the greatest danger, but most of the time the patient will have aching in the leg, a tender cordlike mass when the clot is in the vein, swelling of that leg and occasionally redness, fever and pain on motion. If the patient has already progressed to pulmonary embolism, and it may only be a small blood clot at first, the signs and symptoms include sudden chest pain, shortness of breath, coughing up blood, rapid heart rate and falling blood pressure. If it is a large embolism, shock and death may occur rapidly!

The physician listening to the heart and lungs can sometimes hear abnormal sounds with pulmonary embolism. If a patient has symptoms even remotely suggestive of thrombus or embolism, the nurse should immediately notify the physician and certain diagnostic tests should be done immediately. Better to have several negative tests than miss a positive one! There are several tests, but three are of major importance. The first, for blood clots in the veins, is called ultrasonography, a sound wave study that can show blood clots in a vein. The second is a lung scan in which a picture of normal and abnormal lung can be determined by injecting and breathing in radioactive materials with very low radioactivity and studying a special x-ray afterwards. The third test is the most specific for embolism and consists of doing an arteriogram, or x-ray of the vessels in the lung using intravenous dye.

If any of these are positive, then anticoagulation therapy is started immediately unless there is a contraindication to using a blood thinner, such as bleeding in an organ such as the brain, abdomen or intestine. In that case, the physician may opt to place a filter in the big vein in the abdomen to prevent large blood clots from getting to the lungs. This filter can either be placed by a radiologist through a vein in the neck or groin called the Greenfield Filter, or can be applied through a surgical incision, the Adams-DeWeese or Miles inferior vena caval clip.

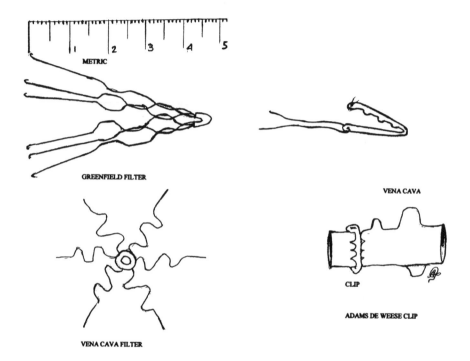

GREENFIELD VENA CAVA FILTER AND ADAMS DE WEESE CLIP

DIAGRAM 1

Chapter 20
DIABETES MELLITUS
AND SURGERY

In your pancreas, there dwells,
An area filled with Langerhans cells.
These cells called islets, so very small,
Produce insulin, as you may recall.

This insulin is what your body needs,
To use the sugars in tiny beads.
Without the insulin, you may be sweet,
But your cells are getting nothing to eat.

In diabetes the islet cells,
For some strange reason, don' work so well,
And if insulin is not produced.
Glucose in your blood's not used.

So let's give three cheers to Banting and Best,
The two researchers that made the test,
And discovered insulin in dogs one day.
So you can enjoy a hot fudge Sundae.

Diabetes Mellitus is a strange disease, and it affects 2-3% of the populace. Whether you have childhood or adult onset diabetes, your body has a problem with the islet cells of the pancreas and they don't produce enough insulin, a word derived from the Latin word "insula" for island or islets. The insulin helps metabolize and mobilize sugars from your blood into your tissue. Some diabetics may be entirely diet controlled because they apparently have some insulin, whereas others are reliant on daily injections of one of the many types of insulin available or, they may take some other medication that mimics the effect of insulin.

Just to digress for a moment, when a person has high blood pressure or hypertension, controlling the blood pressure with medications completely corrects the problem. If there is no high blood pressure, it usually means there are no problems related to hypertension!

Unfortunately the situation with diabetes mellitus is more complex than just elevation of the blood sugar. Even if the diabetic patient maintains his blood sugar at a normal level with diet, or other means such as insulin, the disease of diabetes mellitus may still progress, affecting different organs in your body. It is in the latter context that the diabetic patient becomes of concern to the surgeon. Diabetes affects the small blood vessels, narrowing them and decreasing the blood supply to the hands and feet or the vessels in the heart and may lead to tissue damage in these areas necessitating bypass surgeries (*see* Vascular Surgery). If very severe and not well managed, amputations of the toes or even a leg may be necessary. Because of the injury to microscopic vessels in the skin, the diabetic may have poor healing of skin wounds and surgical incisions may heal more slowly and with greater chance of infection and wound separation. Somehow the effect on the skin also involves the sensory nerves and diabetic patients may develop abnormal nerve function and numbness, called neuropathies, in the toes and feet.

If the diabetes effects the eyes a condition called diabetic retinopathy can occur and lead to poor vision or blindness.

Diabetes mellitus is a strange and wide effecting disease. What are the surgical considerations and why do I give a whole chapter to the subject? First, the surgeon and anesthesiologist must carefully monitor the blood sugar during the stress of surgery; surgery is a stress both emotionally and physiologically! If the blood sugar gets too low, hypoglycemia, then not enough sugar is getting to the brain cells and seizures or brain damage can occur. If the blood sugar gets too high, hyperglycemia, then a serious condition called diabetic keto-acidosis can occur with severe tissue consequences and even death.

The surgeon knows that because of the diabetic effect on tissue, there is poorer blood supply to tissue and skin and thereby a greater chance for wound infections (*see* Wound Healing chapter), slower healing and more complications. Whereas we usually take out skin sutures after seven to ten days, in the diabetic I may wait twice as long! Sores and ulcers that heal rapidly in the non-diabetic may become a complex lingering problem in the diabetic patient and even skin grafting will have poorer results.

Patients who have blood vessel problems from hardening of the arteries or arteriosclerosis, or secondary to smoking will have even more problems if they are diabetic. In the diabetic patient with vascular disease, if they don't stop smoking, the outlook for saving a foot or leg is very poor! The diabetic needs to take exquisite care of his skin, and whenever there are even minor cuts or bruises, he should seek out medical attention immediately.

New research with pancreas transplants may offer some wonderful treatment options in the future but this work is still embryonic in the transplantation field.

If you have diabetes mellitus, you probably know much about what I have spoken, and it is important that you continue to educate yourselves in all the new treatment possibilities on the market. Sometimes a general physician may not have the time to be up-to-date on these types of advances and as a second opinion you may want to consult an endocrinologist, a physician who specializes in endocrine disease of which diabetes mellitus is one!

Chapter 21
WOUND HEALING

I wish we'd find a magic way,
For scars and deformity to go away.
Unfortunately though, the process of healing,
Leaves scars and deformities and some bad feeling!

Healing a wound is like building construction,
It starts with site cleanup and tissue destruction.
Certain cells, the WBC's, remove all the dead and poor tissue,
And then bring equipment to rebuild the issue.

And like any construction, it takes time for achievement,
And depends on the needed equipment receivement.
The roads for supply in the body are arteries.
If you have em in plenty, the work soon gets starteried.

But also you need all the building materials.
Which you get in your body with all the right cereals,
With proteins and lipids and good carbohydrates.
And vitamins, minerals and adequate heart rates.

And all this assumes you're in top peak condition,
Without Diabetes or heart aches or malnutrition,
Or aged, or fat, or have cancer or infection,
Or jaundice or trauma or lost an election.

In other words, the ideal state is just what it says,
Since most are not perfect in so many ways,
So I have to advise you, and it's not all my fault,
Take this information with a small grain of salt!

HTe healing process is a very sensible and orderly one, much like building a home. After an injury, which may be traumatic or surgical, the wound, like your building site, has to be cleansed of debris and the body sends in white blood cells (WBC's) to do this function. The WBC's come in by small arteries, arterioles, and much like in construction, the body has to build new roads to bring in the heavy building materials. In the body this is called angiogenesis (angio=vessel, genesis=creating) and this allows the entire "repair" team to get into the area for repair.

Most texts describe wound healing in stages, but in actuality many of these processes are happening at the same time. First comes hemostasis and coagulation, stopping the bleeding and sealing off the area from further bleeding. Then comes inflammation, which is a somewhat misunderstood word because many of us equate inflammation with infection. Not so. Inflammation is actually the process of bringing white blood cells or leukocytes into the area of a wound. They have many roles, but mainly to clean up debris and bring in raw materials for healing. The next stage is the growth of fibroblasts called fibroplasia which will go on to form the building block of a strong wound, collagen. During this time another process called epithelialization is occurring in the skin which means the growth of skin or epithelial or epidermal cells.

Now how does the body know what to do and how to do it? Recent studies have shown that substances called cytokines appear in the blood stream after an injury or surgery, and these somehow act as messengers to organize this redevelopment process.

A lot of factors will effect your ability to heal properly, as mentioned in the poem, and I will repeat them here for you. If you have any of these factors you will heal more slowly and you should understand that the healing process in each individual is different. With a procedure as simple as an appendectomy, some individuals will be ready to go back to normal activity in a few days whereas others may be incapacitated for a month or more.

The factors are age, general health, whether you have local wound problems such as: hematoma or seroma, anemia, presence of malignancy, obesity, trauma, vitamin deficiencies, medications you are on, such as steroids which markedly inhibit normal healing, diabetes mellitus, chemotherapy and chronic liver disease to name a few. Also, if your surgeon treats the tissue badly, it won't heal well. It's also important to keep the wound clean and probably best not to go bungee jumping or play football for a two to four-week period.

In conclusion, I should emphasize that as of yet there is no way to make an incision and not end up with a scar. Certain individuals may be scar formers with development of thickened, unsightly scars at the incision site called hypertrophic scars or keloids. These can sometimes be lessened by the injection of a steroid substance such as Kenalog into the wound, but it usually does not completely eliminate the problem. If you have to have elective surgery, discuss the location of the incision with the surgeon and he may be able to place it in such a way that it won't ruin your social life!

Chapter 22
ANESTHESIA

Though this profession has its class,
These Docs are known for passing gas.
But you won't know it cause they keep,
All their patients fast asleep.

Actually that statement is only partly true. Anesthesiology is a profession requiring several years of training after medical school and these physicians have a whole armamentarium of ways to keep you from experiencing pain during a surgical procedure.

The advent of practical anesthesia in the mid eighteen hundreds opened the doors for tremendous advances in surgical technique which were impossible in awake or sedated patients. In the last fifty years the advances have progressed to safer and more esoteric methods of dealing not only with eliminating consciousness and pain during surgery, but also to a subspecialty of pain management which allows them to help patients with chronic pain from benign or malignant disease.

The anesthesiologist will take a history from the patient, review the records and do a limited appropriate physical exam. If you are having a surgical procedure, he will discuss with you the various options including full general anesthesia, where you are put to sleep, heavy sedation plus local anesthesia, or some type of spinal or regional anesthesia. Except for the completely local anesthetics, most anesthesiologists will need to have an IV started for administration of medications and he or a nurse will start this in the pre-op area. Once you have gone into the operating room, you will be hooked up to an EKG monitor. Depending on the seriousness or location of the surgery, he may want to place an arterial line, an IV line in an artery to better monitor your blood pressure and a place to draw blood samples if needed, and give antibiotics. After you are asleep, he could place a nasogastric tube down your nose into your stomach and a Foley catheter in your bladder to measure urine output. While the surgeon is called the captain of the ship in the operating room, the anesthesiologist is certainly the second captain and manages the patient's vital signs and any non-surgical problems that might arise during the case. This includes a host of medical problems including heart abnormalities, respiratory problems, paralyzing the patient when needed, and looking for any untoward reactions to the abnormal state of anesthesia.

The patient is usually sedated prior to entering the operating room to allay anxiety, and some of the drugs, like Versed, may cause total amnesia from the time it is given until you wake up in the recovery room. Once in the operating room the anesthesiologist administering a general anesthetic will give more medications by vein followed by a combination of intravenous medications and gases, the last of which are given either through a mask held or strapped over the patient's mouth and nose, via an endotracheal tube inserted into the trachea, or a special laryngeal tube fitted into the throat. The anesthesiologist may either breathe for you, if you are completely paralyzed, or connect you to a machine which will breathe for you at a fixed rate and give you a fixed volume of oxygen mixed with several anesthetic agents. We don't need to discuss the specific agents except to say that ether and chloroform, two old standbys, are no longer used.

Some patients may develop headaches, nausea or dizziness after a general anesthetic, but this is all treatable with medications and rapidly passes away.

For those patients who do not need or want a general anesthetic, the anesthesiologist can give a heavy sedation in combination with the surgeon injecting a local anesthetic like marcaine or xylocaine. Many surgeons do hernias, breast biopsies, removal of skin tumors and many other general and orthopedic surgeries under combined general sedation and local anesthesia.

A third method of anesthesia is the regional block. In this type the anesthesiologist injects local anesthetic agents around specific nerves to block or temporarily deaden the area. The patient feels no pain although he may still retain a sense of pressure or vague touch.

Still another type of block is the spinal or epidural, another location near the spinal cord, such as used in delivering babies or even to do abdominal or lower extremity surgery. This is usually augmented by some sedation, again to decrease the anxiety during the surgical procedure.

In many medical centers, the anesthesiologists are giving what is called a continuous epidural block which involves placing a very fine tube in the epidural space in the back and delivering a set amount of medication such as morphine even after the surgery is completed. This takes away most of the discomfort after a major abdominal or lower extremity surgery and can be kept in place for several days. It's certainly the way I want to go if I have to have any major surgery, but it takes a specially trained physician to place the tube and to monitor it carefully afterward.

The anesthesiologist and pain management specialist has a large number of procedures he can do to permanently block sensory nerves in individuals with severe pain from chronic diseases and from cancer. There is practically no situation where pain cannot be alleviated and these specialists are the ones a surgeon will turn to when that expertise is needed. But, remember, it is necessary and important for the patient or the family to be "proactive" and ask about all these types of procedures.

Chapter 23
BURNS

Somehow, with whatever happens inside,
We can retain some personal pride.
Because when our faces and smooth skin are left
We're somehow not completely bereft.

The tragedy with burns appears to be
They can harm our personality,
We can tolerate an inner pain, you'll discover,
But destroy our looks, and we may not recover!

Today most major burns are handled in comprehensive burn centers, with dedicated nurses, internists and surgeons familiar with this subspecialty. Some estimates indicate that there are more than 200,000 major burn victims in the United States each year, and more than a third require hospitalization. Burns are graded as first, second and third degree depending on their depth of penetration and injury to the skin. Most of us are familiar with first degree burns which are essentially like sunburns causing redness, pain and occasional swelling. This type of burn may result in superficial peeling but does not cause any permanent scarring.

Second degree burn is a more extreme extension of this with blister formation, severe pain and partial sloughing of the outer layer of skin. It takes regular cleansing and care not to get infected and yet it will heal on its own without skin grafting. However, depending on the depth and location, it will probably leave some scarring and deformity.

Third degree burns indicate full thickness destruction of the skin and are often initially not painful because the skin and its nerves have been destroyed. If the area involved is more than a small percentage of the body surface area, there can be severe loss of fluids and the body chemistries called electrolytes, high chance for infection locally and throughout the body, a shock-type state with possible damage to the lungs and kidney. The involved skin will never recover and these areas have to be covered with eventual skin grafts or rotation of skin from adjacent or other areas of the body. These situations will result in severe scarring and disfigurement, often very difficult to correct with plastic surgery.

The treatments for advanced burns in a burn center consists of cleansing the areas, debridement and removal of dead tissue in what is often a painful process because of the live skin remaining next to the dead skin, vigorous fluid and electrolyte replacement, antibiotic therapy and a very strong psycho-social support program.

The skin is the largest organ in our bodies and if you didn't already know it, it is a vital organ, keeping infection out of your body and keeping fluids, heat and chemicals inside. Loss of even a small amount of skin can therefore be very dangerous requiring intensive treatment. In spite of this many burn patients die. The problem is more severe in children because they can deteriorate very quickly and don't have the body "reserves" of fluid to withstand such a major insult.

Often, the survivability of a burn patient is dependent upon two factors: The percentage of the body burned and the amount of second and third degree burns. The following diagram shows the percentage of body surface areas and is used by a doctor in determining these factors.

RULE OF NINES

REGION	PER CENT
HEAD AND NECK	9
UPPER EXTREMITIES (ARMS)	18 (9 X 2)
LOWER EXTREMITIES (LEGS)	18 (9 X 2)
FRONT OF BODY	18
BACK OF BODY	18
GROIN (PERINEUM OR GENITALIA)	1
TOTAL	100

DIAGRAM 2

Also important is whether the patient has sustained lung damage, thermal or heat damage and whether there is damage to the kidneys. Underlying other conditions, such as diabetes mellitus, heart disease, kidney disease, and lung problems, such as emphysema from smoking as well as advanced age and poor general physical condition, may cause an increase in the mortality rate.

Burn care is a very complex problem of management and my best comment is to insist that any significant burn should be treated in a burn center by specialists. It's better to take all burn victims to the experts at once, rather than a day or two after the incident when complications have already started. It is no longer a condition that a family doctor or general surgeon can manage with anywhere near the acuity of specially trained nurses and doctors in a burn facility and the needed isolation units, debridement tanks, special large holding tanks for bathing and debriding, and specially trained anesthesiologists to control the pain management. The plastic surgery required for even the most basic reconstruction is beyond the expertise of the average plastic surgeon.

When confronted by a severe burn - think only BURN CENTER!

Chapter 24
SUTURES, STAPLES
AND DRAINS

Sutures, staples and drains, I contend,
Are all a means to a surgical end.
And to dispel any bizarre surgical rumors,
They're just to close wounds and drain evil humors.

The choices we have to close wounds are as varied,
As the tomb you can choose if you want to be buried.
You can suture the skin with nylon or silk,
Or use something else of a polymer ilk.

And of drains, there are plenty for blood or infection,
You'll find in the hospital, a massive collection.
The only big choice is just when to use 'em,
And how to place 'em and not to abuse 'em.

The first question many of my patients have before elective or emergency surgery is: "Will there be a big scar?" It's almost as if it doesn't matter what goes on below the skin level.

Vanity, Vanity - the touchstone of humanity!

Well let's move on. In the past one hundred years we have developed all kinds of suture materials, each with its own particular advantages and disadvantages. Some are non-absorbable like the old silk and wire to the newer Prolene, nylon, Nurolon, polypropylene, Ti-Cron and other chemical polymers, while others are absorbable, which means they dissolve in the body's tissue anywhere from a few weeks to a few months after usage. Among the absorbable sutures are the old catgut which comes in plain or chromated varieties, to the newer synthetic materials like polyglycolic acid (PDS) sutures and vicryl. Some sutures used on the skin have to be removed while other used just under the skin in the subcuticular later, are placed like hem stitches and never have to be removed; they eventually dissolve. Nowadays the thread comes attached to the needle and it's very rare that the nurse has to thread a needle for the surgeon. This saves time, and because the thread is amazingly fitted into the back end of the needle, the atraumatic needle, the hole made while suturing is exactly the diameter of the needle itself.

For suturing the fascia, the strong structure holding in your abdomen, and for suturing tendons and heavy structures, we use heavy suture material, whereas for delicate structures like facial skin, children's skin or blood vessels we use finer material that leaves less scarring. Sutures are grades numerically from the very thick #2 to the very fine, thinner than a human hair, 10-0 used for some types of eye surgery.

Using too weak a suture material may result in wound breakdown and the surgeon must take the overall wound healing into consideration as we have discussed in Chapter 21. When an area is under tension, the sutures need to be left in longer, and when there is no tension and a more plastic closure is desired, the sutures may be taken out earlier and replaced with paper strips called Steri-Strip to hold the wound together without leaving suture marks.

There are several types of wound closures as illustrated. Simple sutures are for the run of the mill closures, mattress sutures for coapting the skin edges a little more securely, and retention sutures for holding large areas together with huge sutures which can be loosened or tightened as needed. There are subcuticular sutures and Steri-Strip as mentioned above. In deep wounds such as the abdominal wall, a layered closure is performed as shown in Diagram 3 (next page).

Now let's move on to drains. Why do we use them? The simple answer is just as it sounds, to drain something out of a wound, whether it is blood, serum from a seroma, bile, infection, pus, or the expectation that there will be an infection or pus. Examples are as follows: with a ruptured appendix, many surgeons will place a drain in the area of the rupture to drain off debris and infected material with the expectation that pus will form and need to get out of the body. With some extensive cancer surgeries, there may be large raw areas which may drain small but steady amounts of serum or blood for a short time. After certain plastic surgery such as breast implants, reduction mammoplasties or mastecto-mies, tube drains may be placed to assure an absolutely dry operative field and prevent formation of hematomas or seromas. These may be Jackson-Pratt drains, Davol sump drains, or Hemovacs. Sometimes the surgeon will place a soft rubber drain called a Penrose in a wound or in

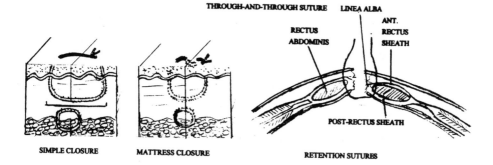

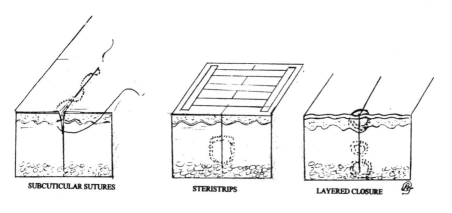

TYPES OF WOUND
CLOSURES

DIAGRAM 3

the subcutaneous tissue to keep a wound open and allow infection to dissipate. Drains, if left long enough, will form a tract so that when they are removed, an opening is still left through which fluids such as bile or pus can drain if needed. It usually takes about seven to ten days to form a tract, so that's how long we usually leave drains in an area of infection.

Sometimes a seroma, which is a collection of watery fluid, or hematoma may form several days after surgery and a patient will need to have this aspirated with a needle and syringe. If the fluid collection recurs then a drain can be placed under a local anesthetic. This can happen in areas such as the axilla or armpit after lymph node dissection, or after some big hernia operations when artificial mesh is used to close a weak abdominal wall.

When drains, small or large, are removed, the surgeon will usually give the patient some pain medication before pulling the tube, although most times the procedure is almost painless.

Another method of closing skin or connective tissue is by the use of staples. These may vary tremendously in size and shape, but for the most part they look like staples in a paper stapler. They can be used for closing skin incisions, especially when infection is present, and generally they leave a very clean incision.

Whereas years ago intestines had to be sewn together in two layers in a tedious procedure, today we have stapling apparatus that can connect one loop of intestine to another in less that a minute, and do so in a more exacting fashion than a surgeon could accomplish with a needle and thread. In laparoscopic surgery (*see* Chapter 15), special staplers have been devised to clip off blood vessels and the gall bladder duct, to amputate the appendix, and staple off the fallopian tube in a tubal ligation. Neurosurgeons use staplers to clamp off aneurysms in the brain, and general surgeons routinely use staplers to occlude blood vessels in many types of surgery such as thyroid resections, hernias, liver and spleen surgery. There is even a special device that ligates or ties off, divides and staples tissue in one motion, called the LDS stapler. There are staplers that can connect two loops of colon together end-to-end and even connect blood vessels end-to-end.

The field of mechanization continues to improve each year and makes surgery safer, more rapid and less risky for the patient and the surgeon alike.

Chapter 25
LABORATORY VALUES

You may not want to be a number
But you are, ain't that a bummer.
And if you don't have pretty data,
Well, you're just a second rater!

Face it. We're just a large accumulation of chemicals. Suffice it to say the status of our bodies is often wrapped up in laboratory values, so you might as well know what the major ones stand for! It's not my intention to describe all the laboratory data, but rather to give you the most common ones and show how they reflect what's going on in your body. It may seem boring, but then, give it a try. If you don't like it, go on to the next chapter!

First, there's the CBC or complete blood count. This includes the hemoglobin and hematocrit which measure the amount of red blood cells, RBC's, in the blood stream. These cells carry, among other things, oxygen to the cells to keep you alive. Normal values of hemoglobin, Hg, range from 13-15 grams and all these values will vary with sex, age, and body habitus, and hematocrit, Hct, should be about three times the hemoglobin or 39 to 45%. Lowered Hct and Hg will indicate acute or chronic blood loss or other conditions including malnutrition, cancer, or deficiency in the bone marrow where blood is made or in the building products of blood such as calcium, Ca. It is usually the first laboratory data which your doctors looks at. The sedimentation rate of red cells, sed rate, is a vague estimation of disease but can be used to monitor certain illnesses, recurrent disease or responses to medications; it is normally in the range of 10-20.

Included in the CBC is the WBC or white blood count which is a measure of many different types of blood cells, as long as they're not red, including polys, monocytes, eosinophils, and basophils. The important thing is that when there is an elevation of the WBC above the normal range of 3,000-9,000, it may mean something's going on such as infection or acute or chronic disease. Usually, the higher the WBC, the more serious the situation. As an example, in appendicitis the WBC may be anywhere from normal to 14,000 or more; with a ruptured appendicitis where the appendix has burst and caused peritonitis and severe infection, the WBC may be into the 20,000 range. Certain malignancies can cause marked reduction or marked elevation of the WBC. The WBC level is used to monitor the cancer patient's response to some chemotherapeutic agents. The WBC is one measure of our ability to fight off infection and in patients with AIDS or on chemotherapy, the level may drop below 1000 and place the individual at high risk for severe systemic infections. The CBC also includes the platelet count (*see* Chapter 18) which should normally be in the range of 200,000 to 400,000/mm3. When levels get below 40,000 then bleeding can occur and the patient may need platelet transfusions!

Other blood studies also relate to blood clotting. The bleeding time should be about 4 minutes. If it's prolonged, you may have a bleeding problem. The PT and PTT are special measures of coagulation and all that's important is that PT should be about 12-14 seconds and PTT should be about 45 seconds. Anticoagulants such as coumadin will cause the PT to be elevated and heparin will cause the PTT to be elevated. The physician must monitor these values to make sure that your blood is not too thin when you are taking these medicines.

Urinalysis is another important blood study and includes measurement of blood in the urine, since normally there should be none; this may indicate lab error, infection, kidney stone or malignancy. Pus in the urine indicates a urinary tract infection. BUN (blood urea nitrogen) and creatinine, Cr, help us evaluate kidney function with normal BUN about 7-18 and Cr about 0.2-0.8.

Bilirubin is one of the breakdown products of blood and measures the ability of the liver to function properly. An elevated bilirubin may mean liver disease but is also elevated with gall bladder disease when a gall stone is blocking the main bile duct (*see* chapter on Gall Bladder and Bile Ducts) or leakage of bile after gall bladder surgery. Normal bilirubin is about 0.1 to 1.1, although there are certain people who have elevated bilirubin because of a strange, otherwise asymptomatic disease called Gilbert's disease. Your doctor knows all about these things. Calcium, Ca, and phosphorus, P, are important chemicals in bone strength and Ca is important in blood clotting. The blood levels of these elements are controlled by small glands in the neck behind the thyroid gland called the parathyroid gland. There are several benign and malignant diseases of these glands which may be indicated by an elevated Ca and a lowered P. Also, since Ca is used in blood coagulation, when there has been a lot of bleeding and blood clotting, the Ca level may fall. Normal Ca is 9-11 and normal P is 2-4.

Amylase and lipase are enzymes or chemicals in the blood secreted predominately by the pancreas. Elevations of these may indicate pancreatitis (see Pancreas) or inflammation in an organ near the pancreas such as the liver or gall bladder. Amylase normally is 25-125 but may rise into the thousands with pancreatitis and similarly, lipase, which is normally about 23-208 can get as high as 20,000 in active disease.

We have already discussed blood type and crossmatching in Chapter 18. We can get blood samples and obtain specific blood products which a person needs rather than just giving "whole" blood. These products include fresh frozen plasma, platelet concentrate, cryoprecipitate, and other complex blood products - that's why we have special physicians called hematologists to sort out the problem.

SGOT, normal level 5-40, SGPT, normal 7-56, and LDH, normal 100-190, are substances which indicate liver disease. It is a complex subject and all you need to know is that when they are elevated the physician has to determine which of many diseases are present such as hepatitis, cirrhosis, malignancy, bile duct obstruction or a whole host of other diseases. Alkaline phosphatase, normal range 20-90, may be elevated in several diseases but is important as an indicator of bile duct obstruction either from inflammation, stones or malignancy. Prostatic acid phosphatase is secreted by certain cells in the prostate gland and elevation may indicate disease of the prostate and prostate specific antigen, PSA, may indicate cancer of the prostate gland.

There are hundreds of other laboratory tests which physicians order to help in the diagnosis of disease and not only blood is used in these tests. We can obtain spinal fluid for infections and malignancies and other diseases of the brain and spinal cord, paracentesis fluid, fluid from the abdomen, to be analyzed for infection, malignancy or chronic diseases, pleural fluid, or thoracentesis fluid from inside the chest for the same type of determinations, and finally fluid aspirated from cysts anywhere in the body for diagnosis, including breast cysts, sebaceous cysts, and ganglion cysts. There are many blood studies for rare metals such as magnesium, zinc and mercury.

The term C&S refers to culture and sensitivity, when samples are taken of possibly infected areas. The culture part means that the bacteria are grown outside the body on a special plate called a Petri dish in a nutrient called Agar. When the bacterial colonies grow, special laboratory workers can identify the organism, such as staph or strep or T.B. The bacteria is then tested for sensitivity to certain drugs and a report is then sent to the doctor indicating the name of the bacteria and the antibiotics which will be most effective in eradicating it.

Other laboratory tests you have heard about and their normal levels are cholesterol <200, serum proteins, albumin and globulin, and blood sugar, 60-100. The laboratory can also measure blood and urine levels of many drugs such as digitalis, chemotherapeutic agents, and alcohol and street drugs. Arterial blood gases, ABG's, measure the amount of oxygen in your blood, and pulmonary function tests measure how much air you can take in your lungs and can determine lung function problems caused by smoking, infection or other diseases.

Now you have a brief overview of diagnostic laboratory tests - I hope it hasn't been too boring and that it has given you some insight into the adjunctive measures your doctor can use in making a diagnosis.

Chapter 26
RADIOLOGY AND DIAGNOSIS
FOR THE SURGEON

I won't go so far as to offer an apology
That surgeons are in bed so to say, with radiology.
But we are quite dependent on what they can show,
And we're often enamored with that which they know.

You see to find answers and make diagnoses
We often need x-rays, from head down to toesies.
They get complex angiograms and CT Scans rolling,
Sometimes I'm not sure if they're coming or going.

T
he surgeon is often deeply indebted to the radiologist for assistance in making diagnoses and for therapeutic radiological procedures. You may think of the radiologist as the physician who just reads chest x-rays, but you'd be quite mistaken. These physicians have a huge armamentarium of procedures involving x-ray, nuclear medicine, ultrasound, computerized scanning, interventional angiography, inserting catheters into blood vessels for diagnosis, treatment, dilating narrowed areas, placing drains, doing x-ray guided needle biopsies of the lung, liver, or breast, and magnetic resonance imaging, to name a few. They have a detailed knowledge of anatomy, pathology, surgery, and medicine and often discuss with the surgeon what studies should be undertaken to make a diagnosis.

I want to describe some of the studies listed above just so you will have a better idea what you're in for should you need their diagnostic and therapeutic acumen.

First, there are the contrast studies of the intestinal tract, such as the upper gastrointestinal and small bowel series, where you swallow a special liquid and the radiologist can examine your esophagus, stomach, duodenum or the first part of the small intestine where ulcers sometime occur, and the entire small intestines. A barium enema is an exam of the lower intestinal tract via the rectum. All these studies can identify benign and malignant pathology, sometimes in anticipation of surgical intervention.

Angiograms are studies of blood vessels using contrast or dye. The uses are extensive. From studying vessels in the brain, to those in the heart, the coronary arteries study is done by cardiologists, and may include the aorta, the vessels in the arms and legs and any other organ such as the kidneys, liver, as well as the veins in the body. When pathology is found it may need surgical intervention, but in the last twenty years radiologists and other specialists have developed techniques for percutaneous angiography and angioplasty. Catheters are placed through the skin without a big surgical incision, opening up closed vessels, dilating narrowings, placing filters in veins (*see* Pulmonary Embolism chapter), and saves patients from large incisions in the operating room. These procedures are done in the radiology department under a local anesthetic and often with sedation.

The radiologist has access to special techniques for visualizing the inside of the body, and among these are computerized axial tomography, the CAT scan, and the magnetic resonance imaging, the MRI scan. This complex machinery can reproduce images of your body on a computer screen showing almost every part of your anatomy, and sometimes do it in an almost three dimensional way. They can see pathology such as tiny lung, brain or abdominal cancers, abscesses, bowel obstructions, and many other abnormalities. They can also tell when there isn't anything wrong, and that's important for the surgeon also. You may have all the signs and symptoms of appendicitis, but with negative radiological studies, the surgeon may decide to hold off on surgery and the diagnosis actually may be as simple as food poisoning or gastroenteritis.

Another modality is nuclear medicine. In this field the patient is given radioisotope material, though not radioactive enough to cause any damage, which frequently localizes in a special organ or special tissue, and radiologists are thereby able to make specific diagnoses. Examples are special scans for pulmonary embolism, for thyroid and parathyroid disease, brain tumors, and infections, to name a few. These are painless studies which give the surgeon a lot of information. For example, when I first started in surgery, we often had to spend hours in surgery exploring the neck for a 3 millimeter parathyroid gland tumor. Now the parathyroid scan can often localize the tumor so that the surgeon can find it rapidly, saving the patient extra time under anesthesia and saving the surgeon from getting ulcers looking for a tumor, like a "needle in a haystack".

Ultrasound is another modality used by the radiologist where sound waves create an image on a screen. The trained technicians and radiologists can diagnose cysts in breasts, liver, pancreas or anywhere else in the body, gallstones in the gallbladder and common bile duct (*see* Gallbladder), and hematomas, seromas and abscesses. The radiologist can also insert tubes and drains in these cysts if indicated, using ultrasound, CAT scan or MRI scan. On numerous occasions radiologists have inserted drains in intra-abdominal abscesses, saving the patient a complex and difficult operation.

The radiologists have been working hand in hand with the surgeons since the end of the nineteenth century when Wilhelm Roentgen first discovered the x-ray, and each year new procedures evolve which will continue to aid in diagnosis and hopefully simplify procedures for the patient.

Chapter 27
ALCOHOLISM, DRUG, AND OTHER ADDICTIONS AND SURGERY

Yo mamma, would you like a hit?
You won't have to worry the least little bit.
A little vodka, some "bennies" or a "toot",
'Cause the doc will fix ya up, room and board to boot!

We have a wonderful system, health care for the addicted
Even if your complications aren't fully predicted,
No matter how sick you get, just another refrain,
You can just go right out and do it again.

It's always remarkable for me to know that upwards of 40% of all hospital admissions are related directly or indirectly to drug, alcohol, tobacco and other addictions. It is a subject rarely well dealt with by the medical schools, residencies and hospitals. It is a serious problem and yet it is apparent that less attention is paid to this topic even in the medical texts than to relatively obscure diseases such as Myasthenia gravis and lupus erythematosus.

With international programs such as Alcoholics Anonymous, Narcotics Anonymous, Smokers Anonymous, and many support groups, and with the individual, nursing, physician and hospital discharge facilities, we are still sorely lacking in appropriate management of this tremendous problem. Smoking alone is responsible for many thousands of deaths each year from lung cancer.

I mention this topic in a surgical text because so many of my patients have this addiction problem to one degree or another. The availability of treatment programs is far below the need, and the HMO and insurance companies shy away from the diagnosis and treatment because it is so expensive and the success rate is so poor.

Let us just run down a few of the problems associated with addictive disease:

1. Smoking can cause bronchitis, pneumonia, emphysema, cancer of the throat, mouth, lungs, stomach, esophagus and pancreas leading to extensive surgeries and morbidity, vascular disease leading to bypass surgery and amputations, and heart disease which may lead to open heart surgery.

2. Alcohol (associated with mouth) can cause esophagus and stomach cancers, or severe liver disease with liver failure, ascites or fluid in the abdomen which may require surgery, heart disease, and severe neurological disorders. There are a host of directly related problems due to excess drinking including auto accidents, spousal abuse and injury, and knife and gun wounds, and kidney failure.

3. Drug abuse can lead to sudden death, abscesses, liver failure, and bizarre behavior leading to trauma and death to oneself and to others.

Many of these problems require surgical intervention and yet the addiction is so strong that the patients keep returning and returning, sicker each time until the problems compound and they die. It's a massive public health problem, yet the public all but turn its back on it. It has taken over a hundred years to make a dent in the tobacco industry in the last few years, and unfortunately, it may take many years to impact the drug and alcohol problem.

If you or a loved one has an addictive disease, you will understand that these are diseases of denial, unlike cancer of the breast or colon. In spite of a deteriorating life in all areas, professional, social, and economic, these diseases destroy the body, often in a slow progressive fashion.

Wake up America! Get yourself or your family member the help needed; don't just treat the sequelae and symptoms of the disease. Too often the patient will gladly undergo surgery, but balks at taking care of the problem which has resulted in the need for the surgery.

Chapter 28
CONTRIBUTIONS
FROM THE SUBSPECIALISTS

It seems in most predicaments,
Someone puts in his two cents,
But if you get enough of tuppence,
Soon you'll have a pound of uppance.

As a surgeon I'll accept,
As much good help as I can get,
So I will get a complete list,
Of every well known specialist.

I want to acknowledge that, as a surgeon, I am continually reliant upon the expertise of a number of subspecialists who have helped me in the diagnosis and treatment of patients over the years. We no longer stand as the independent physicians of the nineteenth century. They were the horse and buggy doctors who visited homes and accomplished their remarkable feats of diagnosis and treatment with only a skeletal outline of what we have today. They often failed and yet they usually did the best they could with the support and tools they had.

With the twentieth century, we saw the emergence of specialties and then subspecialties of medicine because of the complexity of diagnostics and the vast increase in information and interventional procedures. This gave rise to the surgical subspecialties, as we will see in Part II, and also gave rise to the medical subspecialties, among which are the gastroenterologists, pulmonologists, intensivists specializing in caring for patients in the intensive care unit, oncologists, hematologists, cardiologists, infectious disease specialists, radiation therapists, pain management experts, psycho-social support teams, and many others. I will mention a few of the ways these experts help the surgeon and let your own imagination lead you to understand how invaluable all these physicians are to the surgeon and thereby to the patient.

The gastroenterologist, in addition to his medical diagnostic expertise, uses several types of endoscopes; these are lighted tubes that can be inserted into the intestinal tract through the mouth or rectum. They can examine the stomach and duodenum, and the entire colon, identifying lesions, taking biopsies, removing some tumors, checking for recurrence of malignancy and even using special devices to stop bleeding that in the past required operative intervention. They give the surgeon more information and thereby help us do our work in a more prepared and educated manner. They can visualize bile ducts and remove stones, obviating the need for most common bile duct surgery. They can place tubes in the stomach through the abdominal wall for tube feedings and are trained in giving total parenteral nutrition, TPN, to support the pre- and post-operative patient who cannot take food by mouth.

The pulmonologists use bronchoscopes to examine the lungs and take biopsies, as well as managing peri and post operative lung problems from pneumonia, to mucus plugs (mucus that gets stuck in the bronchi or tubes in the lungs which prevent a patient from breathing adequately), and managing respirators and all pulmonary problems with the latest medications.

We have discussed infectious disease doctors and hematologists in prior chapters. Their contributions to the support team is invaluable. The oncologists manage the cancer patients. Many years ago the surgeons would manage all aspects of cancer therapy, but this is rarely the case today.

So, the surgical care of a patient is a comprehensive one, and the surgeon who uses all the help at hand, will be doing his patient a great service.

Chapter 29
CHEMOTHERAPY AND RADIATION THERAPY FOR CANCER

It's important that we say enough,
That cancer treatment's sometimes rough.
In this chapter I'll be brief:
It ain't all roses, but it's not all grief!

L et me make it clear at the outset: This is not a book about cancer and cancer therapy. It is about surgery. But many times the patient undergoing a surgery for cancer will have preoperative or postoperative chemotherapy or radiation therapy. I want to give you at least an introduction as to what you can expect in terms of side effects and treatment of these side effects.

Chemotherapy is very strong medicine and is designed to kill cancer cells. Unfortunately most chemotherapeutic agents are not completely and solely specific for the cancer cells and attack and destroy some healthy normal cells during the treatment of the cancer. Of course the pharmaceutical companies and your oncologists understand this and have to weigh the benefits of the drug with the disadvantages and side effects. Although most of the side effects are transient such as hair loss, anemia, rash, bleeding possibilities and tiredness, there are some that may be more permanent. Some of the strongest drugs may have toxicity or injury potential to the heart and the kidneys and even the liver, but when there is no alternative, then these potential problems have to be explained to the patient and a decision has to be made about their use. I have outlined the function of an infusion center, a place where chemotherapy and other medication therapy is given, in my book on "Comprehensive Breast Care", and it outlines the prevention and treatment of side effects such as nausea, vomiting, low red blood count, white blood count and platelet count. The other complications of chemotherapy include lethargy or tiredness, headache, depression, weight gain, skin changes, mouth sores, tingling of the hands and feet and others. But remember that some patients develop minimal side effects and the side effects are directly related to the type of medication you receive and the dosage. In the past few years, there has been tremendous progress in treatment of these side effects with new medication for all but eliminating nausea and vomiting. And there are drugs to increase your blood count. It is beyond this chapter to go into all the side effects and their treatment, but your oncologists will explain this to you in detail prior to starting the treatment. The American Cancer Society has wig banks and "Look Good, Feel Better" programs to help with the changes during chemotherapy, and most good cancer treatment programs have strong psychosocial departments to help the patient cope with the stresses of the disease and the treatment. Every surgeon should make his/her patient aware of all the programs available in any comprehensive cancer program.

Radiation therapy may last for up to eight or ten weeks, usually taking a few minutes each day. The radiation therapist will explain to you about the treatment and the side effects. The one I hear about most frequently is tiredness and rest is very important while going through this therapy. The other side effects will depend on the area being treated. Skin can develop a sunburn or rash which may be painful. Abdominal radiation may cause nausea and vomiting, diarrhea, urinary symptoms of burning and pain and, if near the pelvis, can cause rectal pain and vaginal dryness. Radiation to the head and neck can cause pain, ulcers and irritation to the throat and tongue. Again, the physician will clearly outline the course of therapy, the side effects and the treatments available and then you can discuss this with all your doctors and decide if you want to go through with it. I find that most of my patients tolerate radiation therapy very well as long as they understand what is going on and get the appropriate psychosocial support and medications to treat the side effects.

Let us now move on to Part II and an in-depth discussion of the surgical specialties and some of their more common cases.

PART II

The objective of Part II of this book is to present twelve surgical specialties and describe in a few concise pages the most common major procedures that are performed by physicians, telling why they are done, how they are done and some of the possible problems and complications that can be encountered. Obviously this is not a text for surgeons, but for the general public to get a clearer idea of what physicians do and what you can expect if you are undergoing a surgical procedure. I have tried to present this material in a medically sound, yet pleasant read so that you may understand the beauty and fascination of surgery.

A

General Surgery

Chapter 30
HERNIAS

Inguinal, Femoral, Umbilical, Ventral and Esophageal

A hernia or rupture, has as its goal,
To push something out of an abnormal hole.
It's usually caused by a weakness of tissue,
And how to repair it remains the main issue.

If tissue is stuck, it is incarcerated,
Which means, like the inmate, it's not liberated.
And if it's so stuck that its arteries are mangulated,
We say that the hernia has become strangulated!

If you draw a line from your hip to the center of your groin we will call that line the inguinal ligament. Everything just below is called femoral area and everything just above is called inguinal. Men and women can develop hernias in both areas which means that there is a weakness or widening of the tissue of the abdominal wall or deep pelvic wall. As seen in the diagram, the inguinal hernia can either come through the area where the spermatic cord in men or the round ligament in women exits the abdomen, called the indirect space, or from the tissue just adjacent to this called the direct space. The femoral hernia appears as a bulge or sometimes a pain in the femoral area. If you place your fingers along that inguinal line and feel the pulse, keep moving inwards and that's where a femoral hernia will be (*see* Diagram 4, next page).

A hernia can appear as a transient bulge with pain or aching, or sometimes a sharp twinge. It will form a sac or bag where it comes out. What's in a hernia? Actually anything in the abdomen that is loose enough to drop into it such as the fatty apron or omentum, the intestine or even the appendix and in women even an ovary. If it comes and goes it's called reducible, which means it can be put back, and if it stays out

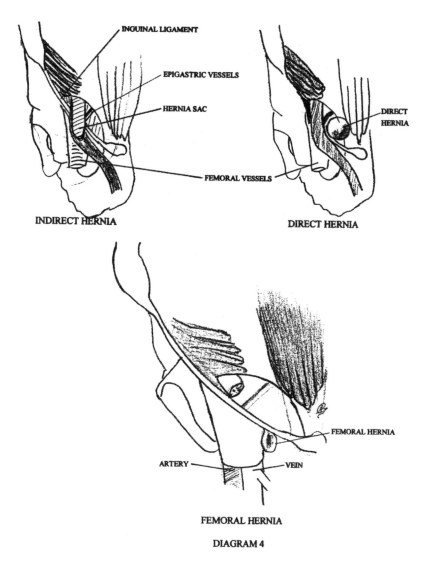

INGUINAL LIGAMENT

EPIGASTRIC VESSELS

HERNIA SAC

FEMORAL VESSELS

INDIRECT HERNIA

DIRECT
HERNIA

DIRECT HERNIA

FEMORAL HERNIA

ARTERY

VEIN

FEMORAL HERNIA

DIAGRAM 4

it's called irreducible or incarcerated. When a hernia is incarcerated and the neck, where it exits the body, is too tight, the blood supply to whatever is in the hernia sac can get shut off and become strangulated, like with the hangman's noose, and unless surgery is immediate, the contents may die resulting in dead intestine or dead fat. Many patients think that because they have a small hernia it doesn't need to be fixed. Well, when talking about inguinal or femoral hernias, it may be just the opposite, the smaller ones may be more dangerous because the openings are smaller and incarceration and strangulation can occur, whereas with the larger ones the opening may have stretched so much that the contents go back and forth easily. However, this is not always true, and hernias should be repaired unless there are medical contraindications to surgery.

Why do hernias occur? Usually there is a weak area aggravated by some heavy work or lifting, sometimes you're just born with it and sometimes it's caused by trauma to the area. The repair may be open or laparoscopic. The open repair consists of: (1) reducing or pushing the contents of the hernia back into the abdomen, (2) sometimes tying off the neck of the sac and cutting away some of the sac if it's large and (3) sewing closed the defect. Sometimes when the tissue is weak an artificial piece of mesh is sewn or stapled in place to reinforce the repair. Laparoscopic hernia repairs (*see* Laparoscopy) are preferred by some surgeons and frowned on by others, but consists of basically closing the hernia defect from inside the abdomen with sutures and mesh. The open hernia repairs can be done under local or general anesthesia; the laparoscopic procedures require a general anesthetic.

This type of hernia surgery is done as an outpatient and the complications are bleeding, infection and breakdown of the repair (*see* Complications). You should not do any heavy lifting or vigorous physical activity for at least three to four weeks after the repair and if you have other medical problems, your physician may tell you to rest for even longer. Occasionally the patient may get ecchymosis and appear black and blue in the groin and in the penis and scrotum in men; it looks awful but goes away in a week or two.

There is a nerve, the ilioinguinal, that goes through the area of the hernia, and if injured it may cause pain radiating into the groin and thigh. This usually resolves in a few weeks but sometimes, if the discomfort is bothersome, a nerve block has to be done if it persists for several months. If the nerve is completely divided, which can occur in the best of surgeon's hands, then the patient will have some numbness in these areas.

I had a hernia repair as a child and had some mild numbness, but it's minimal and I only remembered it because I'm writing this chapter.

Let's move on to umbilical hernias. Some are congenital around the umbilicus or bellybutton. In children they will often close off by themselves and we don't operate on them in the first couple of years unless they are very large, greater than two centimeters or symptomatic.

When you have any hernia as an adult, think of it as a balloon. It's difficult to start blowing it up, but once it's started it's easy for it to get larger. It's the same with hernias, especially the umbilical type. These hernias are very easy to repair when small, just sew the two edges together with strong suture, but the larger they get, the more complex the surgery and possible need for mesh. They usually occur in overweight people and sometimes in women after several pregnancies; they are also found in individuals with chronic liver disease who develop ascites or fluid in the abdomen.

Another type of hernia is the ventral hernia occurring anywhere in the abdominal wall. These develop after previous surgery and are usually found when there has been prior wound infection, chronic illness, obesity or co-morbid conditions such as arteriosclerosis or diabetes mellitus. The repairs may be very complex because of the prior complicating factors and may involve dissecting intestine out of the hernia and finding good tissue to approximate. Since these hernias usually develop in individuals with other problems, the healing may be slow and frequently an artificial mesh may be used. Drains may be needed to prevent blood and fluid from accumulating, and complications includeing breakdown of the repair, infection, and incisional pain. Overweight patients should try to lose weight before a repair. As with the other hernias we described, incarceration and strangulation can occur which may demand urgent repair.

Other hernias in the abdominal wall are basically described by their location such as epigastric in the upper abdomen, spigelian in the lower outer abdomen, and flank or lumbar. An annoying hernia for the patient and the surgeon is the parastomal hernia. Individuals who have colostomies or ileostomies where the intestine is brought to the abdominal wall and a bag is attached, may develop hernias with pain and bulging around the stoma. This requires a general anesthetic and exploration and repair by suturing the opening.

Now let's move on to the esophageal and diaphragmatic hiatus hernia, which is an opening in the diaphragm where the esophagus passes through just before it connects with the stomach; hiatus means gap. We'll talk more about acid reflux or heartburn and esophageal movement problems in chapter 34; I want to focus on the hernias of the diaphragm at this time. As in the diagrams below, there may be several areas where hernias occur in the diaphragm and these are repaired with special sutures. Those not near the esophagus are closed completely, but those around the esophagus have to be done carefully so as to prevent a narrowing at the end of the esophagus and difficulty swallowing. The esophageal hiatus repair includes sutures in the diaphragm as well in two medium sized muscles on either side of the esophagus called the crura (*see* Diagram 5 next page).

Esophageal hiatus hernia repairs may be done for associated symptoms of acid reflux and motility or swallowing problems, gastroesophageal reflux disease, GERD, and other problems so that a simple repair of the opening in the diaphragm is combined with anti-reflux procedures as we shall discuss in a later chapter. The only point I need to make is that a complete gastroenterological, GI, evaluation must be done prior to the surgery so that all problems can be taken care of at once. The diagnosis can be made by endoscopy, x-rays or CT scans, and the indications for surgery are usually dependent upon the severity of the individual's symptomatology. Complications of this type of surgery are usually related to the esophagus and stomach more than the simple repair of the hernia in the diaphragm. The repairs are usually done from the abdominal side, either as an open operation or laparoscopically, but with recurrence or complex problems, repairs done through the chest are occasionally undertaken.

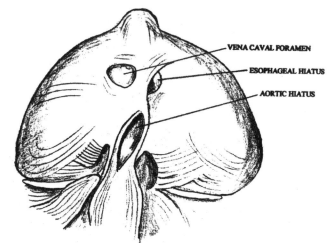

DIAPHRAGM VIEWED FROM BELOW

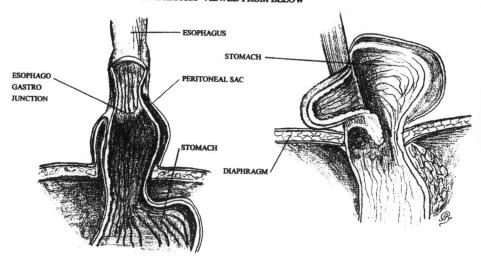

SLIDING HIATUS HERNIA

PARESOPHAGEAL HIATAL HERNIA

ESOPHAGEAL HIATUS

DIAGRAM 5

Chapter 31
THE BREAST

I think it really would be best,
If you'd buy my book about the breast.
But if you're cheap, or beyond your budget,
I'll give you some facts and won't begrudge it.

Instead of a book of four hundred pages,
I'll condense it to six and tell you in stages,
About all the changes benign and malignant,
And if you don't like it, just don't be indignant.

I have written so much about the breast, it's difficult to give a meaningful short version, but I'll try. The important concept to understand is that the female breast undergoes tremendous changes throughout a woman's life and that about one in every eight to ten women in the United States will develop a breast cancer at some time in her life. The incidence increases sharply after age fifty.

One hundred years ago a woman would come to her physician only when she had a large mass in the breast, and it was usually an advanced cancer. The only procedure was radical mastectomy, removing the entire breast and the axillary lymph nodes in the armpit, the underlying chest wall muscles, the pectoralis major and minor, and the prognosis was poor and the cosmetic outlook grim. Women now are urged to examine their breasts monthly and get a yearly mammogram after age forty. Breast disease has come out of the closet and we're making earlier diagnosis, doing breast conservation surgery, and are having better cosmetic and survival results. Women are taught about their breasts and understand that most lumps that they feel are not cancer but that new lumps must be evaluated by their physicians. To understand the anatomy, physiology and history of the breast I must really refer you back to my book on "Comprehensive Breast Care", but for now let us divide the discussion into benign and malignant disease, the diagnostics, the surgery and a few comments about diet, genetics, hormones and risk assessment.

Male breast cancer is very rare and lumps in the male breast are usually a benign disease called gynecomastia, which only needs to be removed if large or symptomatic. Male breast cancer is generally treated by mastectomy.

As I mentioned, female breasts change throughout the course of their life and are directly affected by several factors. The most important is the constant stimulation by estrogens from the onset of menstruation, menarche, to the end of menstruation, menopause, and we know that obesity, high fat diet, family history, pregnancy and age of first child all are contributing factors. Diagnostics include self examination, which you can learn from a free video at the American Cancer Society or from your physician, mammography, ultrasound and more recently MRI studies, although the latter are not available everywhere at the time of this writing (*see* Diagram 6 next page).

The breast anatomy, as in the diagram, consists of acini, lobules, ducts, supporting tissue, and the nipple and areola; there is the associated axilla with its normal lymph nodes and the underlying muscles, nerves and vessels.

Benign diseases include fibroadenomas, rubbery masses often found in very young women, fibrocystic disease which has cavities filled with fluid that may get larger and smaller during the month or may just remain the same, or a whole host of non- cancerous conditions including atypical ductal hyperplasia, adenosis, scarring, infections, huge uncomfortable breasts called hypermastia, underdeveloped breasts, hypomastia, and marked discrepancy in size between the two breasts, and I'm talking about major size difference. Most women have one breast a little larger than the other!.

When an x-ray is done, radiologists compare the new films with previous films if possible and look for masses, changes in architecture and microcalcifications, which are small white dots which can represent abnormalities in the breast but which the radiologists can differentiate into benign, suspicious or cancerous. For further help in clarifying what he sees on x-ray, the radiologist may want enlargement films, ultrasound or when available in some breast centers, MRI. We have been getting farther and farther away from making the diagnosis by open biopsy and now prefer to do needle biopsies with large core needles, done by the surgeon if the mass can be felt. If the mass cannot be felt, and, if there is asymmetry or suspicious microcalcifications, special stereotactic x-ray

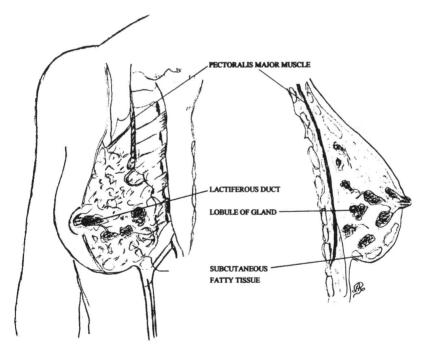

ANATOMY OF THE BREAST

DIAGRAM 6

guided biopsies are done by the radiologist using a computer guided x-ray apparatus on a special table.

There are many different types of breast cancer. The earliest form is ductal carcinoma in situ, DCIS or stage 0 cancer where the cancer is confined to a duct and apparently does not have the ability to spread or metastasize and is essentially 99% curable. Invasive cancers increase in stage by their size and by the presence or absence of cancer in the lymph nodes in the armpit, or the presence of metastatic disease where the cancer has spread beyond the breast and axillary lymph nodes. The TNM system is used with T standing for tumor size, N for presence or absence of cancer in the lymph nodes and number involved, and M for presence or absence of metastases. Surgical and oncological treatment depends to a great degree on staging as we shall see. The survivability of breast cancer is such a complex subject that it is more appropriate for women to discuss this with their surgeons or oncologists.

Stage 0   is DCIS

Stage I   is T1, N0, M0 (with T less than 2 cm)

Stage II   is T2 or 3 (T2 is a tumor larger than 2 cm but less than 5 cm; T3 is a tumor larger than 5 cm), N0 (or N1 in certain cases), M0

Stage III   is T0-3, N2 (matted nodes - fixed to one another), M0

Stage IV   is any T, N with M1 (distant metastasis)

STAGING FOR BREAST CANCER
DIAGRAM 7

Comprehensive breast care is recommended which means that each cancer case is discussed at a tumor board conference where the x-rays and any biopsies are discussed by the board members including oncologists, surgeons, radiologists, pathologists, radiation therapists, plastic surgeons and general physicians. The patient is essentially getting many second opinions and a course of treatment is recommended.

Let us go on to surgery of the breast. Simple cysts can be aspirated by the surgeon in his office using a syringe and needle, and similarly infections of the breast can be opened and drained, usually with a local anesthetic and pain medicine. Simple biopsies can be done as mentioned above but large benign tumors are usually removed in the operating room under local with sedation, or under general anesthesia.

When a core or needle biopsy has been done, if it shows atypical ductal hyperplasia, ADH, which is a benign disease but one occasionally found with cancer nearby, DCIS or invasive cancer, then a surgical excision of the area is needed as recommended by the tumor board. For almost seventy five years, starting in the 1880's with Dr. William Halsted, the radical mastectomy was the procedure of choice for any cancer of the breast. But due to the work of Dr. Bernard Fisher and others, it was found that in many cases removal of the tumor alone with a generous margin of uninvolved breast tissue in conjunction with axillary lymph node dissection and post-operative radiation therapy gave the same results as the radical mastectomy. This was the beginning of breast conserving surgery, and we have continued to progress even more since then. Sometimes a modified radical mastectomy, removal of the entire breast and node dissection but leaving the big pectoralis chest wall muscles, or skin sparing mastectomy, a procedure with smaller incisions removing the nipple and areola but leaving most of the skin for plastic reconstruction, is indicated for extensive disease. Generally we are moving toward breast conservation surgery which includes lumpectomy, quadrantectomy, and partial mastectomy along with axillary node dissection.

The latest progress is that of sentinel node biopsy, possibly eliminating the need for the axillary node dissection. The sentinel node is the first lymph node that a tumor will spread to from a cancer and can be found by radioisotope and/or blue dye injection methods. It requires special training, but most surgeons are starting to learn the technique. If the sentinel node is negative for cancer, there may be no need for axillary dissection; if it is positive, there is still a debate as to whether further dissection is indicated. Clinical trials are being done to answer this question.

When the axillary nodes are removed or the area is radiated, there is a 15-30% incidence of the woman developing lymphedema of the arm on that side. Lymphedema is a swelling of the arm secondary to blocked lymphatic channels and this can vary from mild to severe and sometimes can occur up to ten or fifteen years after surgery.

When mastectomy, axillary dissection and some lumpectomies are performed, the surgeon may place drains to prevent hematomas or seromas. The complications of breast surgery are skin flap problems, some skin may die, infections, hematoma and seroma. In untrained hands, there may be significant deformity associated with breast biopsy and lumpectomy, and plastic reconstruction by specially trained oncoplastic surgeons may be needed. Oncoplastic surgery is a new area of plastic surgery more popular in Europe but which will eventually be part of the training of the general surgeon who wants to specialize in breast cancer surgery.

The nerves in the armpit can be damaged causing a winging of the scapula, the large bone on your upper back, and some weakness around the involved shoulder, but this is uncommon. Some numbness on the upper part of the arm and the back of the armpit can occur if the intercosto-brachial nerve is injured. Many plastic surgical procedures are used to reconstruct the breast after mastectomy and even after lumpectomy (*see* Plastic Surgery).

I will not go into a discussion of chemotherapy (*see* "Comprehensive Breast Care" book) except to say that there is still discussion as to whether patients with large tumors greater than 4-5 cm should have preoperative chemotherapy to shrink the tumor and make breast conservation surgery possible, and then have surgery. Your surgeon will have his own opinion on this matter, but it is a subject on which the experts have differing opinions.

Much of the other surgery on the breast is cosmetic including augmentation mammoplasty, making them bigger with saline implants since silicone has been banned except in selected cases, and reduction mammoplasty, making them smaller. We'll talk more about this in the plastic surgery section.

Finally I want to emphasize that, as with other cancers we will discuss, the patient should be sent home with all types of information to help her deal with having cancer. In our medical center we have a breast discharge packet that includes pamphlets about the American Cancer Society information center, Reach to Recovery, where breast cancer survivors talk with newly diagnosed patients, wig banks, and cosmetic programs. There are psychosocial support groups and therapy, physical therapy to prevent lymphedema in patients who have had axillary node dissection, and other information to help the newly diagnosed patient cope with the stress of the diagnosis and treatment. It's all part of Comprehensive Breast Care. Now go out and get the book!

Chapter 32
GALL BLADDER
AND BILE DUCTS

If you're forty, female and getting fatter,
You may have stones in your gall bladder,
And will have pain in your upper belly,
If you eat fat foods and spicy deli.

But surgeons love your crazy diet,
(Whatever you eat, be sure you fry it)
'Cause how can we send our kids to college,
To fill their heads with useless knowledge?

Unless you have a cholecystectomy,
Either open...or laparoscopically,
Surgeons and their families will "die on the vine"
And live in a hovel and drink a cheap wine.

So eat up, you ladies and gents fat and forty,
Gain weight and be happy, dietetically naughty.
Don't mind if you're temporarily sickly,
You have a disease we can cure very quickly.

The gall bladder was made for surgeons to remove. It is a saclike structure which stores bile from the liver. Because of some metabolic problems, it may concentrate the bile so much that it may crystallize into small or large stones. When this happens the gall bladder is diseased and may give symptoms of pain in the right upper abdomen, especially after eating fatty and spicy foods. The diagram shows the anatomy of the gall bladder and surrounding organs.

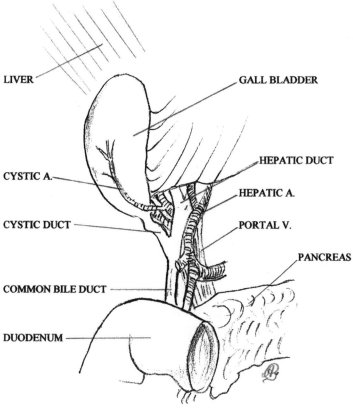

LIVER

GALL BLADDER

HEPATIC DUCT

CYSTIC A.

HEPATIC A.

CYSTIC DUCT

PORTAL V.

PANCREAS

COMMON BILE DUCT

DUODENUM

GALL BLADDER AND SURROUNDING ORGANS

DIAGRAM 8

Bile flows from the liver down the common bile duct into the duodenum, the first part of the small intestine right after the stomach, where it helps dissolve and absorb fat and vitamins A, D, E and K. There is a small muscle called the sphincter of Oddi at the ampulla of Vater and normally this is closed tight. Bile refluxes back up the cystic duct into the gall bladder where it is stored. When you eat fatty or spicy food, the sphincter muscle relaxes and the muscles in the gall bladder wall contract sending bile into the intestine to help with digestion. If you have a diseased gall bladder, and you can have a diseased gall bladder without stones, when it contracts it causes pain, nausea and vomiting. If you have your gall bladder removed, the common bile duct functions like a gallbladder, and you have no more pain, nausea or vomiting.

The symptoms of gall bladder disease are right upper abdominal pain, occasionally going to the back, nausea, and vomiting, but sometimes your brain gets confused and refers the pain to the chest. Some people and their physicians think they are having a heart attack. Now, it's possible to have two problems going on at once, so if you are over 40 we generally get an EKG just to check you out. The diagnosis of gall bladder disease is made by an x-ray called the gall bladder series, by ultrasound (showing the stones) or by a CAT scan or a HIDA scan. The latter is a study where a weakly radioactive substance is injected into the blood stream, is taken into the liver and excreted into the bile duct and gall bladder to show abnormalities. It is important to realize that many patients with gall bladder disease do not have gall stones called acalculous cholecystitis and this is diagnosed by a study called kinevac which measures the function of the gall bladder.

The surgery is the removal of the gall bladder and the cystic duct. Until the early 1980's, all gall bladders were removed under general anesthesia through an oblique incision just below the right rib cage margin. The muscles had to be divided, the abdomen entered and the gall bladder duct and its blood supply tied or clipped and divided. The gall bladder was then removed from its bed in the liver by dissection with instruments, stopping small bleeding vessels with cautery. Since about 1984, most surgeons have learned how to do the procedure laparoscopically through small incisions as shown below. Whereas the patient who has an open cholecystectomy usually stays in the hospital a few days, the laparoscopic procedure may be done as an outpatient with much less pain and quicker recovery. The complications of gall bladder surgery are bleeding, infection, bile leakage, and injury to bile ducts and other organs. Patients usually return to normal activity within one to two weeks after a laparoscopic cholecystectomy and a little longer after the open procedure.

Cancer of the gall bladder is rarely diagnosed early in the course of the disease and this makes it difficult to cure unless it is found incidently with the removal of the gall bladder for stones or cholecystitis. The problem with gall bladder cancer is that by the time it's diagnosed it has already spread to the liver and is difficult to cure unless the surgeon can remove large portions of the adjacent liver. There is a higher incidence of gall bladder cancer in patients with gall stones.

Let's move on to the diseases of the common bile duct. There are three basic problems aside from congenital abnormalities; they are stones, infection and cancer. The stones are usually from the gall bladder and if they're small, they will pass down the common duct into the intestine. But if they are large, they may get stuck in the common bile duct and block the passage of bile into the duodenum. Backup of bile causes elevation of alkaline phosphatase but the most visible finding is yellow jaundice. The treatment is removal of the stones by the gastroenterologist who can place a scope at the sphincter, open it widely and get the stone out with special balloon catheters. Rarely if the stone is large or stuck, a surgeon will have to remove it with an open operation. Occasionally infection, called cholangitis, gets into the bile duct from the intestine or gall bladder and this requires antibiotic treatment, removing the underlying cause, and placing a temporary tube called a t-tube in the common duct to drain off any infection. Associated with gallstones is the problem of gallstone pancreatitis, an inflammation of the pancreas due to blockage of the pancreatic duct by a gall stone. The treatment is removal of the stones and the gall bladder along with vigorous medical management with antibiotics and intravenous fluids.

Now for cancer of the common duct and sphincter. As opposed to gall bladder cancer, this cancer causes very early symptoms because the bile duct becomes blocked and the patient presents with yellow jaundice. This factor makes it potentially curable. The diagnosis can be made by endoscopy, and endoscopic retrograde cholangiopancreatography, ERCP, where the gastroenterologist injects contrast material directly into the bile duct and gets a picture of the pathology. The only problem is that to do an adequate cancer operation, the surgeon has to remove a portion of the bile duct, part of the duodenum, pancreas and stomach, in other words, a big surgery. This is called the Whipple procedure. It is a complex procedure only done well by a limited number of surgeons and should not be done if there is any evidence of spread of the tumor. If the cancer cannot be completely removed, it is best to do a palliative operation, bypassing the blockage. There are many ways to do this; sometimes a radiologist or gastroenterologist can pass a firm tube through the blockage to allow the bile to pass. The complications of these procedures are infection, leakage of bile or intestinal fluid and all the other potential complications of major surgery.

Chapter 33
APPENDIX

With "Found a Peanut" there to guide us,
It was our earliest story of appendicitis.
"It was rotten, it was rotten" so they say,
But you ate it anyway!

The only part, I have to say,
Is that most patients don't "die anyway"
Appendectomy today without hesitation,
Is the commonest surgery throughout the nation.

Appendectomy is indeed the most common major surgery performed in the United States today. The appendix, I must explain, is not a "plural" thing, as some patients believed. Many patients have thought that when they had their appendix out that it refers to more than one organ. Sorry there is no "appendick". It's just one plain old appendix, a worm-shaped structure that hangs off the end of the cecum part of the colon (*see* Diagram 9 next page).

What used to be an extremely dangerous and often fatal disease has now become a very treatable, operable and curable problem. Remember Rudolph Valentino, the actor and heart throb of the twenties...he died of a ruptured appendicitis. With today's armamentarium of diagnostic tools, surgical techniques and antibiotics, he'd most probably be alive and still "heart throbbing". The patients who die of appendicitis usually have ruptured appendicitis and have other major medical problems related to old age, diabetes, liver, kidney or lung problems.

The appendix gets infected when something such as food, stool, a parasite, etc., gets stuck in the opening resulting in progressive disease and the signs and symptoms we see. Classically these are the gradual onset of pain in the mid abdomen around the bellybutton, periumbilical pain, which moves into the right lower quadrant of the abdomen into an area under McBurney's point as the disease progresses. The pain becomes

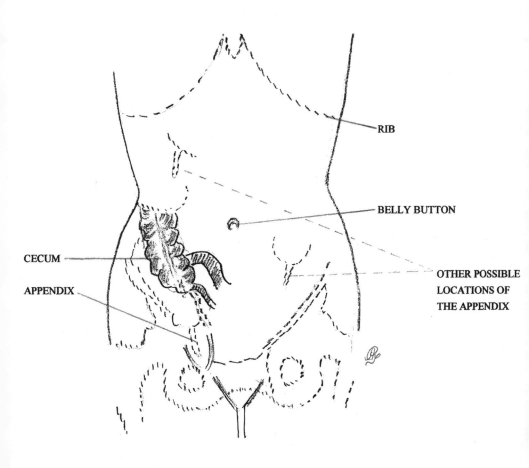

RIB

BELLY BUTTON

CECUM

APPENDIX

OTHER POSSIBLE
LOCATIONS OF
THE APPENDIX

THE ABDOMEN AND THE APPENDIX

DIAGRAM 9

more severe and crampy as the appendix distends from infection and possibly pus; distention of the intestine and colon frequently causes pain like that of severe constipation. Sometimes, when the appendix gets too swollen, it ruptures and breaks and the pain of distention goes away for a short while. That's why patients with ruptured appendicitis think that they're getting better when the pain goes away, only to have more severe pain of peritonitis when the appendiceal fecal contents spill into the peritoneal cavity.

It is important to note that although nausea, vomiting, pain and fever are the usual classical signs and symptoms of appendicitis, there are all kinds of other symptoms of appendicitis. It has been known as the great mimicker of other diseases including that of the gall bladder, intestine, colon, heart, lungs (i.e. pneumonia), back and spine. Without going into much detail I'll give the differential of the other diseases that a surgeon must consider when given several symptoms for appendicitis. The most common are acute mesenteric adenitis, usually in children and essentially swollen glands around the area of the appendix, ruptured corpus luteum ovarian cysts usually two weeks after the last period in females, gastroenteritis and food poisoning. Also there is Meckel's diverticulitis, an extra, appendix-like structure which occurs in 2% of people and can have the same symptoms as appendicitis. Then there are diseases of the testicles, inflammatory bowel disease called regional enteritis, perforated ulcer, kidney stones, and pelvic infection in women.

I hope you can understand that the accepted error in diagnosis of appendicitis is 15%. That means that 85% of the time the surgeon will find appendicitis and the remainder he will find something else and occasionally, no pathology. There is a good rationale that one should operate on a patient when it is suspected. If you were to wait until you were absolutely sure, several cases would go on to rupture with more problems and complications. For a surgeon, waiting is aggravating.

The diagnosis in the very young and very old is sometimes difficult and it often takes the surgeon with gray hair to make the early diagnosis. The laboratory work usually shows an elevated WBC with what we call a shift to the left with an increased number of polymorphonuclear leukocytes. Diagnosis may also include CAT scan, ultrasound which can see fluid and ruptured ovarian cysts or may show a mass indicating appendicitis. However I need to stress that this remains a clinical diagnosis based on the history and physical by your surgeon. He feels your abdomen and looks for several signs, including psoas sign which is lying on your left side and pulling your right leg back to cause right sided abdominal pain, and Rovsing's sign, pressing on the left side of the abdomen and moving in an upward counterclockwise direction towards the appendix causing severe pain. He will also look for a sign of peritonitis such as rebound tenderness which means that when you press on the left side of the abdomen and let go suddenly, there is pain on the same or other side indicating irritation of the peritoneum (*see* Peritonitis).

Appendectomy can be done as an open procedure or laparoscopically depending on you or your surgeon's preference. They both cause scars and the laparoscopic procedure takes a little longer, but in my hands both are equally good with similar recovery rates. The exact methods of the procedures are not important. If you have a ruptured appendix, your surgeon will probably want to place some drains and you will be hospitalized for several days. In severe cases I usually consult an infectious disease specialist to manage the antibiotics since the higher the antibiotic doses, the greater the chance for drug related problems of kidney failure, nausea, vomiting, diarrhea and even hearing loss.

As you can see, probably anyone with a little training can do an uncomplicated appendectomy, but only the well trained surgeon can manage the problem cases.

Chapter 34
THE COLON

I wish that I could make a pact,
With my entire colonic tract,
I'd forego all its pain and sass,
If it would stop producing gas.

The colon does just what it oughter,
When it conserves minerals and water.
But it oft does just as it pleases,
And gives us many bad diseases.

I think God Just went out bowlin',
And that other guy designed the colon.

The colon is a large tubelike structure in your abdomen that extends like a question mark from the right lower side of your abdomen, clockwise up, to the left and down towards the rectum with a sigmoid, S-shaped segment just before it exits at the bottom (*see* Diagram 10, next page).

As in the diagram, it has several parts, the cecum with the appendix attached, the ascending, transverse and descending colons, the sigmoid colon and the rectum and anus. It has a fairly good blood supply unless as you get older you develop narrowing of the vessels or severe diabetes, vascular disease effecting the vessels.

It is a complex organ with many disease processes, many of which may require surgery, and although there are some physicians starting to do laparoscopic procedures for non-cancerous disease, and a few attempting a good cancer operation laparoscopically, most surgeons do open operations for the multiplicity of diseases we shall discuss here.

The main function of the colon is to reabsorb water and electrolytes from the intestinal fluid and to have motility which is peristalsis to move your waste through the colon and out through the rectum. The colon contains many bacteria, some of which produce gas and result in flatus.

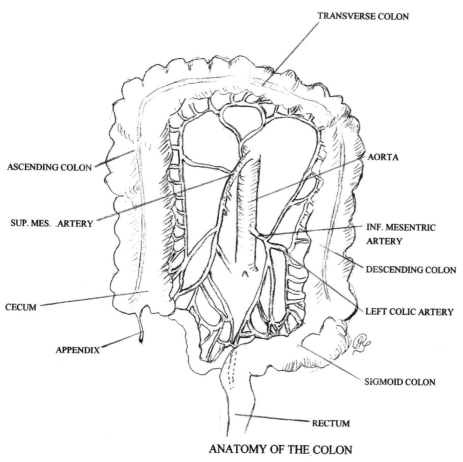

ANATOMY OF THE COLON

DIAGRAM 10

Changes in the normal flora or bacteria of the colon may cause diarrhea, and dehydration or diet change may result in constipation. Distention of the colon causes cramping abdominal pain which can be very severe. In the right side of the colon the intracolonic contents is liquid whereas in the left colon and below it becomes solid.

Before we discuss diseases, I want to spend some time talking about ileostomy (bringing a loop of small intestine to the skin level for drainage and application of a pouch) and colostomy (bringing a loop of colon to the skin for external drainage and applying a pouch). Initially the emotional and physical impact of having a pouch for bowel movements is tremendous, and requires gentle counseling and frequent psychosocial and medical support and help. Some patients become very depressed and need anti-depressant medications. But the patient should understand why there is no other option and should realize that many individuals lead near normal lives with ostomies. I personally know of many actors and public celebrities who have lived years with a colostomy or ileostomy, and usually the public does not know about it. It frequently takes a patient as long as three months to learn all the ins and outs of living with an ostomy and there are many support groups that are helpful in this regard. In spite of all this I can tell you I have had patients who would rather die than have a colostomy and these decisions have to be fully discussed with an understanding, patient and knowledgeable surgeon.

Let us first discuss the benign diseases of the colon...volvulus, ischemia or decreased blood supply, hemorrhage, radiation induced colitis, pseudomembranous and infectious colitis, diverticulitis, Crohn's Disease, ulcerative colitis, benign tumors, and Ogilvie's syndrome.

Volvulus means twisting of the colon around itself causing an obstruction. It occurs in the parts of the colon that are moveable, the cecum and the sigmoid colon. It causes severe pain, nausea and vomiting and elevated WBC. It is diagnosed by abdominal x-ray and can frequently be resolved by barium enema or colonoscopy, which may de-rotate the bowel. If the volvulus recurs or cannot be corrected, then an open surgery is performed and the volvulus part of the colon is either sewed into the correct position or the intestine is removed possibly requiring a colostomy.

Ischemia means decreased blood supply and this may be due to several factors which might cause occlusion or blockage of the major arteries to the colon such as thrombosis, embolization, blood clots coming from somewhere else, i.e. the heart, or complications of aortic aneurysm surgery. This presents with pain and occasional rectal bleeding and can be diagnosed on abdominal x-ray, CT scan and endoscopy by the gastroenterologist. Sometimes, if mild it will resolve spontaneously in a few days, but if symptoms worsen and WBC rises markedly, a surgery may be needed and the involved bowel may have to be removed either with or without a diverting temporary colostomy.

The whole category of infectious colitis may be secondary to external bacteria or an unusual reaction to high dose antibiotics. These diseases rarely need surgery and are treated by the gastroenterologist and infectious disease specialists. In rare instances temporary colostomy or colon resection may be needed.

Hemorrhage or bleeding from the colon may be microscopic, where no blood is seen grossly but is found in special stool tests, or gross bleeding. All rectal bleeding needs to be checked out by a physician. Most of it is from hemorrhoids, but even if hemorrhoids are present, the physician must make sure that there is not a second problem somewhere else in the colon. Inflammation of the colon, benign and malignant tumors, volvulus, and diverticulitis are the main causes and depending on the amount of bleeding, a rapid evaluation may be needed to find the source. Blood from the rectum may be bright red, meaning it's coming from somewhere low down in the GI tract or even from a rapidly bleeding duodenal or gastric ulcer.

Dark rectal bleeding is usually pathognomonic of upper gastrointestinal bleeding when the blood is older and turns purplish. The workup consists of a complete physical exam, and passing a temporary nasogastric tube through the nose into the stomach to determine if there is any blood there; then a colonoscopy and if needed for massive bleeding, special scans or even an angiogram to show the bleeding vessel. Bleeding can usually be stopped with medications and local treatment by the gastroenterologist, but in recurrent or severe cases emergency surgery may be needed and sections of the colon removed. Obviously if the bleeding is stopped, the etiology must be treated electively at the appropriate time.

After patients have had radiation treatment to the lower abdomen for cancer, they may develop radiation colitis and this may either respond to medical management with rest and antibiotics or maybe so severe as to necessitate partial colon resection. Pseudomembranous colitis is a disease of severe diarrhea caused by extensive antibiotic treatment, resulting in an overgrowth of dangerous colonic bacteria, usually Clostridium, and usually responds to medical treatment. It is the rare case that needs surgery.

Diverticulitis is an inflammation of the diverticulae or outpouchings in the colon that occur in most people as they get older, into their 40's and 50's or beyond. The symptoms are pain, fever, elevated WBC, occasional bleeding, and some alteration in bowel habit, usually constipation and sometimes diarrhea. Although the cause is unknown, it is often associated with a low fiber diet. Diverticulitis is diagnosed by colonoscopy, barium enema or by clinical exam and history, and usually resolves with proper antibiotics and placing the bowel at rest and giving IV fluids. If the attacks become frequent or if a diverticulum bursts and causes peritonitis or an abscess, then surgery is indicated. If a colon operation is elective (not an emergency), then the bowel can be prepared or cleansed with special solutions and antibiotics prior to surgery which will evacuate all the stool and kill most of the bacteria making it safe to perform an operation. These include "bowel preps" with oral liquids such as GoLYTELY - a remarkable name for something that makes you go anything but lightly, and rectal enemas. When the bowel is prepared, then the abnormal segment can be removed and the bowel connected back together. However, in most areas of the colon, in an unprepared bowel emergency such as perforated diverticulitis, in addition to removing the diseased segment of intestine, a temporary diverting colostomy must be performed, bringing out the proximal colon as a temporary colostomy. If the involved segment is in the right colon near the cecum, either a direct connection is made after the resection or a diverting ileostomy, bringing out the distal ileum, is done at the discretion of the surgeon. This is sometimes possible because the cecum and right colon have liquid stools and may be fairly clean. The colostomy or ileostomy is closed in three to six months with a second operation. The complications are deep and superficial wound infections along with the other potential complications of major surgery can occur.

The next topic is inflammatory bowel disease, which basically includes two major diseases, ulcerative colitis and Crohn's disease, regional enteritis or segmental colitis. Ulcerative colitis involves the inner lining of the colon called the mucosa and Crohn's disease involves all layers of the bowel wall and can occur, not only in the colon, but throughout the intestinal tract from the mouth to the anus. The full name of the latter disease is Crohn, Ginzberg, Oppenheimer disease after three physicians at Mt. Sinai Hospital in New York. When I did my internship there,

Crohn was no longer alive, but Ginzberg was. We had to call it Ginzberg's disease! The exact causes of the diseases are unknown although it has been suggested that there are genetic and autoimmune implications with the body's immune system working against itself, and environmental factors including, of course, smoking, alcohol and sugar. Ulcerative colitis is more common in men and Crohn's more common in women, especially those of Jewish heritage.

The symptoms are somewhat similar with pain, diarrhea, and fever in both, more bleeding in ulcerative colitis and more pain, vomiting and general wasting and weight loss with Crohn's. There is also marked malnutrition. There is the potential for severe disease around the anus and anal skin in Crohn's disease. Inflammatory bowel disease can effect the bones and joints, arthritis and osteomyelitis, lungs, heart, kidneys, liver, blood system, eyes, and skin with it severe acne and mouth sores.

I won't go deeply into the diagnostics except to say the gastroenterologist uses endoscopy to make the diagnosis, along with barium enema and CAT scans. Both diseases are initially treated with antibiotics, steroids and immunosuppressive agents which are special medicines that suppress your body's immune system which is supposed to be partially responsible for the disease.

When is surgery indicated? Well it may be different for the two diseases. In ulcerative colitis, surgery is indicated when the patient has continued severe symptoms in spite of maximal medical management, in case of severe bleeding, or when there are changes suggesting a high risk for impending cancer. The surgery is removal of part or all of the colon. Because it is a disease limited to the inner lining of the colon, the anal sphincter muscles (those muscles that help control your rectal function so you don't leak stool below) are not affected and all the colon can be removed completely eliminating the disease. If this is done, the end of the small intestine is then made into a rectal pouch which is hooked to your anus keeping the muscles intact. A temporary diverting ileostomy is frequently done to protect the lower connection for a few months to allow it to heal well. The entire surgery is a delicate procedure usually requiring special training and frequently done by colon and rectal specialists. The complications are many including inflammation, breakdown of the pouch and eventual need for conversion to permanent ileostomy (*see* Diagram 11 next page).

Crohn's disease is usually more difficult to manage because it may skip

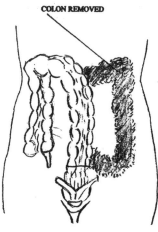

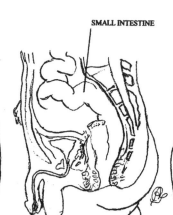

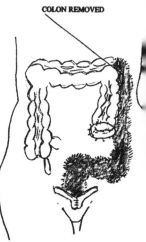

COLON REMOVED

SMALL INTESTINE

COLON REMOVED

LOW ANTERIOR RESECTION
OF RECTOSIGMOID WITH
COLORECTAL ANASTOMOSIS

PARTIAL COLECTOMY

COMPLETED J-POUCH ILEOANAL
ANASTOMOSIS AT DENTATE LINE

TOTAL ABDOMINAL COLECTOMY
WITH ILEORECTAL ANASTOMOSIS

ABDOMINAL- PERINEAL
PROCTOSIGMOIDECTOMY WITH
PERMANENT END COLOSTOMY

ABDOMINOPERINEAL RESECTION
AND COLOSTOMY

TYPES OF SURGERY ON THE COLON

DIAGRAM 11

throughout the intestinal tract. Surgery is only done when there is severe unrelenting disease or direct indications for surgery including massive bowel distention, ruptures, sepsis, obstruction from stricture which is a narrowing secondary to inflammation, abdominal abscess and perianal fistulas which means drainage of infection in tracts from the colon through the anal area skin. The medical treatment is similar to ulcerative colitis. When the disease becomes intractable, surgical intervention is needed, removing as little diseased intestine as possible. In severe cases the disease may reoccur anywhere else throughout the intestinal tract and requires constant monitoring and recurrent treatment. Usually the rectal area is spared in Crohn's disease so the entire colon does not have to be removed. However, because of the severe perianal disease, temporary diverting ostomies may have to be performed and if the rectal segment is involved, because the disease involves all layers, the rectal muscle usually has to be removed, leaving no possibility for "rehooking up" below. These patients may need a permanent ileostomy.

In conclusion, inflammatory bowel disease can be considered pre-- malignant, in that after ten years there is a 1% per year incidence of cancer of the colon, and needless to say, these patients need to be watched carefully for this problem whether or not they have undergone surgery.

Benign noncancerous tumors of the colon include adenomatous polyps, villous adenomas, and familial polyposis and they may develop into cancers if left long enough and should be removed. This can usually be done by gastroenterologists from below, but if the tumor is very large, an open surgery may be needed. Frequently the surgeon does not need to remove any colon, just opens the area, removes the tumor and sutures or staples closed the colon!

Now let us move on to colon cancer. We now know that there are many genetic abnormalities leading cells to change from normal to abnormal or adenosis, cancer cells to metastatic cancer cells. Further work on etiology is continually being done but we still don't have definitive answers. It is the most common cancer of the intestinal tract, and is second only to breast cancer as cause of death from cancer. The symptoms are varied but usually include rectal bleeding, abdominal pain, or some change in bowel habit such as constipation, narrow stools, diarrhea, etc. As we have mentioned, the contents of the right colon are liquid so it takes longer for signs of partial obstruction to occur. Right sided cancers are often detected because of bleeding, whereas left colon tumors may have all the above symptoms and may cause obstructive signs earlier. Another presentation may be bowel perforation and peritonitis.

Diagnosis is made by sigmoidoscopy or colonoscopy, barium enema, and CAT scan, and a full evaluation must be done to evaluate the full extent of the disease, to see whether there is any spread beyond the colon to the liver, lungs, etc. The surgery involves an open operation and removal of the involved segment of colon and its supporting tissue with wide margins or normal tissue on either side. Usually a bowel preparation can be done and no colostomy is needed. In emergencies, the cancer is removed and a temporary colostomy is placed, to be closed is three to six months. If the cancer involves the lowest portion of the rectum and anus, then this portion must be removed, including the anal muscles in a procedure called an abdominal perineal resection and a permanent colostomy established.

We have mentioned the TNM, Tumor Size, Lymph Node Involvement, Evidence of Metastasis, staging methods in another chapter and I will outline it for colon cancer.

STAGING FOR COLON CANCER

TUMOR	LYMPH NODES	METASTASIS (SPREAD BEYOND COLON AND NODES)
T1-tumor in inside layers	N0-No node involvement	M0-no distant spread
T2-tumor into midpart of colon wall		M1-metastasis
T3-tumor through wall but not beyond	N1-3- Nodes involved	
T4-tumor through wall into other structures		

Stage	T	N	M
Stage I	T1 & 2	N0	M0
Stage II	T3 & 4	N0	M0
Stage III	Any T,	N1,2,3	M0
Stage IV	Any T	Any N	M1

DIAGRAM 12

The staging is important to determine future therapy and to indicate the seriousness of the disease and will be discussed with the patient by the surgeon or oncologist.

One last thing I want to discuss is what type of surgery you do for colon cancer if it has already spread distantly. As opposed to some other cancers, colon cancers always have to be removed to prevent future bleeding, pain and obstruction. These are called palliative operations and are done even if we cannot do a surgical cure. When to leave the primary tumor may cause serious discomfort or life threatening problems in the future. It requires full discussion with the patient and family. This entire concept is discussed in Chapter 47.

Chapter 35
THE STOMACH

To eat or not to eat, that is the question,
When thinking seriously about our digestion.
"If music is the food of life, play on,"
But really, food is the music of life, anon.

So we must worship that utmost cavity,
Spoken of often with such depravity.
The stomach of course, the way to a man's heart,
And if you don't believe it...you're not very smart.

The stomach has been in literature, song and history for thousands of years. People probably knew vaguely about the stomach before they even had a name for it. It personifies eating, health, social status, cultural background as well as several disease entities.

The stomach is a large pouch-shaped organ that begins just below the diaphragm which is the muscle separating the chest from the abdomen, and extends from the esophagus above to the first portion of the intestine, with the duodenum, below. Just for interest I'll name a few of the cells found in the stomach and their functions: The cardiac gland cells produce mucus, antral cells produce mucus and gastrin, parietal cells produce acid, and chief cells produce a precursor of pepsin. The mucus protects the stomach wall from the acid, and obviously substances that interfere with mucous production will leave the stomach open to irritation and destruction by its own acid. There are also substances that cause increase in acid production and eventually may lead to peptic-ulcer disease. Among these substances are certain bacteria such as H. Pylori, alcohol and smoking (*See* Diagram 13 next page).

It has several arteries and veins and two important nerves called the vagus nerves. The stomach produces acid, hormones and enzymes that help in the digestion of food and then passes it into the intestines for absorption. The antrum produces gastrin, a hormone that causes release

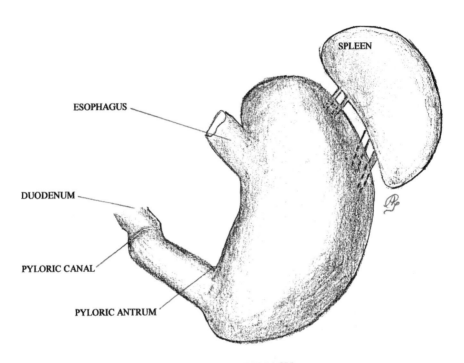

ANATOMY OF THE STOMACH

DIAGRAM 13

of acid by the body of the stomach. There is a muscular ring at the end of the stomach called the pylorus that can contract, keeping contents in the stomach, and relax to allow emptying of the stomach.

There are three phases of acid secretion in the stomach. The Cephalic phase means that the brain, when stimulated by the smell, sight, or taste of food, sends a message down the vagus nerves to the antrum, stimulates the production of gastrin which in turn causes acid production. The Gastric phase, including gastrin, results when food enters the stomach, causing distention and release of several substances in addition to gastrin, which leads to acid release. The third phase is the Intestinal phase. When food enters the intestine at the duodenum, it causes the release of gastrin from the duodenum which in turn stimulates gastric acid release.

First let me talk about my fluffy, black, long haired cat, Sara. Not related to the subject you say...wrong! If you have a cat like Sara, who is sitting next to my word processor, you know that hairballs can be a big problem. Similarly, humans can develop a "hairball" type mass in the stomach call a "bezoar", which may get stuck in the stomach and not be able to pass into the duodenum. This used to require surgery, but now can be removed by a gastroenterologist or a surgeon who does endoscopy, putting a lighted tube into the stomach and removing the bezoar or cutting it into smaller pieces so it will pass by itself.

Other problems, usually medically or endoscopically managed, are severe gastritis or Menetrier's disease, severe inflammation of the stomach, foreign bodies such as when some crazy man swallows a spoon, and sometimes a tear at or near the junction of the esophagus and stomach called a Mallory-Weiss tear.

Next let's talk about acid reflux disease which we mentioned briefly in the chapter on the esophagus. These patients have reflux of acid from their stomach into the esophagus causing severe acid indigestion and burning mid-chest pain often mistaken for heart disease. The pathology is that the normal muscle or sphincter at the gastro-esophageal junction is not working well and needs to be repaired. Prior to this procedure, many tests of esophageal movement, acid production and special acid studies need to be done. The treatment is initially the same as for peptic ulcer disease. The surgery includes hiatus hernia surgery as well as an anti-reflux procedure where the upper part of the stomach is wrapped around the end of the esophagus at the gastroesophageal junction to create a new sphincter. The procedure can be done laparoscopically or open, depending on your surgeon, but can have many post-operative problems including breakdown of the repair, post operative infection, chronic nausea or, vomiting, if the wrap is too tight and resumption of symptoms if the wrap is too loose.

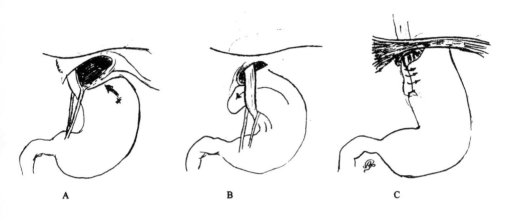

A   B   C

NISSEN FUNDOPLICATION

DIAGRAM 14

Twenty five years ago the most common surgical disease of the stomach was the ulcer. Today with all the medications, antacids, H2-receptor antagonists, substances that prevent the production of acid, antibiotics and other substances with strange names such as prostaglandins, anticholinergics and benzimidazoles, we rarely see severe ulcer disease unresponsive to medical management and surgery is only rarely needed. Basically, an ulcer is a hole in the wall of an organ. If it's only part way through the wall it can be treated medically; if it bleeds it can usually be cauterized by a gastroenterologist, but if it goes all the way through, perforating the wall freely into the abdomen, or if the bleeding can't be stopped, then surgical intervention is indicated. I emphasize that instead of two or three stomach operations I did each month for ulcer disease twenty years ago, I now see only a few each year.

There are many surgeries as shown below including (1) oversewing the ulcer by using stitches in the same manner you might mend a sock and sometimes taking a biopsy to rule out cancer, (2) cutting the branches of the vagus nerves that go to the stomach to decrease the cephalic phase; this surgery also causes a slowing of gastric movement and will usually require opening the end of the stomach more widely to facilitate emptying, (3) removing the antrum of the stomach to eliminate gastrin production and thereby cutting down on acid production; frequently this is done with stapling machines and in severe cases removing most of the stomach and making one of three reconnections.

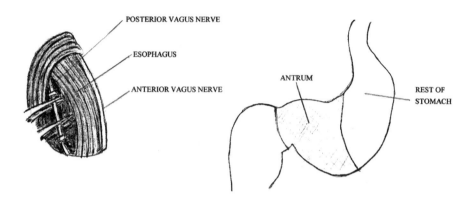

SURGERY FOR PEPTIC ULCER DISEASE

DIAGRAM 15

Tumors of the stomach can be either benign or malignant. They may present with pain, bleeding, nausea and vomiting or in the case of some cancers, with severe weight loss or intestinal blockage. Workup includes endoscopy and biopsy, upper GI series, and sometimes CAT scans. CBC and coagulation workups may be needed along with the usual preoperative evaluations.

The benign tumors, lipomas, and polyps (non-cancerous growths in the stomach) can either be removed by the endoscopist or in an open surgery where an opening is made in the stomach, the mass removed and the stomach closed, usually with a stapling device.

Cancers of the stomach can be adenocarcinoma, a gland forming tumor, lymphomas, cancer of the lymph glands which can occur just about anywhere, and the rarer leiomyosarcoma, cancer of the muscle wall of the stomach. Extensive cancer of the stomach is sometimes referred to as "linitis plastica". The lymphomas, after diagnosis is made, can usually be treated with chemotherapy and sometimes radiation therapy for a complete cure, and rarely do they need surgery except to make the diagnosis. The other cancers require removal of most or all of the stomach, subtotal or total gastrectomy, and do best with the Roux-en-Y gastro-jejunostomy as shown above. The survival rate depends on the TNM rating, with similar staging to that of colon cancer.

Another area of surgery on the stomach is called bariatric or surgery for "morbid obesity" - at least 100 pounds over ideal weight. Initially surgeons would bypass large portions of the intestine, making it essentially shorter; they felt less food would be absorbed and thus weight would be lost, but liver failure and other complications led then to give up the intestinal bypasses. In recent years much work has been done in gastric bypass procedures using staples and minimizing the amount of stomach left for receiving food. There is excellent weight loss in many cases but there are many potential complications unless done by experts who are well versed in the technical, psychosocial and comorbid conditions. With weight loss the patients have significant improvement in many health conditions such as diabetes mellitus, lung problems, high blood pressure called hypertension, arthritis and "just getting around"; there is no long term data to show that these patients will actually live longer. The studies are now in progress. Bariatric surgery is best discussed in detail with bariatric surgeons! (*see* Diagram 16 next page).

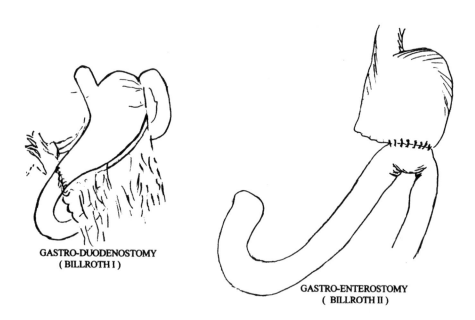

GASTRO-DUODENOSTOMY
(BILLROTH I)

GASTRO-ENTEROSTOMY
(BILLROTH II)

ROUX -EN- Y GASTROJEJOUNOSTOMY

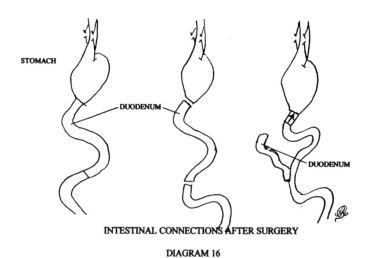

STOMACH

DUODENUM

DUODENUM

INTESTINAL CONNECTIONS AFTER SURGERY

DIAGRAM 16

Chapter 36
THE ESOPHAGUS

The esophagus was not designed,
With just sword swallowing in mind.
Nor would it seem the best creation
For man to use for eructation.
(belching)

T he esophagus is a tubelike structure extending from the back of
the throat, the pharynx, down to the stomach, and is divided into
the upper, middle and lower thirds, the cervical, thoracic and
abdominal. It has a complex muscle function to allow swallowing
and progressive propulsion or motility of food and fluid down to the
stomach and usually prevents reflux which means backflow, emesis or
vomiting.

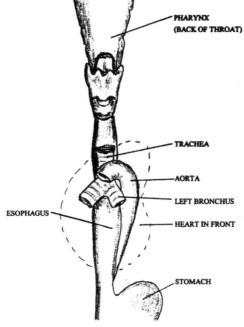

ANATOMY OF THE ESOPHAGUS

DIAGRAM 17

Problems with motility are often difficult to manage and require an extensive workup with endoscopy, acid studies, and manometry which measures the sequential pressures in the esophagus. This rarely requires surgery except for severe reflux disease which may require anti reflux procedures such as the Nissen fundoplication which we have discussed and outlined in the last chapter.

In the neck or cervical portion of the esophagus, a small outpouching can develop as a result of a motility disorder called Zenker's diverticulum. This can cause difficulty swallowing and may actually fill with food, which is vomited up several days later and is foul smelling. It is relatively easy to remove surgically through an incision in the neck, a small muscle cutting and a sewing or stapling off of the diverticulum. It is done under a general anesthetic with minimal postoperative problems or complications.

There are a number of benign processes such as lipomas or fatty tumors and muscle tumors called leiomyomas, which can be removed endoscopically or with a small incision in the esophagus. A number of syndromes produce painful swallowing called dysphagia and abnormal swallowing or dysmotility, as well as pain, and are treated medically, rarely requiring surgery. I'll give you the names but unless you have need to know, they're too obscure to discuss; they are Plummer-Vinson syndrome usually associated with iron deficiency, brittle nails, chronic anemia and spoon shaped fingers, Schatzki's ring, a band of tissue in the distal esophagus which can cause partial obstruction and reflux, Scleroderma, a systemic vascular collagen disease which causes acid reflux, inflammation and stricture, and Mallory-Weiss syndrome.

Perforation of the esophagus by food or the local "knife and gun club" will require appropriate operative intervention with suture, rest and usually decompression with an NG tube.

The most common major surgery of the esophagus is for cancer. The symptoms include partial or complete obstruction to swallowing, bleeding, pain, nausea and vomiting, weight loss, and swallowing disorders. The cancers can be of two types depending on the tissue of origin, squamous and adenocarcinomas, and cancer is found more commonly associated with alcohol, certain food additives, certain mineral deficiencies, zinc and molybdenum, tobacco smoking and certain long standing swallowing disorders. Unfortunately, cancer of the esophagus can extend up and down the esophagus from the site of origin requiring extensive surgical resections for attempts at cure. The diagnosis is made by endoscopy and biopsy and the extent of the tumor may be further evaluated by UGI series and CAT scan.

Surgery may be undertaken initially to confirm that a tumor is completely removable. If extensive disease, metastases and extensive lymph node involvement is found, palliative treatment may be indicated rather than putting the patient through extensive surgery with potential serious complications when a cure cannot be hoped for. While the criteria for possible resection differs among surgeons and in different countries, suffice it to say that the surgeon must be skilled and experienced not to result in extensive blood loss and serious morbidity such as leakage, infection and death. Some surgeons will not attempt a surgical resection if several lymph nodes are involved with cancer. If surgery is not indicated, a rigid tube can sometimes be placed through the area of the tumor so that the patient can swallow. The patient can then be treated with chemotherapy and radiation; I have one patient who is alive and doing well (though not cured) six years after diagnosis, radiation and chemotherapy.

The surgery frequently involves an abdominal and thoracic operation and the entire esophagus and surrounding nodal tissue is removed. The gap created is filled by either bringing the mobilized stomach up to the pharynx or using a segment of cleansed colon as an interposition. Although the TNM staging has been widely discussed and changed frequently, it is enough to say that with the esophagus, the cure rate is not good and the wisest surgeon is the one who in certain cases will recommend good palliation rather than surgery with high morbidity for probable incurable cancer. Because of the complexity of the subject, it is best left for further discussion by the oncologist or surgeon.

Chapter 37
SMALL INTESTINE

As a spokesman for the small intestine,
I will pose to you the following question,
You see, we're concerned about lack of respect,
For this excellent organ, as you might expect.

How often you treat it as the GI tract slut.
Why must you use that atrocious word "Gut"?
We have gut impressions, and guts and glory,
"Gut it out" and others to add to the story.

But this organ protects us and makes many hormones,
Absorbs food and water from sodas to corn pones.
Here's a blue chip that you ought to invest in:
Three cheers and a bow for the unsung intestine.

The small intestine is a large snake-like tubular structure that extends from the stomach to the colon. It has three distinct sections: first portion--the duodenum, about 20 centimeters long; the second--the larger jejunum, about 100 centimeters; the third--the ileum, about 150 centimeters, but the length varies with the height of the individual. The small intestine makes up about 50% of the GI tract, and has a mucosa, submucosa, muscularis and serosa. When I was in medical school, we knew little about the nature and function of the small bowel. Now we know that the functions and cellular makeup are multiple. The small bowel's function includes absorption of nutrients, motility for moving things through, multiple hormonal functions, producing substances which affect other organs, and major immune functions protecting the individual against infection and small intestinal cancer.

The small intestine has a tremendous internal surface area made up of fold or fronds called microvillae through which absorption occurs after digestion. Through these intestinal wall villae, the body absorbs water, fats, carbohydrates, protein and electrolytes in complex manners.

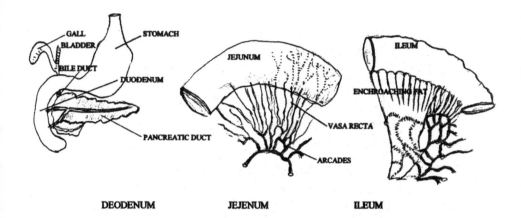

ANATOMY OF THE SMALL INTESTINE

DIAGRAM 18

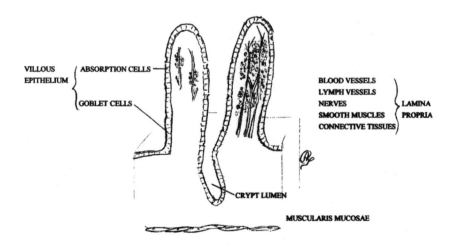

MICRO ANATOMY OF THE SMALL INTESTINE
(GIVING LARGE ABSOPTIVE SURFACE))

DIAGRAM 19

SMALL INTESTINAL CELL TYPES AND FUNCTION

Goblet Cells - produce mucous the help protect the mucosa
from breakdown
Paneth cells - secrete enzymes and tumor necrosis factor
Epithelial cells - lining cells of the stomach
Entero-endocrine cells - produce many substances such as gastrin
which stimulates stomach acid production, secretin which stimulates
pancreas secretions, cholecystokinin which stimulate gall bladder
contraction and many others such as somatostatin,
and enteroglucagon.

DIAGRAM 20

The small intestine also has a major immune function which prevents bacteria from entering the blood stream and also somehow reduces the incidence of cancer in this part of the body.

Inflammatory disease in the small intestine is Crohn's Disease which can cause obstruction, perforation, pain, hemorrhage, abscess, growth retardation and a higher incidence of cancer. Crohn's Disease is not curable and therefore the only surgery indicated is for alleviating symptoms when they don't respond to medical management. This may entail removing the involved segment of intestine using special staplers or sutures. The important thing to remember is that surgeons should not operate on Crohn's disease of the small bowel unless the symptoms are severe, or perforation and obstruction are present.

Other noncancerous pathology are Tuberculosis, diverticular disease, Meckel's diverticulum which is an outpouching of the small intestine occurring in 2% of people, two feet from the cecum and occasionally mimics appendicitis, and a host of congenital problems beyond the scope of this book. Surgery for these problems usually involves taking out the diseased segments and reconnecting the bowel. Benign tumors include adenomas, leiomyomas, and lipomas all of which may cause bleeding or obstruction and are diagnosed by small intestinal x-rays or small bowel endoscopy.

Let us now move on to malignancy. It is fairly rare in the small intestine (forty times less than in the colon!), but is usually difficult to cure because it is not completely removable when diagnosed. The symptoms are similar to the benign tumors with nausea, vomiting, bleeding, crampy abdominal pain and anemia, and the diagnosis is made with endoscopy and x-rays.

Surgery entails removal of the tumor along with uninvolved margins and with the lymph nodes. Unfortunately it does have a poor prognosis. There are several types of cancer including adenocarcinoma, a tumor from glands, sarcoma, a tumor from supporting tissue and muscle, lymphoma and carcinoid. The last two are the least serious and most common. Lymphoma is usually a systemic disease that frequently responds well to systemic chemotherapy by oncologists after surgical resection. Carcinoid is a strange cancer that can present with hypertension, diarrhea, and flushing of the face and after resection may linger for many years without recurring. It is diagnosed, in additional to the above studies by a specific urine test called 5HIAA which can also be used to follow the patients and determine the recurrence or extent of the disease.

Occasionally we refer to an upper abdominal segment of distended small intestine as a "sentinel" loop when seen on x-ray which results from partial paralysis of motion of the small bowel due to disease in an adjacent organ such as the pancreas, liver, stomach, spleen or colon.

Another whole area is the problem of adhesions, often involving the small intestine and this will be fully discussed in the next chapter.

Chapter 38
ADHESIONS

My doctor says I've got adhesions,
And he gives me many reasons,
Why he will not operate,
To make my insides nice and straight.

I'm having pain and my belly's distended,
But my surgeon insists that it cannot be mended,
He says it's not because he's lazy.
It's cause dad's an attorney and I'm crazy!

Here's another topic that's minimally discussed in the surgical texts yet it is a significant problem for both the surgeons and the patients.

What are adhesions? They are a kind of fibrin, platelet scar that develops into collagen or firm scar, that can occur on most wounds, but we will discuss mainly the ones that occur in the abdomen. Think of it as a sticky substance passed into the abdomen; it takes seven to ten days to solidify and upwards of six months to mature and soften. This sticky stuff, fibrin, platelets and collagen, may be very localized or may be very diffuse. It may occur after any surgical incision such as hysterectomy or cholecystectomy, or only after severe infections such as ruptured appendicitis, diverticulitis or cancer. Organs in the abdomen which are usually unattached to adjacent structures, may become intimately adherent making surgery very difficult and in some cases impossible.

The adhesions may involve a single loop of intestine with a string-like band or be so extensive that all the intestines and other intra abdominal structures are intimately stuck together and cannot be separated without tearing the bowel wall and making irreparable tissue damage.

From one to seven days after an operation it is still safe to re-explore the area - the adhesions and connections, if they are forming, are soft and can be pushed down with a sweep of the fingers; but from about ten days to three months the adhesions may be so severe that the surgeon can't even open the abdomen without serious damage to adherent organs. As time passes, the adhesions soften and surgery becomes possible.

What causes adhesions? Certainly there is an individual body tendency; two patients undergoing the same surgery by the same surgeon may have radically different postoperative adhesion formation. Other things that can cause more adhesions are blood in the abdomen, infection and repeated abdominal operations. Some professors feel that surgeons can help avoid adhesions with delicate handling of tissues and preventing blood loss, and by irrigating the peritoneal cavity with saline to eliminate blood and contamination after surgery. Often though, no matter what is done, adhesions will form.

The most common cause of intestinal obstruction is adhesions secondary to prior surgery; the second cause is cancer. Once the surgeon has ruled out cancer and determined the cause with CAT scan and other x-rays, he should always be very conservative about operating to relieve pain or bowel obstruction secondary to adhesions unless there are signs of ischemia which means lack of blood supply, or dead intestine called strangulation usually shown by markedly abnormal blood tests and x-rays. When the intestine is put at rest with IV fluids, nasogastric tube in the stomach for decompression and rest, a good percentage of small intestinal obstructions will resolve spontaneously. If the problem doesn't resolve, if the obstruction remains complete or if the patient has several hospital admissions for the same problem, a surgical exploration and lysis of adhesions may be indicated. But, the surgeon knows and the patient should be made aware that it may be necessary to remove some intestine and that the underlying process causing the adhesions often is not cured, just ameliorated. Adhesions are a major problem and be sure your surgeon has gray hair or gets a second surgical opinion before resorting to surgery.

Chapter 39
THYROID AND PARATHYROID

Last week I had to reconnoiter,
With Heidi, who had a very large goiter,
She lived all her life in an Alpine hut,
And she didn't have iodine while she grew up.

She was slow, with coarse hair, and a little bit chubby, Arriving by
plane with her "goat herding" hubby.
It took several months to reverse the disease,
But the goiter stayed large; she appeared ill at ease.

She was now much more active and lost twenty pounds,
And wanted to "look good" while they "made the rounds",
So I "lopped" out her goiter, which caused a great rancor,
When she dumped the goat herder and married a banker.

The goiter or enlargement of the thyroid gland in the neck, was described on papyrus in Egypt 4000 years ago. There wasn't much known and it wasn't until the 1800's that it was found that iodine deficiency was the main culprit.

The thyroid, with its adjacent parathyroid glands, is in the front of the neck partially surrounding the trachea in the midline, and it moves up and down with swallowing called deglutition. The thyroid is about the size of an average butterfly with two lobes on either side of the trachea connected by an isthmus or narrow strip connecting the two sides. It weighs about twenty grams. The parathyroids are tiny yellowish brown glands, only 40-50 mg., the size of a large pinhead and usually in two pairs, are situated behind and intimately attached to the upper and lower poles of the thyroid gland on each side. The anatomical variations occurring in the location and size of the thyroid and parathyroid are numerous and the surgeon needs to know these intimately before attempting surgery on either organ.

Let us first discuss the thyroid gland. The anatomy is depicted below with the blood supply from the superior and inferior thyroid arteries and the middle thyroid vein, the proximity to the carotid arteries, the trachea and the all important recurrent and superior laryngeal nerves.

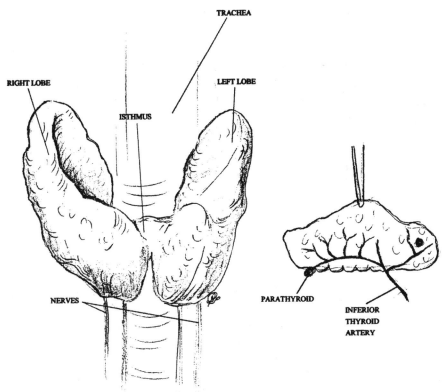

ANATOMY OF THE THYROID AND PARATHYROID GLANDS

DIAGRAM 21

The recurrent laryngeal supplies the voice box or larynx and injury to one or both nerves causes severe hoarseness; if both nerves are cut, which never happens, the vocal cords are paralyzed and the individual would be unable to talk or breathe. I was once told the story and I think it is true, that almost 70 years ago the famous Metropolitan Opera singer Amelita Galli-Curci had thyroid surgery. Apparently the superior laryngeal nerve on one side was injured. She was not hoarse, but could never hold a sustained high note after this and her career ended. These tiny, superior nerves are tremendously variable in position and result in weakening of the voice which usually doesn't cause much problem in non-singers.

The thyroid gland consists of cells which produce thyroid hormone, thyroxine or T4 and tri-iodothyronine, or T3, which effects metabolic activity in the body, and iodine is important in the production of this hormone. If you are hypothyroid, you don't have enough hormone; if you are hyperthyroid, you have too much hormone. The production of this hormone is controlled to a certain degree by a back and forth mechanism with the brain which produces a substance called thyroid stimulating hormone, TSH. If you have enough hormone in the blood, it shuts off the brain's production of TSH; if there's too little hormone, that causes the brain to produce more TSH which causes the thyroid to produce more thyroid hormone.

What are the symptoms of thyroid disease? There are essentially three types of thyroid disease: hyperthyroidism, hypothyroidism and tumors, benign and malignant. Hyperthyroidism, also known as thyrotoxicosis in severe cases, can be caused by too much thyroid hormone such as in Grave's disease, where there is a diffuse toxic goiter, a big thyroid in the neck and many symptoms. Plummer's disease means there is a solitary nodular goiter, or a benign tumor of the thyroid. Hyperthyroidism can also be caused without increase in hormone, in conditions such as cancer and others called Hashimoto's thyroiditis and Reidel's struma. Paradoxically, the thyroiditis patients may initially present with hyperthyroid symptoms and later when the thyroid gland becomes "burnt out" in the later stages of these diseases, they become hypothyroid!

The symptoms of hyperthyroidism are weight loss, intolerance to heat, fast heart rate or tachycardia, fatigue, agitation, goiter or enlarged thyroid and exophthalmos ("bug eyes" - Bette Davis exaggerated). These are the major signs and symptoms; there are many more. The diagnosis is made by inspection, thyroid function blood tests such as T3, T4, and TSH, by radioactive iodine scan and occasionally a CT scan. Most patients with

Grave's disease can be treated with radioactive iodine and medical management, but some patients do need surgery once they have been medically stabilized or if the medical treatment has not been successful. The surgeon never operates on a patient who is hyperthyroid - it's too dangerous. The patient must be made euthyroid with normal levels of T3 and T4 before going to surgery to avoid a terrible disaster called thyroid storm where the patient can die in surgery; this can usually be accomplished by giving iodine or other medications for ten days before surgery. The surgery technique for thyroid disease is much the same for all it's diseases, however the amount of thyroid removed varies from disease to disease. In cancer most surgeons do a complete or nearly complete thyroidectomy. The diagram below shows the stages of thyroid surgery.

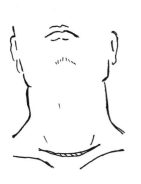 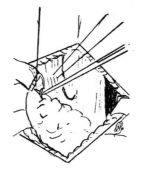 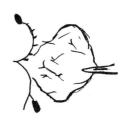

LOCATING THE GLAND   IDENTIFYING THE   REMOVING THE
                           ARTERIES AND NERVES   THYROID

THYROID SURGERY

DIAGAM 22

Hypothyroidism need only be mentioned as a medical entity since it does not require surgery. These patients do not have adequate circulating thyroid hormone. Some may be born with inadequate thyroid tissue or have strange autoimmune problems, marked mental retardation and severe neurological deficits called cretinism. In adults, hypothyroidism results from thyroidectomy, radiation to the neck and chronic thyroiditis. It's treated with thyroid hormone replacement.

Thyroiditis (Hashimoto's, Reidel's, etc.) can produce an enlarged thyroid with signs of mild inflammation. There is no surgical therapy unless tumor is suspected in conjunction with the thyroiditis.

Goiters are enlargements of the thyroid, often caused by iodine deficiency, but also by other more obscure causes. Most goiters respond to medical treatment, and surgery is not indicated except when they are so huge that they cause symptoms by pressing on the trachea, or when veins cause tremendous deformity. I have had the opportunity to remove goiters in several women because they were large, unsightly and the women wanted them removed.

Next we come to the major indications for surgery on the thyroid gland...nodules and tumors. When a patient is found to have a mass in the thyroid it needs to have a workup consisting of thyroid function tests, T3, T4, TSH, and a thyroid scan with radioactive iodine. It may show a "hot" or "cold" nodule depending on whether the nodule takes up the iodine. Generally, cold nodules are suspicious for malignancy, but could be cysts or benign tumors, and hot nodules are either benign tumors or hyperthyroidism. Then a needle aspiration of the nodule is done. The material removed with the needle is sent to a pathologist who evaluates the tissue for possibility of cancer. It is a relatively painless procedure and the only problems I have seen relate to a small amount of bleeding in the area of the needle puncture. If the report is benign with no suspicious tissue, no surgery is indicated. If definite cancer or suspicious tissue is found, then exploration and possible subtotal or total thyroidectomy is indicated. Some physicians will treat suspicious nodules with thyroxine to see if it regresses; if it does they will just follow it; if it doesn't then surgery is probably indicated.

Of the three major cancers of the thyroid, papillary cell type is the most common; this accounts for 75-80% of the tumors, is twice as common in women as men, and may spread to lymph nodes in the neck. If lymph nodes are involved, removal of some neck nodes is done in a procedure called a lymph node dissection. The second most common malignancy is called follicular, occurring in about 10% of thyroid cancers, is three times more common in women than men and very rarely spreads by blood to the lungs, liver and bones. The third cancer is called medullary and is relatively uncommon. Another much rarer cancer, the anaplastic type, occurs only in elderly persons (70's and 80's) and is very dangerous and difficult to treat.

With papillary and follicular carcinomas, the patient may receive radioactive iodine after the surgery, since it will be taken up by any remaining thyroid cancer tissue and will probably destroy it.

Complications of thyroid surgery include bleeding, nerve injury leading to a husky low voice, and hypoparathyroidism if all the parathyroid glands are removed or injured.

The parathyroid glands have been described above and the anatomy shown in the diagram. These tiny organs produce the hormone parathormone which helps regulate calcium levels in the body. Vitamin D is also important in this process. Calcium is needed for strong bones and too much, due to hyperparathyroidism, can cause kidney stones, ulcers and hypertension. Other symptoms of hyperparathyroidism are weakness, headaches, weight loss, nausea, vomiting, constipation, and muscle and joint pain. The main cause of this is usually a benign tumor of the parathyroid gland; parathyroid cancer is very rare. Other non-parathyroid etiologies must be ruled out such as cancers of the kidney and lungs, and multiple myeloma. The workup includes laboratory tests for calcium, phosphorus, and parathormone, and recently I have been using a parathyroid scan to help localize the involved gland.

The surgical exposure is similar to that for thyroid disease, and the surgeon must be aware of the variations in anatomy and exact location of the recurrent laryngeal nerve. Even in the best hands, it is sometimes difficult to find the diseased parathyroid, and if more than one gland is involved, recurrent hyperparathyroidism may occur necessitating re-exploration of the neck. Each successive surgery becomes more difficult.

Chapter 40
SKIN
AND SUBCUTANEOUS TISSUE

The fatty tissue and the skin,
Is just the stuff we're packaged in
It keeps us warm, keeps out the cold,
And fights off poisons, bugs and mold.

And if you're looking kinda strange,
And need some one to rearrange
The nose, the lips, the face, the hair,
Your friendly plastic surgeon's there.

I remember as a child when someone came up and called "Hey, your epidermis is showing!". It was a moment of awareness as I ran home to tell my mother that something was obviously exposed, and she explained that the epidermis is the skin. And for all of us some epidermis is always showing. This is the outermost layer of the skin, the inner layer being the dermis, which contains a vast network of small blood vessels and nerves. Under this is the subcutaneous tissue containing fat, fibrous tissue, sweat glands, sebaceous glands and hair follicles.

The skin is actually the largest organ in the body and has several complex functions without which we cannot live. These include temperature regulation, and protection from the outer environment such as bacteria, foreign bodies, and solar radiation. It is a very complex organ, varying in its composition depending on the area of the body. For us, it is important to recognize it's makeup and discuss some of the surgical aspects of skin pathology.

Our first interaction with skin is usually as a child with congenital abnormalities. The vascular tumors, such as hemangiomas, are more common, are unsightly and can be very large on a newborn. They often get slightly larger and then slowly regress over the next few years, often disappearing without any need for surgery. Those that do not disappear

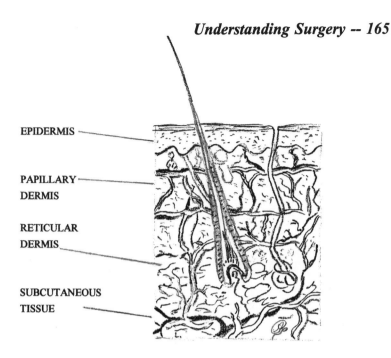

EPIDERMIS

PAPILLARY
DERMIS

RETICULAR
DERMIS

SUBCUTANEOUS
TISSUE

ANATOMY OF THE SKIN

DIAGRAM 23

may be surgically excised later on. Other vascular abnormalities such as blood vessel malformations appear as purplish marks, occasionally very large and can be covered with cosmetics until a child is old enough to undergo a major surgery. Some of these abnormalities have high blood flow as arterio-venous malformations, and surgery can be very dangerous with huge blood loss. The radiologist can often block the artery to the malformation using a special angiogram which may make it smaller or completely disappear. Often surgeons use a combined technique of angiography with arterial embolization clotting off the feeding artery, along with excisional surgery.

Our next contact with skin problems was when we fell off the bicycle or cut ourselves experimenting with a knife; namely, the suturing of wounds. This can be a simple one layer closure or may involve extensive surgery if tissue has been damaged or lost. This may involve rotation of skin flaps into the involved area and closure may be in two or more layers depending on the size of the individual and amount of subcutaneous tissue. The size of the suture used usually depends on the tissue being closed and the under-lying musculature. The smaller the suture, usually the smaller the scar.

I frequently have patients come to me with soft lumps under the skin on the neck, back, chest or anywhere and want them removed because of discomfort, deformity or to be sure there is no possibility of malignancy. They can be removed under a local anesthetic in the physician's office or in an outpatient surgical center without much discomfort.

The most significant area of skin pathology is in the treatment of malignancy. The price we pay for worshipping the sun in our youth is skin cancers as we get older. Of course, there are other etiologies of skin cancers such as immune deficiency, as in AIDS patients, exposure to carcinogens of tars, and nitrogen mustard, certain viruses, radiation, chronic injuries, burns and pressure sores.

The first cancer we will discuss is basal cell carcinoma. It grows slowly and can get very large, almost never spreading beyond the local area and deaths are extremely rare. However they can be locally invasive and can penetrate deeply into underlying tissue causing pain and deformity, and should be completely removed with adequate margins while they are small. Adequate margins means enough normal tissue around the tumor to be sure that it is completely removed, usually at least 2 millimeters.

Squamous cell cancer is the next malignancy, and it is less common but much more serious, with a potential to spread locally and distantly. Extensive squamous cell cancers can even cause death in rare cases. After biopsy and diagnosis, small superficial squamous cell cancers can sometimes be treated with careful radiation therapy or application of topical anti-cancer agents such as fluorouracil, 5FU, but the preferred method of treatment is surgical excision with confirmation of clear margins. Frequently when removing any skin cancer, the specimen has the margins appropriately labeled and sent to the pathologist for frozen section quick staining to determine if the tumor is completely removed. If any margin is involved, namely, has tumor in it, the labeling will allow the surgeon to know where the margin is and re-excise more skin until the margin is clean.

I have purposely avoided trying to describe the appearance of basal and squamous cell cancers because it takes an expert to make the diagnosis. Abnormalities in the skin may be smooth or ulcerated, with a skin breakdown or hole in it, may be pale or dark, brown, purple or beige. As with any skin lesion benign or cancerous, whether it is basal, squamous or melanoma, you should have a physician evaluate it and not try to make the diagnosis yourself. Early recognition and diagnosis cannot be learned from a book or pictures; it takes years of training and experience!

Melanoma is a scary word for most people because they always hear about it in relationship to the worst scenarios, people dying of malignant melanoma. Melanoma is a tumor that can occur in the melanocytes or pigmented cells anywhere in the body, even the eye and intestinal tract, but most commonly in the skin. They are classically described as dark, raised, irregular, occasionally ulcerated lesions, often having rapidly and recently changed in shape and color. But I should emphasize that melanomas can be regular in shape, colorless, nonulcerated and very bland looking. It's not a diagnosis for a novice! See your physician for any skin lesion that is new or changing in any way.

There are several different types of melanomas. I will only mention the four most common just so the names are familiar: the superficial spreading melanoma, the nodular melanoma, the lentigo maligna and the acral melanoma. The seriousness of the melanoma, however, is primarily related to the staging which goes by TNM as in other cancers. It's not important for me to give the whole complex staging criteria except to say that the deeper it goes into the skin, the worse the prognosis, as is the presence of involved lymph nodes and distant metastases. This aspect of the disease needs to be discussed in detail with the surgeon or oncologist. The primary treatment of melanomas is wide excision and if so much skin is removed that primary edge to edge skin closure is not possible, then rotation flaps or skin grafts may be needed. As with breast cancer, the sentinel node, first lymph node draining the area of the cancer, is isolated by blue dye or radioisotope methods and if this node is positive for cancer, a regional dissection of lymph nodes is done. With complex melanoma cases, it is best to have a comprehensive evaluation by a tumor board so that a treatment regimen can be outlined. These tumors are not usually very responsive to radiation or chemotherapy, but immunotherapy has shown some early success. A whole host of new treatments are being evaluated and an oncologist should be able to discuss this with patients having advanced melanoma.

There are many other skin cancers and skin problems which are beyond the scope of this book and these need to be assessed by a dermatologist and treated appropriately.

Chapter 41
THE LIVER

It's long been known, if you love you're a lover,
If you love one too much you may never recover.
For the loved is the lover, the lover the giver,
But the lover who lives is never a liver.

You can live to love and love to live
And your life will flow like sand in a sieve,
You may move in the world like the running of Grunions,
But you'll never be loved like some liver and onions!

The best way to describe the liver is to say it is a brownish red partially rounded huge blob sitting in the right upper aspect of the abdomen. It has a left and right lobe, a large blood supply and a bile drainage system.

The liver helps us metabolize, breakdown and use proteins, carbohydrates and fats and produces bile which flows down the bile ducts into the intestine to help digest food and absorb vitamins A, D, E and K. The liver produces many of the substances needed for blood clotting, detoxifies many substances, and has Kupffer's cells which devour waste products.

Symptoms of liver disease include tiredness, yellow jaundice, intestinal tract bleeding, mental changes, weight loss, pain and fever. Signs of liver disease are similar including jaundice, fever, abdominal distention with fluid called ascites, liver enlargement and tenderness, abnormal liver function tests, male breast enlargement called gynecomastia, intestinal tract bleeding, enlargement of the spleen and loss of armpit and pubic hair, to name a few. The laboratory tests have been mentioned in Chapter 25.

It can be examined by x-rays, CAT scans, ultrasound, liver scans using radioisotopes, liver biopsies using needles, angiograms and venous studies. It is the bailiwick of the gastroenterologist, and the surgeon only gets called in when problems can't be managed medically. The main dis-

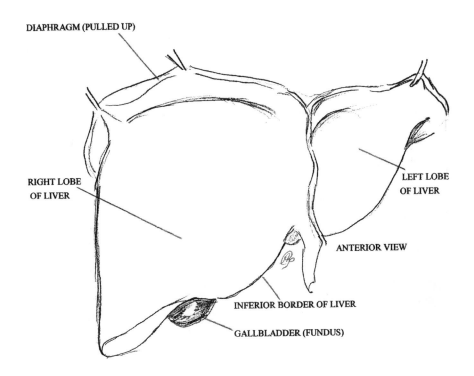

DIAPHRAGM (PULLED UP)

RIGHT LOBE
OF LIVER

LEFT LOBE
OF LIVER

ANTERIOR VIEW

INFERIOR BORDER OF LIVER

GALLBLADDER (FUNDUS)

ANATOMY OF THE LIVER

DIAGRAM 24

eases of the liver in the United States are hepatitis, the name for any inflammation of the liver, cirrhosis, an end-stage deterioration of the liver, most often from chronic alcoholism, portal hypertension, a complex problem where the liver veins aren't functioning correctly and there is a backup of blood behind the liver; it has a long list of causes including cirrhosis, hepatitis, cancer, etc.

The indications for surgery are related to trauma, bleeding caused by portal hypertension, ascites, cysts in the liver, benign and malignant tumors, and blockage of the main bile duct.

Let us approach the most simple procedures first. Frequently a simple cyst of the liver can be aspirated and drained under a local anesthetic by the radiologist, who can also place a drain tube for continued drainage. Abscesses and complex cysts may be handled by the radiologist or require an open surgical operation. The complications of this procedure are infection and bleeding, and the patient requires careful observation after the surgery.

If a patient has trauma to the liver as from an auto accident, knife or gunshot wound, the liver can be evaluated by CAT scan. If the injury is minor, sometimes the liver will heal itself. However, frequently there is massive bleeding accompanying other injuries and the abdomen has to be opened in the midline and the liver injury has to be repaired using special large sutures and pieces of material to prevent the liver tissue from falling apart. Unfortunately, trauma that is severe enough to cause liver injury usually causes other intra abdominal injuries which compromise the patient's recovery.

When there is bile duct obstruction from an impacted gall stone, this can usually be extracted by a gastroenterologist using endoscopy in a procedure called endoscopic retrograde cholangio-pancreatography (ERCP), a big word for looking at the bile duct by putting a tube through the mouth and down into the intestine and actually finding the opening of the bile duct into the intestine, dilating it, and removing the stone. On rare occasions an open exploration of the bile duct is required.

In cases of late liver disease such as cirrhosis there is a backup of fluid in the abdomen called ascites. A fellow named Dr. Harry LeVeen in New York devised a special one way shunt tube, one end of which is inserted into the abdomen and the other is tunneled under the skin from the abdomen to the neck where it is placed in the internal jugular vein. Fluid is pulled from the abdomen into the vein and the increased fluid load in the vein is excreted by the kidney. Since the fluid in the abdomen contains a large amount of protein, just sucking the fluid out of the abdomen is not good idea. With this method, the abdominal fluid filters through the kidneys which retains the good components and excretes the rest in the urine. The LeVeen shunt is placed n the patient under local or general anesthesia and works in about 50% of cases. Complications are mainly secondary to large fluid shifts, bleeding, infections, and kidney malfunction.

Portal hypertension as described above is the backup of blood and thereby elevated pressure in the veins in the abdomen. Patients with this condition can bleed massively. Often the gastroenterologist can stop the bleeding with special cautery or tamponade pressure procedures done endoscopically. If not, in the past it would require a complex operation, bypassing the liver with the huge abdominal vessels shunted into the vena cava, the large vein in the abdomen, but it required a long and dangerous procedure. Now the radiologist can perform the same shunting by a procedure called trans internal jugular portal-systemic shunt, TIPS. All you need to know is that this procedure, now successful in over ninety percent of the patients, has all but eliminated the need for the older operation.

Tumors of the liver can be benign and malignant. The benign ones often don't require surgery unless they are symptomatically painful or bleeding, or premalignant. They include hemangiomas, benign blood vessel tumors, adenomas which are benign growths of liver tissue and several other rarer tumors which I'll name and then you can forget - hamartomas, focal nodular hyperplasia, teratomas and so on.

Cancer in the liver can either be primary, originating in the liver, or metastatic, spread to the liver from another organ such as colon or breast. The extent and nature of a liver cancer is determined by CAT scan or MRI scan and percutaneous needle biopsies can be done by a radiologist to ascertain the diagnosis. The management of liver cancer depends on many factors and these cases are usually discussed at a tumor board where several different specialists are present including radiologists, oncologists, surgeons, pathologists and internists. When a patient has spread of a cancer to the liver, it is usually not a situation where surgery would be recommended unless it is a single or even two solitary areas of involvement that the surgeon thinks he can completely remove in a curative operation. This is only done when a curative operation has been done or can be done on the primary tumor. For example, if a patient has a colon cancer that can be cured with local surgery, but also has a single metastatic tumor in the liver, a decision may be made to attempt to remove the tumor in the liver. However, at the time of the surgery, the surgeon often finds that there is more disease in the liver than was seen on x-ray and the liver surgery is canceled.

The primary malignant tumor of the liver, hepatocellular carcinoma, HCC, is actually the most common cancer in the world today. Its etiology, while not specifically known, is impacted by chronic liver disease, alcoholic cirrhosis, hepatitis B and C and a number of other hepatotoxic agents including to a much lesser degree smoking and oral contraceptives. The diagnosis is similar to that of benign tumors with radiological studies including CAT and MRI scans, and angiography evaluating the blood supply to the tumor and the liver and to determine the extent of the disease. A laparoscopy may be indicated, at which time the surgeon can determine whether the tumor is removable. Large hepatic resections require special expertise and in my community there are a few surgeons who specialize in this complex area; their experience markedly lowers the morbidity and mortality of these operations. However, minor liver resections can be done by most well-trained general surgeons.

Finally, we are now in an age when teams of surgeons can do liver transplants in patients whose liver disease has reached the point where they will die of liver failure if something is not done. Usually this requires the donation of a liver by the family from a brain dead individual after trauma such as an auto accident, or gunshot wound, but now there are incidences where a family member has donated part of a liver to another family member. The demand for liver transplants far exceeds the supply and a careful selection of appropriate recipients is undertaken by special hospital committees. The surgical expertise in liver transplants has improved markedly over the past ten years so that the survival rates, depending on the patient's underlying health varies from 60 to 85% in the best hospital centers. These procedures not only requires specially trained surgeons, but also special nurses, hospital facilities and teams of support personnel to diagnose and manage any of the many problems that can occur after the surgical procedure is over.

Chapter 42
THE PANCREAS

The pancreas looks like a flounder, with a head, neck, body and tail,
It lies transverse in the abdomen looking glandular and quite frail.
Its function is quite complex , making enzymes and some hormones,
To help the body digesting its food from steaks and chicken to scones.

The gland makes insulin to prevent diabetes, and not to dispel any
rumors,
It also makes cysts, and can get bad infections and also can form nasty
tumors.
And when you are dining at a posh restaurant, you'll often get stares
and turn heads
When you order some pancreas, au gratin, known to the upper class
snobs as sweetbreads.

T he pancreas is an elongated glandular organ lying across the back
of the upper and mid-abdomen, behind and below the stomach,
behind the colon and in front of the abdominal aorta. As shown
in the diagram, it is arbitrarily divided into four parts, a head,
neck, body and tail and has a rich blood and lymphatic supply.

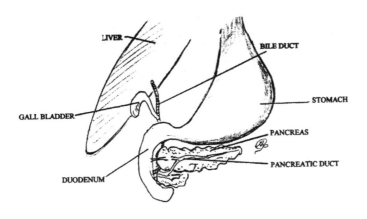

PANCREAS AND SURROUNDING ORGANS

DIAGRAM 25

It has two separate functional divisions, the endocrine and the exocrine. The endocrine consists of small clusters of cells called the islets of Langerhans which contain two cells types: the alpha cells produce glucagon which increases blood sugar or glucose, and the beta cells produce insulin which lowers blood glucose and prevent diabetes mellitus. These hormones are delivered directly into the blood stream and do not go through ducts - thus called endocrine or ductless.

The exocrine pancreas has cells which produce many enzymes including amylase and lipase which are delivered by way of the pancreatic duct system through tubes to the intestine where they help in the digestion of carbohydrates, fats and proteins.

Pancreatitis, an inflammation of the pancreas, is often found in association with gallstone, alcoholism, cancer and unknown etiologies. The gallstone variety usually responds and improves by removal of the gall bladder and extraction of the gallstones blocking the pancreatic duct. The disease is essentially a medical one responding to rest, IV fluids, no food by mouth and antibiotics. In pancreatitis, the very strong enzymes sometimes leak into the pancreas and the organ autodigests itself or eats itself up. In cases of severe pancreatitis not responding to vigorous medical management, surgery may be indicated to remove dead pancreatic tissue and drain off the toxin enzymes. It is a major surgery with many potential complications, including bleeding, infection and death.

One of the long term problems of pancreatitis is the development of pancreatic pseudocysts, which are large fluid filled cavities in the pancreas that may need to be drained surgically. Diagnosis of pancreatic disease is by blood tests, amylase and lipase, blood sugar level and by CAT and MRI scans, and ultrasound.

Tumors of the pancreas are predominantly malignant cancers. When they occur in the body or tail, they usually grow fairly large without causing symptoms, and are thereby diagnosed late in the disease; this makes cure very difficult. On the other hand, tumors of the head of the pancreas and around the ampulla of Vater usually cause early blockage of the common bile duct resulting in yellow jaundice. Any patient that develops yellow jaundice deserves a complete gastroenterological evaluation, and therefore an early cancer of the pancreas can be discovered. Cancer surgery for curable pancreatic cancer is very involved, often requiring the Whipple procedure. This procedure involves removing a large portion of pancreas, part of the stomach, duodenum, and common bile duct and then putting back together what's left. Cure rates are low and potential complications are high so a surgeon doesn't want to operate unless he can offer a fairly good chance for cure. Because pancreatic cancer can often cause obstruction to the outlet of the stomach as well as block the common bile duct, causing jaundice which causes severe itching, palliative surgery is often done in non-resectable or non-removable cases. This consists of bypassing the stomach so it won't get obstructed and bypassing the common bile duct, also so it won't get obstructed. A loop of intestine is usually brought up and connected to these structures.

Patients with pancreatic cancer may have pain related to the tumor invading the nerves in the back of the abdomen and this can be eliminated or alleviated either by the surgeon or by pain management specialists, by doing nerve blocks.

In conclusion, there is now experimental work on pancreas transplants at several university medical centers which may eventually lead to better treatment for diabetes and for the individual whose pancreas has been destroyed by disease.

Chapter 43
LUMPS AND BUMPS

I have a collection of lumps, bumps and scars,
In a closet at home in old Mason Jars,
Some say it is truly a ghoulish collection,
And still others call it a vile vivisection.

So... If you have a brown ugly bump on your nose,
Something that just can't be covered by clothes,
I'll gladly excise it without much to say,
(But I'll keep the lump and I'll throw You away!)

Most every surgeon fills his spare working hours removing "lumps and bumps". It's easy and fun and the patients are always happy. The lumps and bumps are the unsightly, annoying things that everyone has on their skin somewhere on their body and has always wanted removed. There's the five millimeter brown spot on the upper cheek that a fourteen year old just can't stand and wants off, the mole on the back "that rubs on my bra strap!", the lump "on my shoulder that's been there for ten years - but I want it off!"

Most lumps and bumps are lipomas, inclusion cysts or sebaceous cysts, lumps on the scalp and annoying "blemishes" that people can't stand anymore and they are almost always non-cancerous.

I usually remove these in my office with a small amount of local anesthetic (marcaine or xylocaine). A small incision either straight over the area or elliptically around it, and a little dissection with an instrument usually does the job. Then I close the wound with a fine suture of nylon or prolene and leave the sutures in for seven to ten days before removal and steri-stripping, or close with a subcuticular suture that absorbs and never needs removal.

These are very simple procedures and yet I have seen patients who keep a hideous, protruding hairy mole for years. Usually any physician can remove these and at minimal cost; you don't need to go to a plastic surgeon to get a fine result!

Go ahead...treat yourself. Get de-lumped and de-bumped.

Chapter 44
PILONIDAL DISEASE

I have a tiny hole above my rectum, 'tween my "cheeks",
And out of it a small amount of fluid always leaks.
My doctor says it will not heal and needs an operation,
So I have given my consent and my cooperation.

He says that to succeed, he needs to rid me of the tissue
That's causing all my pain and is the basis of the issue.
But he has warned me that the wide excision will be large,
Like something after blowing up a city block long barge.

I'll never understand why such a tiny leaking hole
Will need such awful massive surgery, to save my soul,
It seems that modern surgery should have a bit more class,
Than this immense procedure, truly one pain_____.

Pilonidal comes from the combination of two Latin words: pilus meaning hair and nidus meaning nest. Although the exact etiology of the disease is unknown, it is postulated that it is the result of ingrown hairs in the area between the buttocks. The entire area may become infected and an abscess may occur which is painful and may rupture on its own. Recurrent infections are the usual course until the entire diseased area is removed.

There are many treatments, some of which include wide excision of all the diseased area and allowing it to heal up by itself, usually taking one to two months or wide excision and closure. The later often does not heal well and may have to be converted to the first method. I have had experience with both methods, and have pretty much given up the procedure where the wound is closed. It almost always gets infected and requires the open procedure. Although it initially looks huge and scary, the wound becomes almost painless after a few days and closes quite rapidly. Patients need to take baths twice a day and keep a clean dressing over the open wound until it is completely closed. Once this procedure had been done, there are almost no recurrences.

Chapter 45
HEMORRHOIDS, ANAL FISSURE AND FISTULA IN ANO

When God in his wisdom designed the anus,
There's one particular that he didn't explain us,
And that is just why we have hemorrhoids that pain us
This embarrassing problem that can be quite heinous.

Hemorrhoids are veins. They occur at the end of the anal canal and are either internal or external. Although the hemorrhoidal plexus of vessels is always present, problems arise when they swell and get larger because of static or exertional pressure in the pelvis from pregnancy, straining at stools, heavy lifting or large, hard bowel movements.

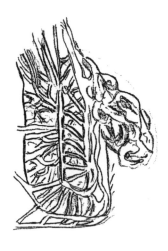

INTERNAL HEMORRHOID

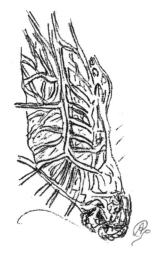

EXTERNAL HEMORRHOID

HEMORRHOIDAL ANATOMY

DIAGRAM 26

The internal hemorrhoids are the kind that are painless but give you a feeling of fullness in the anus and can bleed or prolapse, progressively extending towards the anal verge or even hanging out. They are covered by mucosa, the lining of the upper anal canal.

The external hemorrhoids are in the end of the anal canal and are covered with skin. This accounts for their pain, itching, and inflammation. They can get swollen or engorged and thrombosed which means they are filled with blood clots and even bleed.

The primary management of hemorrhoids is threefold: first, alleviating the symptoms with pain medications such as anesthetic creams or suppositories, second, applying anti-inflammatory medications in the form of suppositories with or without steroids - i.e., Anusol, Preparation H, etc., and third, instruction about bowel habits including increased fiber diet, increased water intake, and avoiding straining at stools or sitting on toilet for a prolonged period.

Most hemorrhoids will improve or resolve on this regimen and surgery should only be reserved for failures at medical management. The diagnosis is made by observation, digital examination, unless too painful and by proctosigmoidoscopic examination. If there is significant pain, heavy sedation may be needed. The important thing is to make the correct diagnosis and for the physician to know that a patient may have more than one problem causing rectal pain or bleeding. I have seen sad cases where a patient has been treated for hemorrhoids only to find out much later that the bleeding was caused by a cancer in the colon. If you have any rectal pain or bleeding, be sure that you have a complete exam by a physician and insist that all possibilities are evaluated including ulcers, fissures, cancer, diverticulitis and of course, psychiatric problems.

For those patients who do not respond to medical management the follow treatments are available.

Internal hemorrhoids can be treated by a special apparatus which places a rubber band at the base of the hemorrhoid. This can be done in a physician's office or an outpatient facility and is relatively painless. Sclerosing agents, lasers or heat coagulation can be used in the operating room or GI lab depending on your hospital's facilities. Large hemorrhoids need to be excised which means cutting them out and usually requires a stay of one or two days in the hospital until the patient is comfortable and having at least the first bowel movement after surgery. The complications after hemorrhoidectomy are mainly pain and occasionally inability to urinate because of spasm and the use of narcotic medications.

Sometimes an external hemorrhoid becomes thrombosed and fills with a blood clot and this is very uncomfortable. It can be lanced (opened) in the doctor's office with local anesthesia which causes a few moments of discomfort and results in tremendous relief. Abscesses of the anal area can develop which are very painful and require opening and drainage in the operating room under a general anesthetic.

The two other areas I want to discuss are anal fissure and fistula in ano, a hole or tract running from inside the rectum to the outside skin.

Anal fissure is a cut injury which occurs in the back and rarely in the front of the anal canal as a result of stretching with bowel movement, diarrhea or secondary to diseases of the anus such as Crohn's disease and problems with the anal muscles called anal sphincters. Fissures cause sharp pain with bowel movements and occasional bleeding and will usually respond to medical management such as stool softeners and adding bulk to the diet. The diagnosis is by visual exam and digital exam is usually too painful. Some physicians have used topical nitroglycerine or local anesthetics with good success. If surgery is required, the most successful method is called lateral sphincterotomy or division of one of the anal sphincter muscles which allows the "split" to heal.

Fistulas result from an infection in an anal crypt with resultant abscess and a tunneling through the perianal tissue to the inside mucosa or the external skin. They can be very simple, single tracts or very complex with tentacles extending throughout the perianal area. The treatment consists of unroofing the tract if possible and treatment with antibiotics. A fistula should be treated when first noticed or it may become complex resulting in extensive surgery. There are several complicated procedures which may be employed for extensive disease and often a colorectal specialist is needed to handle these situations.

Chapter 46
ABSCESSES, INFECTIONS, CELLULITIS, DEHISCENCE AND EVISCERATION

Sometimes, whatever you do, you can't win!
Perhaps it's from too much engaging in sin.
But whatever the cause, it's apparent from the start,
That sooner or later we'll all fall apart.

I just hope it's not with infections and abscesses
(They're so gosh darn dirty, and leave such big messes)
And I pray to heaven that I don't eviscerate
On the way to my funeral I'd probably be late.

This is the potpourri chapter. It's just to emphasize what can happen to the human body when adverse things happen during and after a surgical procedure.

As we mentioned previously, there is always the chance of contamination during an operation, either from the airborne organisms, the abdomen, skin, instruments or unknown causes. People with potentially debilitating medical problems such as cancer, diabetes mellitus, respiratory problems, chronic illness have an increased risk for the complications of wound infection. Bacteria can grow in a wound, cellulitis with bacteria can invade surrounding tissue and cause pain, redness, and swelling, and abscess, a severe infection can produce pus in a closed space as in a wound, or deep in the abdomen, chest, brain etc. Other problems include dehiscence where the fascia of a wound closure breaks down because of infection or weak tissue, chemotherapy, diabetes mellitus, cancer, severe coughing, obesity, malnutrition, post-radiation therapy, hematoma and poor technique, and the wound under the skin opens causing a hernia. Evisceration is when a dehiscence occurs and the skin opens, allowing the contents to spill out; in the abdomen an evisceration may result in the intestines coming out of the belly.

Infection and cellulitis, when recognized, need to be treated with antibiotics. These problems can become severe, even threatening a limb or life. You may recall newspaper accounts of the "flesh eating bacteria" which is actually a kind of streptococcal infection; it needs to be treated rapidly and with the correct antibiotics. The treatment of an abscess is always drainage except in the rare cases when the patient is too sick to undergo any procedure; many of the patients treated only with antibiotics do not survive.

Dehiscence is a situation which needs to be recognized and the patient must be taken back to the operating room for wound reclosure. Similarly, if evisceration has occurred, the patient must go back to surgery to have the intestines replaced into the abdomen and the abdomen closed with special large retention sutures, which are sometimes left in place for months.

Complications are part of the surgeon's life and how soon he recognizes them and deals with them appropriately is the most important thing. The surgeon doing simple procedures will probably have a complication free life; the one treating complex cases will inevitably have problem cases, and his quality as a physician can be measured by how well he handles the problem, the patient and the patient's family, as well as his own emotions. People are not like man made machines and surgery is not like changing a muffler or carburetor!

Chapter 47
CANCER - WHAT OPERATIONS

When we talk of Cancer schmancer
Surgery isn't always the answer!

In the past, one hundred years ago, it was felt by most notable physicians and surgeons that the best treatment for cancer was removing it entirely, and while this philosophy may hold true in many circumstances, we need to go through the various treatments for cancer that may or may not involve complete removal of the tumor. Sometimes your physician may say that the tumor cannot or should not be removed and this is not necessarily an ominous sign. So let us briefly talk about Cancer - the types of surgery.

In many instances complete removal of a tumor is the best way to attempt a complete cure of the disease. In situations such as breast cancer, colon cancer, lung cancer and kidney cancer this is often the objective of treatment. If the cancer is localized to one area and is removable without extreme damage to vital organs, then a cancer operation is performed; this generally means removal of the primary cancer along with normal tissue around it with clear margins and some of the draining lymph nodes included. But in some cases surgery may not be the best treatment. An example is a tumor called squamous cell cancer of the anus. In the past we used to do radical surgery removing the rectum and anus and leaving a permanent colostomy. Today we know that many of these cases can be cured with chemotherapy and radiation treatment and the more radical procedure is only used when there is failure of this more conservative treatment. The only surgery needed then would be the biopsy to determine what type of tumor it is. Another situation is certain types of lymphoma. This is generally a systemic disease. namely all over the body, although a mass of nodes may only appear in one place. It is often sufficient to do a biopsy of the mass, do the appropriate studies on the tissue, and then be treated with radiation and chemotherapy, often times with complete disappearance and even cure of the disease. I have seen patients with extensive lymphoma of the stomach, who in the past might have undergone radical surgical resections, who can be cured by non-surgical modalities today. So, in summary, the second treatment is biopsy for diagnosis, followed by curative radiation and/or, if necessary, chemotherapy.

In some cases we do surgery for palliation. This means that the tumor has grown in a place or to a size or with distant metastases, that makes a complete curative resection impossible. The important thing is to treat the individual's symptoms and make the patient comfortable. In brain cancer, frequently a neurosurgeon will remove 95% of a cancer so that symptoms of weakness, paralysis, pain or other neurological symptoms will diminish or disappear. Even though the cancer can't be cured, the patient can be relieved of symptoms so that he/she can resume a normal life. The patient with colon cancer which has already spread to the liver and lung needs to have the tumor bearing portion of the colon removed to prevent future obstruction, pain and bleeding. The patient with an unresectable or unremovable pancreatic cancer should have a bypass of the common bile duct to prevent jaundice and bypass of the stomach to prevent obstruction. These are palliative procedures and are part of the armamentarium of every surgeon.

No one should suffer with cancer. Pain in almost every case can be treated successfully by palliative surgery or by pain management specialists with nerve blocks and other methodology.

In gynecological cancers such as ovarian cancer, the malignancy may not be detected until it has spread throughout the abdomen. These patients are operated upon by gynecological oncologic surgeons who remove 95-98% of the cancer from all over the abdomen in what is called an extensive debulking procedure. If they remove enough tumor and if it is sensitive to chemotherapy, they may actually cure some patients even with extensive disease.

And even if there is no possibility for cure in many debulking and palliative surgical cases, the patients are given long disease-free or symptom-free intervals of life to live and enjoy.

So, talk with your surgeon and understand the various surgeries that are possible...curative, debulking, palliative, and diagnostic. Each year that I am in practice, new boundaries are broken in the cure of diseases using new chemotherapeutic and radiotherapeutic modalities. When I was in medical school, in my first week in the pathology department, I was in the morgue when a friend from high school was brought in. He had died from testicular cancer. Today, with all our treatment capabilities, he would probably be cured and leading a normal life. Don't compare your or your family member's situation with a past history of someone else because the treatment and outcome today may be very different than it was only a few years ago.

Chapter 48
THE SPLEEN

Even the Greeks knew of the spleen, and apparently vented it often;
I guess what they meant was it housed the emotion that frequently led to the coffin.
The spleen stood for malice and spite and bad temper, an overly evil emotion,
And I don't know why so gentle an organ could ever have started that notion.

For the spleen is the place where your blood gets cleansed, and the old cells go to die,
A place of sadness for tired old blood, that enters and fades with a sigh,
It also can help you to fight off disease by helping your body's immunity,
So please stop your carping and critical words about spleens, that you use with impunity.

The spleen is about the size and shape of a child's baseball glove and is situated in the left upper aspect of the abdomen, just under the lower rib cage, next to the stomach, behind the colon and above the left kidney. In fetal life, in the womb, the spleen contributes to the production of blood, but this does not continue in the adult. The main role of the adult spleen is twofold; first is the cleansing of the blood of old red cells, white cells and platelets along with other debris. The second role is an immunologic one producing substances that help you fight infection and other diseases. The diagram usually shows the location and anatomy of the spleen which we will refer to later when talking about surgery. Of interest is the fact that there can be accessory spleens, appearing around the area of the real spleen. They look like little kidney beans and are of minimal importance other than to note their presence.

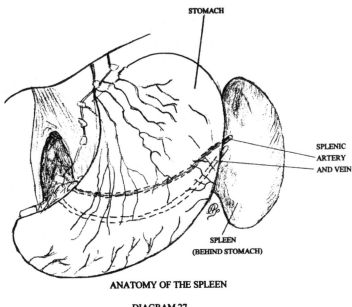

ANATOMY OF THE SPLEEN

DIAGRAM 27

Let us first consider splenic injuries. When an individual sustains a fall or blunt trauma to the left lower ribs or left upper abdomen, there is always the possibility of causing splenic injury. This injury may vary from minor bruising to frank rupture with massive hemorrhage. The spleen has a capsule, but it is very thin and is easily ruptured or injured. Because it is so vascular with many blood vessels, it can cause extensive bleeding and after some accidents with splenic rupture, the patient can actually exsanguinate and die if not brought to a hospital and immediately operated upon. The signs of injury to the spleen may be broken ribs on the left, usually numbers ten through twelve, abdominal pain, falling blood count, falling blood pressure and rising pulse rate. We used to do abdominal needle taps to see if blood is in the abdomen, but now spiral CAT scans can be done rapidly to make the presence and extent of the injury known. Sometimes there is just a swelling inside the spleen, a subcapsular hematoma, and these patients can be observed carefully in an intensive care unit for several days; a delayed full rupture can occur, necessitating surgery. Similarly, sometimes the laceration of the spleen is very minor and is sealed by a blood clot. In the past we would take out any injured spleen but today, knowing the immunological importance of the organ, we try to preserve it if possible. However, if there is a large tear or if bleeding persists, the spleen must be removed surgically. A patient who has a spleen removed must be given pneumococcal vaccine, Pneumovax, to prevent severe infection, and this is standard for this procedure.

If a patient does not have the spleen removed, he/she must be observed carefully for several months after the initial week of hospitalization, because it takes that long for the spleen to heal properly. This sometimes creates a problem for professional athletes and young sportsmen who want to get back to these activities and may impact whether the spleen is removed!

The actual procedure, splenectomy, is carried out under a general anesthetic through a midline or left subcostal incision. The cut is either in the middle of the abdomen from the bellybutton up or obliquely below the left rib cage. The abdomen usually contains blood which is rapidly evacuated and the patient is usually receiving blood and fluids by this time intravenously. The pedicle or hilus of the spleen is located and the splenic vein and artery are carefully dissected out and tied off using strong sutures. Then the other vessels to the stomach and occasionally to surrounding tissue are tied and the spleen is removed. Sound simple? It can be very simple or very complex depending on the patient's anatomy and the size of the spleen. Post-operative complications include bleeding or infection, both of which may require re-operation. Patients may also have partial lung collapse, or atelectasis on the left side which will need vigorous breathing exercises, and there may be transient marked elevations of the WBC, RBC and platelet counts. After surgery, since there is no further chance of rupture, the patient can resume normal activities in two to four weeks.

There are several diseases for which splenectomy may be indicated. A physician will explain these to the patient but I will list them for you. There is idiopathic thrombocytopenic purpura, thrombotic thrombocytopenic purpura, hypersplenism, and certain malignancies. In many cases, abnormalities in splenic function cause too much destruction of the red cells, the white cells or the platelets, and when the spleen is removed, there is an initial rise in the number of these products, and it may take weeks or months to return to normal.

There are cases where the injury to the spleen is not sufficient to require splenectomy but where abscess may develop as a late complication requiring late surgery. There are also many tropical diseases which will effect the spleen causing masses or abscesses or cyst formation. We do not see much of this in the United States.

Most recently, several surgeons have been doing splenic repairs and partial splenic resections, especially in children, to preserve the spleen at least until a child is over two years old. Special suturing techniques and artificial tissue wraps have been devised for that purpose but the patients must be observed carefully for breakthrough bleeding.

Chapter 49
TRAUMA

The alarm had sounded, the crowds had been found,
The onlookers, curious, were holding their ground.
The four paramedics raced in and raced out,
The traffic was halted, police used their clout.

They arrived at the ER and rushed to the room
Where the doctors were ready for all gloom and doom.
I stood for a moment awaiting the news,
It was life and death trauma, from everyone's views.

When the doctor appeared, I started to sway,
Medicine had reached its apex that day.
With acrylics and instruments filling his pockets,
He announced with great pride we should send up the rockets.

Mrs. Lulu Van Snoot's medication won't fail
We've managed to save her indented toe nail.
The crowds became wild, with three hoots and hollers,
Another saved toenail - just six thousand dollars.

Okay, so maybe that's not trauma to you. You'd be surprised to see how many Van Snoot clones appear at the emergency room door complaining of major wounds. Our Emergency Rooms have become the repository for everything from the critically ill to the patient who didn't want to bother the family physician about some minuscule problem. This chapter is about trauma and I want to give you some basic understanding about what the physician and paramedics look for, how they prevent injury to the already injured and how they institute immediate life-saving measures while the patient's condition is being evaluated. I will give a few examples and some general principles for care, since thousands of pages have been devoted to this subject alone.

The American College of Surgeons has an Advanced Trauma Life Support Course for physicians which emphasizes initial treatment of trauma patients. There is a primary survey called the ABC's consisting of: A - maintaining an Airway so the patient can breathe while making sure there is no neck injury, B - Breathing for the patient if he/she is unable, and C - making sure that the heart is beating and that there is Circulation of blood. The paramedics don't want anyone who is not trained working with a trauma victim because they could inadvertently make a situation worse. When the paramedics arrive, stand aside! The paramedics also can determine when the lungs are collapsed and the physician may need to place a tube in a chest to help re-expand the lung. If many ribs are broken, the patient may need continuous respiratory assistance. You have heard about CPR, cardio-respiratory resuscitation, and I can't give you a class in this chapter. It is always helpful for anyone who is able, to take a brief class in CPR and I know many who have saved lives when seconds and minutes have meant the difference between the life and death of a loved one.

One of the first important things when resuscitating a patient is finding IV access, namely a place to put an intravenous needle for giving fluids and medications. While someone is seeing to the ABC's, usually a nurse or physician is starting an IV, with fluids and lifesaving medications.

When there is severe trauma with blood loss, the pulse will be fast and thready, the blood pressure will be low and the patient may have lost consciousness. Often a CVP or central venous pressure line is placed to help monitor the fluid replacement and blood loss. The patient will be undergoing a complete examination by the emergency room physician and will probably have appropriate x-rays, CAT scans and angiograms as needed. If there is no abdominal injury or chest injury and the leg is broken, then obviously the focus will be on the leg, but the physician must be sure not to overlook a potentially catastrophic injury which is not visible just because there is a major injury which IS visible. The job of the emergency physician is to ascertain and correct heart, lung and hemorrhage problems as quickly as possible and determine whether surgery is needed. If so, then the operating room personnel need to be ready. Let us look at some of the areas of focal interest.

The head evaluation is done with an initial assessment of brain function based on what is called the Glasgow Coma Scale which assesses eye response, verbal response and motor or movement responses. The scale ranges from 3 (the lowest response) to 15 (normal) and depending on the rating will determine what types of tests are needed and with what urgency. When x-rays and CAT scans of the head are done, bleeding can be evaluated and a decision made as to whether emergency surgery is needed.

The neck comes next and must be evaluated for cervical spine fractures, spinal cord injury, injuries to vessels and to the trachea or airway. Stabilization is important to prevent causing further injury and that is why you frequently see trauma patients immediately placed in a neck brace.

The chest, as we have discussed, can have injuries to the lungs, heart and great vessels which the ER physician will immediately assess by physical exam, EKG, and appropriate x-rays.

The abdomen and pelvis are next and must be evaluated for bleeding, rupture of organs such as liver, spleen, intestines, and pancreas, and determination must be made whether exploration is needed.

At this point I'll digress for a moment to discuss the mode of injury. Blunt trauma such as an auto accident and falls are handled as we have discussed. Penetrating injuries are often more difficult because the entry point often will not indicate the location or severity of the injury. This is most often the case with gunshot and knife wounds and often necessitates exploration to assure that the area involved is not severely damaged. All gunshot wounds of the abdomen have to be explored and any knife wounds that have penetrated into the peritoneal cavity will probably have to be explored. Small injuries to the intestine can result in terrible infections, sepsis and death if not handled appropriately from the start. I have seen patients shot in the chest with the bullet seen on x-ray in the pelvis and similarly I have seen patients shot in the chest or abdomen where the bullet missed every vital structure. When there is injury to an extremity, either arm or leg, the physician must assess the nerves, arteries and veins, sometimes using angiography or vessel x-rays with dye to determine whether surgical repair is indicated.

This brief outline is just meant to show you what must be done by the physician evaluating the trauma patient. The bywords are training, experience, excellent paramedical teams, excellent emergency room facilities with nurses, aides and a whole host of backup experts who know exactly what to do. For the layman, the best approach is education, specifically CPR and basic first aid. I recommend this for everyone especially if you have small children or elderly persons living with you.

The other trauma areas are insect, snake, animal and fish bites, minor trauma, and specific injuries to the kidneys, ureters, bladder, urethra, or genitalia, both male and female, and other organs. Many medical centers have specially trained trauma teams and in larger cities, the major trauma patients are directed to these facilities greatly increasing patient survival and decreasing patient morbidity.

Chapter 50
THE DIAPHRAGM

You may think that the way to a man's heart is through his stomach
But you can't get to the heart from the stomach without traversing the
diaphragm.
Now you may ask why I wrote a poem where diaphragm was supposed
to rhyme with stomach.
It's cause I can't think of a word that rhymes with stomach except
lummock or dummock.
Ho hummach!

I want to begin by saying that there's not a lot to say about the diaphragm. It's just that I have found most patients really don't know what it is and where it is and the general consensus is that a diaphragm is contraception, which it can be but that's another subject entirely.

The diaphragm is the muscular and tendinous structure that separates the abdomen from the chest. It is innervated by two important nerves, the right and left phrenic, which cause the diaphragm to move in such a way that it assists the lungs in expanding and contracting, thereby helping you breathe. Above the diaphragm are the lungs and heart in the chest. Below the diaphragm is the stomach near the center, the liver on the right and the spleen on the left. Below this is the rest of the abdominal cavity.

There are three holes in the diaphragm as shown below, one for the esophagus, one for the vena cava, the largest vein in the body, and one for the aorta, the largest artery. The diaphragm has the potential for several hernias, two congenital, Bochdalek and Morgagni, and then several different kinds of esophageal hiatus hernias. We have discussed the surgery for the latter, and the former are usually closed only when large and symptomatic, by using sutures and small cotton or Teflon pads as bolsters. Surgery on the diaphragm is otherwise unusual unless there is massive trauma requiring closure of a tear.

Chapter 51
TRANSPLANTATION

Heart, pancreas, lung or liver,
I'd rather receive, than be a giver.
Lung, liver, pancreas, heart,
If you're a donor, you're dead from the start.

But to donate a kidney, you may be
Alive or dead, it seems to me.
Thankful people throughout the nation
Hail as their savior, Transplantation.

The entire field of organ transplantation has blossomed over the past thirty years. Starting with the simplest skin grafts at the turn of the twentieth century, it was discovered that skin could be taken from one part of the same body and transplanted to another site. However, a skin graft could not be taken from another individual without immediate rejection; the body refuses the skin as foreign and the skin dies, often creating a severe reaction in the recipient. Let us define a few terms regarding transplantation. Transplants or grafts between genetically identical persons, identical twins, is called syngeneic, same genes, while that between different persons, not twins, of the same species is called allogeneic, other genes. Transplants between different species are called Xenogeneic, foreign or strange genes as between pig and human, and the skin graft from one part of an individual to another part of the same individual is called autotransplantation. The site or the individual who gives the transplanted tissue is the donor and the receiver is called the recipient. Sometimes a transplant is placed in the normal position in the body such as a heart transplant being placed in the exact position from where the nonfunctioning heart has been removed. This is called orthotopic transplantation. When the organ is placed in a different position as with a kidney transplant which is placed in the pelvis, it is called heterotopic transplantation.

For centuries people tried to transplant organs without success because the body's immune system rejected the transplanted tissue as foreign. Although the techniques for transplanting organs was well known for many years, the problem of rejection was not understood until the 1940's when Dr. Peter Medawar and others made inroads into the problems of immunological rejection and medications were discovered that would suppress the body's natural tendency towards rejection of foreign tissue. The human lymphocyte was found to be the prime carrier of the immune response and medications at suppressing lymphocyte activity were successful in the 1960's so that kidney transplantation became much more frequent. This was followed by liver, pancreas and in 1967 by heart transplantation by Dr. Christian Barnard in South Africa. The discovery of the drug cyclosporine by Dr. Jean Borel in 1974 radically improved the success of transplantation. Since then tremendous advances have been made in our ability to prevent organ rejection and opened the door to all types of allogeneic organ transplants. The biology of transplantation and the complexities of the human immune response are certainly beyond the scope of this chapter, but it is important that you have a basic understanding of why it was so difficult to take a kidney from A and put it in B.

Because most transplants such as heart, lung, pancreas, kidney and intestine come from "donors" that have died, the tissue is removed when the donor is declared brain dead and the heart is still beating, keeping the organ alive, the availability of donor tissue is limited and frequently doctors have committees to decide who are the appropriate recipients. These transplants are usually reserved for those individuals in whom their own organ has failed, such as with the kidney where the patient can be placed on an artificial kidney while waiting for a transplant or where there is severe disease and the individual is in the last stages of survival. Attempts are made to salvage your own organ before sights are turned towards transplantation. The individual requiring an organ transplant usually has several coexisting problems and the surgery and the post-operative care is very demanding. The complications following these surgeries are rejection, organ failure, infection, and because of the immunosuppression, an increased risk for developing cancer and blood vessel disease. Then you must add to these the usual potential complications of surgery which are exaggerated by the patient's general condition and immunosuppression, such as pulmonary problems like pneumonia, infections and leakage from one of the several anastomoses between blood vessels to attach the organ.

In all, transplantation offers survival for many individuals who in the past faced progressive medical deterioration and death. Like many highly specialized areas of medicine, it should only be done by trained surgeons working with cohesive teams of nurses and support experts in a facility that is operating on the cutting edge of medical and surgical care.

B

Vascular Surgery

Chapter 52
VASCULAR ACCESS

No one ever loved in artery, though many have loved in vain,   And
some have loved with a hot blooded ardor, and some have loved in
pain.
But to love with an artery is to go with the flow,
Love in vein is in vain, cause the flow is so slow.

I'm sorry I started this vascular poem,
I should have just packed up and gone back hoem.

At the outset, let me give you a little background on blood vessel surgery. It started many years ago with the tying off of bleeding arteries, but little advance was made until the twentieth century when vascular anastomosis techniques, connecting one vessel to another using sutures, were perfected. This had to wait until the development of aseptic surgery, anesthesia, and the pioneering work of Dr. Alexis Carrel in the early 1900s, for which he received the Nobel Prize. Surgeons became adept in suturing damaged arteries and connecting arteries together as well as using veins to replace missing or damaged segments of arteries. Later came the development of artificial material which could be used in place of the patient's own artery and from the 1950's onwards there have been steady improvements in this field of surgery.

In this chapter I want to talk about vascular access. This means, basically, getting to the vessel or the blood stream, either for removing blood or blood products or for administering blood, fluids or medications. Giving fluids and medications directly into the blood stream is often the most rapid method of institution of treatment and yet often the veins are not accessible and the physician is asked to find appropriate access sites.

Let us now go through a list of the access sites and by that I mean places to put intravenous (IV) lines.

First, there is the standard IV site used to draw blood or start an IV line. A nurse or technician will usually place a tourniquet around the arm or occasionally the lower leg to dilate the veins. Once a suitable vein has been found, the skin may be anesthetized with a spray such as Cetacaine or local xylocaine injection, cleansed with alcohol, and a needle is inserted into the vein for its purpose. If the vein is missed, punctured through and through or injured, blood may ooze into the surrounding tissue causing pain, and ecchymosis leaving a black and blue mark, but this heals fairly rapidly, usually in a few days. This type of IV is called a peripheral line and is the standard method in most cases. However, when there are no good veins found, because of chronic use, or just small veins, or when an IV will be needed for a long period of time (weeks or longer) other access is needed. The physician can place a peripherally inserted central line called a PICC line in an arm vein with a catheter that extends into a large vein in the chest. This will usually last for a long time and blood can be drawn from this catheter for tests, and fluids and medications can be given. It is a relatively painless procedure when local anesthetics are used.

In patients who need long term IV's and/or who have no peripheral arm or leg veins, a central venous catheter must be placed. These come in many brands, names and sizes, the most common being an Arrow central line for shorter term use and a Hickman or Groshong catheter for longer term usage. These catheters or tubes can be placed into any moderate sized vein, but the most frequently used site is the subclavian vein in the chest. The physician uses a sterile technique, local anesthesia and a specially prepared tray to place these catheters which are inserted through the skin and then under the collar bone, clavicle, into the large subclavian vein. The catheter is then directed into the superior vena cava. A subclavian central line can be placed in the emergency room or at the bedside, but the Groshong and Hickman catheters should be done in the operating room, often with x-ray fluoroscopy. These procedures leave the patient with large IV access and may be important for resuscitation when large amounts of blood, fluids or medications are needed. However, the procedures are not without risk and the complications of pneumothorax or lung collapse requiring placement of a chest tube to re-expand the lung, hemothorax which means blood in the chest which may have to be withdrawn or inability to find a vein are not rare. These lines can also be placed in the jugular vein in the neck or in the femoral vein in the groin. Central lines are often placed by emergency room physicians when treating massive trauma, bleeding or other major illnesses when the peripheral veins have collapsed.

Another type IV access is called a port-A-Cath where a small round port or container attached to a IV catheter is placed in a pocket made under the skin. This eliminates the tubing of a catheter hanging outside the body, but it needs to be accessed with a special needle to withdraw blood or inject fluids. It is basically a question of doctor or patient preference whether there is a port-A-Cath or a Hickman/Groshong Catheter placed.

When a patient has kidney failure, whether transient or permanent, he needs to have hemodialysis. This means he/she is placed on an artificial kidney which rids the blood of toxic agents and breakdown products which would normally be taken care of by the kidney. In order to place the patient on dialysis, the technician must either find large veins in which to stick the two needles needed for this procedure, or have artificial catheters to hook up to. The temporary dialysis catheters are known as Quinton or Tessio Catheters and are inserted much the same as the Hickman or Central line catheters, usually in the subclavian vein. This procedure is more difficult because the catheters are much larger. The complications are the same.

For long term dialysis, a patient can either have a graft placed in the arm or have an artery and vein sewed together, a Cimino Fistula. The graft is usually a synthetic tube placed under the skin in the arm and connected on one end to an artery and on the other to a large arm vein. This procedure can either be done under local or general anesthesia in the operating room. The Cimino fistula is a delicate operation where an artery and vein are sewn together using fine suture material and often the surgeon uses loops or magnifying lenses if the vessels are very small. Because these procedures create an increased (arterial) pressure in the usually low pressured venous system, the veins dilate over a few months and then the patient's veins can be used for inserting the dialysis catheter needle. The complications of graft and fistula are the same as for IV and subclavian central lines; these are infection, bleeding and some new ones - occlusion of the graft with blood clots and causing too much blood flow to the heart or too little blood flow to the arm beyond the fistula called a steal. In the latter cases, the graft or fistula sometimes has to be removed. Grafts and fistulas for dialysis may last for years or may intermittently become occluded with clots and the patient is then either taken back to surgery to declot the graft or has special substances injected into the clot which dissolves it. Removing clot or thrombus from a graft requires an operation under a local anesthetic where the occluded graft is opened and a special catheter called a Foley balloon catheter is inserted. This has an inflatable balloon at the tip which can be blown up after the catheter is inserted past the blockage. By pulling back on the inflated balloon catheter, all the clots are pulled out of the graft. The opening in the graft is then sutured closed and blood flow reinstituted. For vascular techniques, see the next chapter. During these procedures the blood is thinned by giving intravenous blood thinners such as heparin so that new clots won't form while the old ones are being removed.

Should recurrent clotting of the graft occur, the original anastomoses, graft to vessel connections, may have to be examined and occasionally the old graft has to be removed and a new graft inserted.

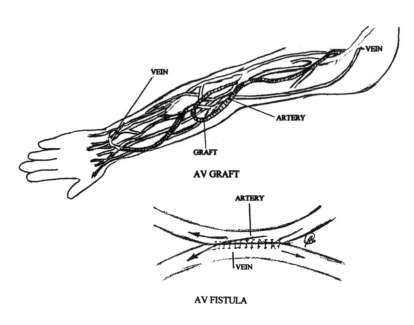

AV GRAFTS AND AV FISTULAS; DIALYSIS ACCESS

DIAGRAM 28

Chapter 53
CAROTID ARTERY SURGERY
AND STENTING

Carotids comes from the Greek word karohtis
If you push them too hard, you may not even notice...
You'll drift off to sleep in a coma or stupor,
And a little bit more and its "adios trooper!"

The carotids are lifelines of blood to the brain,
To keep the cells happy, so they can maintain,
The thoughts that you have, the loves that you cherish;
If you don't keep 'em clean, all your brain cells will perish!

Just a few words about blood vessels in general, then we'll talk more specifically about the carotid arteries. The arteries come from the heart, carrying oxygen-rich blood to the tissues and the veins carry the less oxygenated blood from the tissues back to the heart and the lungs. The arterial system is a high pressure one, and the venous system is low pressure. The arterial system is susceptible to many diseases. Atherosclerosis (athero meaning nodule, sclerosis meaning hard or thickened) is a disease of arteries where there is material laid down in the wall called plaque. This can cause narrowing, or if the plaque is disrupted or dislodged it can flow beyond the area and clog a smaller portion of the artery, essentially shunting off blood flow to that area and causing tissue death. Also, blood clots can form at or around plaques and sometimes the blood clots dislodge and embolize, traveling through the blood stream to other areas and causing tissue ischemia; decreased blood flows mean decreased tissue oxygenation and can lead to tissue death. Nicotine in tobacco apparently has a very strong effect in producing arterial narrowing as do certain diseases such as diabetes mellitus which effects smaller vessels, obesity, and collagen diseases such as lupus erythematosus, periarteritis and Raynaud's disease.

Now when we are talking about the carotid arteries, we are focusing on the two vessels which are the primary suppliers of blood to the brain. The vertebral arteries do supply some but generally the brain cannot survive if both carotid arteries are occluded. And if there is plaque formation with marked narrowing or if there is embolism, the brains cells will be deprived of some oxygen and may not function optimally.

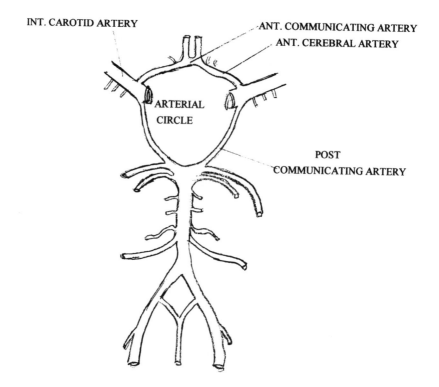

INT. CAROTID ARTERY

ANT. COMMUNICATING ARTERY

ANT. CEREBRAL ARTERY

ARTERIAL CIRCLE

POST COMMUNICATING ARTERY

CAROTID ARTERIES AND CEREBRAL (BRAIN) CIRCULATION

THE CIRCLE OF WILLIS

DIAGRAM 29

As seen in the diagram above, the brain has a network of arteries called the Circle of Willis. It's not always as complete as in the picture, but if it is it means that the blood supply to the brain from one carotid artery may be good enough to take over supplying that part of the brain usually supplied by the other carotid. When an individual does not have an intact Circle of Willis, then occlusion of one carotid may shut off most of the blood to one portion of the brain and that will result in that part of the brain dying, called a stroke. As you can see, this is a complex area involving an in depth understanding of the brain blood supply. The important thing to understand is that when symptoms of decreased blood flow occur, a complete workup must be done and some measures taken to correct the situation before an irreversible stroke occurs.

Arteries may be acutely occluded, immediately blocked, or gradually occluded and the symptoms may be very different. Complete occlusion of an artery is usually a catastrophic event and the organ or tissue supplied by the artery will live or die depending on whether there is collateral circulation, namely other blood vessels supplying the area. We usually speak of the 5 "P's" associated with acute deprivation of arterial blood supply. These are Pain, Paleness, Paralysis, Paresthesia which means change or absence of sensation, and the absence of a Pulse. In the legs this would mean pain in the calves, feet or toes along with the other signs. In the brain, the signs may be loss of consciousness, partial paralysis, blindness or death depending on the extent of the disease and the presence or absence of collateral circulation. Chronic arterial ischemia means gradual onset of signs and symptoms over weeks or even months.

We will talk more about this in Chapter 54, but in connection with the carotid arteries, the symptoms may be very subtle. Physicians use the abbreviations TIA, standing for transient ischemic attack, to denote reversible neurological changes that occur with deprivation or decrease in brain blood flow. These patients may have all the symptoms of a stroke but the symptoms will clear completely, usually within minutes or up to twenty four hours. Next comes a RIND or reversible ischemic neurologic deficit, just a longer lasting TIA taking up to three weeks to resolve. A CVA, cerebrovascular accident, is another word for stroke where many of the deficits such as weakness, paralysis, loss of speech, vision and intellect may not be reversible.

One of the symptoms of a TIA may be amaurosis fugax, a transient loss of vision in one eye; others include aphasia, the inability to talk or understand words, confusion, weakness and paralysis, and a whole host of other neurological signs and symptoms which a neurologist is specially trained to identify. The most important thing is to recognize that something is wrong and see a physician who will make the diagnosis and determine if the cause is related to disease in the carotid arteries.

On his physical exam he may find absent pulsation or weak pulsation in a carotid artery in the neck, or he may hear a bruit which is a noise over the artery. Diagnostic studies will include a Doppler study or duplex ultrasound study, a sound evaluation to determine if there is flow and if so how much flow, and angiography, a special x-ray study done by injecting dye into an artery which will show a picture of the area of disease. The surgeon can then evaluate the problem and decide if surgery is indicated. If he decides on surgery, the procedure is known as carotid endarterectomy.

I will go through the steps in this surgery briefly for you, but remember this is a gross simplification!

1. Under an anesthetic, usually general, but sometimes local, an incision is made obliquely on the involved side of the neck and the carotid sheath is identified containing the carotid artery, the jugular vein and the vagus nerve.
2. The common, internal and external carotid arteries are dissected out and rubber strands are placed around them for mobilization.
3. The patient is given a systemic anticoagulant, heparin, to preventblood clotting in the vessels during the procedure.
4. Clamps are placed on the three vessels.
5. The artery is opened.
6. A shunt or tube is place in the internal carotid artery, the vessel going to the brain, and the common carotid arteries and clamped in place. Then the other vessel clamps are removed from these two vessels to allow blood to once again flow to the brain and leave the operative site bloodless.
7. The plaque is dissected out.
8. The vessel is sewn up most of the way.
9. The vessels are clamped again as the shunt is removed.
10. The remainder of the vessel is sewed up.
11. The clamps are removed restoring blood flow to the brain.
12. The wound, including the skin, is then closed.

This surgery is highly successful in trained hands, but it does have some potential serious complications, the worst of which is a stroke. There may also be bleeding and a re-exploration to control bleeding occurs rarely. Patients are usually sent home in two days.

Currently at my primary hospital, several physicians are doing carotid stenting. This is a procedure where the cardiologist or surgeon places a special catheter into an artery in the groin and from there up into the carotid artery. They then dilate the narrow area and place a special stent or tube in the artery to keep it open. This procedure is still in the investigational stage, only being done in a few centers and will probably eliminate the need for carotid endarterectomy in most cases in the future. If you have carotid disease, you may want to ask your physician whether there is anyone who performs this procedure in your area.

Chapter 54
AORTIC SURGERY
AND ANEURYSMS

When we talk about vessels we think about ships, sailing the seven
seas,
And don't even think about arteries, and how they can be hit by
disease.
But like those ships, the vascular vessels, can't function if there is a
hole,
The seaships will sink and so will the bodies unless all these rents are
made whole.

The aorta's the body's main ship of state, and it's open to many
diseases,
And like an old ship, as we age, it may fail us in as many ways as it
pleases.
The surgeon and shipwright have much work in common repairing the
vessel and sloop,
And both must act quickly before it's too late, or both ships will end
"in the soup".

It's better to fix a damaged ship before rupture can occur,
So careful inspection and attention to details, is the best way to
insure...
That a hole won't work through, and sink the whole crew,
Or if surgeons, won't devastate you.

The aorta is the largest artery in the body and arises from the
heart, arches to the left and then plunges down the back of the
chest and the abdomen until it divides into the smaller iliac
arteries, which in turn continue to divide into progressively
smaller tributaries supplying blood to all the organs. The diagram shows
the three main divisions of the aorta; the arch, the thoracic aorta and the
abdominal aorta.

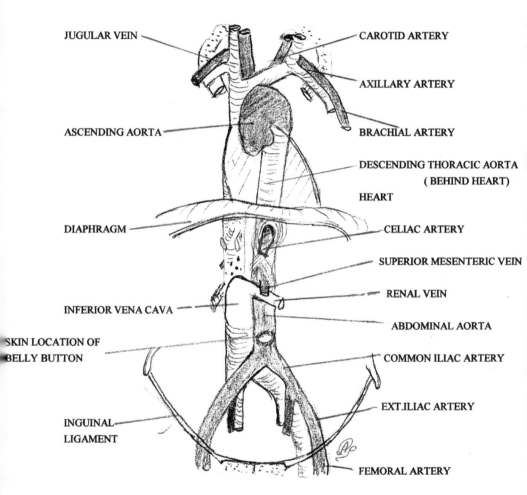

JUGULAR VEIN

CAROTID ARTERY

AXILLARY ARTERY

ASCENDING AORTA

BRACHIAL ARTERY

DESCENDING THORACIC AORTA
(BEHIND HEART)

HEART

DIAPHRAGM

CELIAC ARTERY

SUPERIOR MESENTERIC VEIN

RENAL VEIN

INFERIOR VENA CAVA

ABDOMINAL AORTA

SKIN LOCATION OF
BELLY BUTTON

COMMON ILIAC ARTERY

EXT. ILIAC ARTERY

INGUINAL
LIGAMENT

FEMORAL ARTERY

ANATOMY OF THE AORTA

DIAGRAM 30

The main diseases of the aorta that we will discuss are aneurysm, a localized enlargement or pouching out of the artery, narrowing and occlusion. The usual cause for these diseases are lumped under the category of arteriosclerosis, although there are some other, more esoteric causes such as syphilis, fungus infections, post-operative aneurysms and trauma. The problem with the aneurysm is the risk for rupture leading to almost immediate exsanguinating hemorrhage or bleeding to death. Although the rare patient may survive a ruptured aneurysm, it is much better to operate and repair the disease before this happens. Although over four to six centimeters in diameter has been mentioned as the dangerous size, any aneurysm can be dangerous and rupture.

The symptoms are generally back and abdominal pain and the signs are a pulsating mass in the abdomen when palpated by the physician. Further workup can include an ultrasound or a CAT scan. When the diagnosis is made, a plan of action should be made and if the patient has a moderate sized aneurysm it should be repaired. The pre-operative workup is standard (*see* Chapter 9), but must include monitoring of the heart and preparation to save the blood lost during the procedure using a "cell saver" and then giving the patient back his own blood. The patient needs to be well hydrated prior to the operation which has a two to five percent mortality in the best of hands.

For an abdominal aortic aneurysm, the procedure consists of opening the abdomen or going into the back of the abdomen, a retroperitoneal approach, and placing loops around the aorta proximal and distal to the aneurysm. The patient is anticoagulated and the clamps are placed on the normal vessel above and below the aneurysm. The aneurysm is then opened, the inside debris removed and part of the wall removed. A tube of artificial material, dacron or other synthetic material, is then sewn in place and the clamps are removed to restore blood flow. It sounds simple but can be very complex with many potential complications including bleeding, infection, colon injury, embolism, kidney failure and death.

Thoracic aneurysms are handled similarly in the chest but complications may include damage to the blood supply of the spinal cord resulting in weakness or paralysis, and in general these aneurysms have a higher morbidity and mortality rate. The arch of the aorta is the domain of the cardiac surgeon (*see* section H cardiac surgery).

The other problem of the aorta is disease causing narrowing or occlusion and this is managed by replacing the abdominal aorta in the same way as with an aneurysm. The surgery is less dangerous and many different types and shapes of graft may be used depending on the nature of the disease and surgeon preference. Sometimes the surgeon will replace not only the abdominal aorta, but also the diseased iliac and femoral arteries.

As with the carotid disease, the latest advances in the management of abdominal aortic aneurysm is stenting or placing a tube through the diseased aorta and attaching it above and below with special stapling devices. This can be done by making small incisions in the groin and passing special catheters into the artery through which special stents or tubes can be placed. This is called endovascular surgery and may replace much of the open operative procedures we do today. Whereas the open aortic aneurysm patient will be in the hospital about a week, the endovascular patient may come in one day and go home the next without an abdominal incision. It's certainly the way I would want an aneurysm fixed if I had one! (*see* Chapter 57)

Chapter 55
PERIPHERAL VASCULAR PROCEDURES

At thirty I ran a six minute mile,
At forty I walked the same, with a smile,
At fifty I walked a mile and a half,
And at fifty-five I began to have pain in my calf.

It's called claudication, my specialist said,
From not enough blood in the vascular bed.
Your arteries are clogged, so please stop your yelping,
Your diet and weight, and smoking aren't helping.

It appears that the vessels are not doing well
Some people would say that they've all gone to____.
And now I've a meeting with Dr. McSwain
Who's going to replace all my vessels again.

In this chapter I will focus mainly on the peripheral vessels from the iliac arteries down to the feet, and the arteries in the arm down to the fingers. Arteriosclerosis, diabetes mellitus and several other diseases can effect these vessels and the patients will present with symptoms of intermittent claudication which is cramping with activity which goes away with rest, coldness, pallor, loss of sensation and on to gangrene or death of tissue, i.e. black toes, fingers, or feet (*see* Diagram 31 next page).

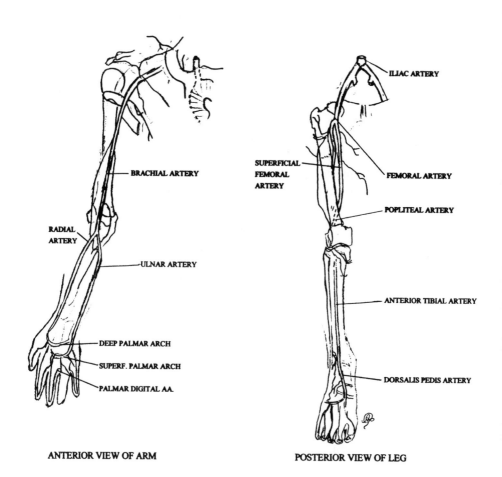

ILIAC ARTERY

BRACHIAL ARTERY

SUPERFICIAL
FEMORAL
ARTERY

FEMORAL ARTERY

POPLITEAL ARTERY

RADIAL
ARTERY

ULNAR ARTERY

ANTERIOR TIBIAL ARTERY

DEEP PALMAR ARCH

SUPERF. PALMAR ARCH

PALMAR DIGITAL AA.

DORSALIS PEDIS ARTERY

ANTERIOR VIEW OF ARM

POSTERIOR VIEW OF LEG

ANATOMY OF THE PERIPHERAL VASCULAR SYSTEM

DIAGRAM 31

Patients are evaluated by Doppler ultrasound and angiography to elucidate the location and extent of the disease. If vessels are narrowed but not completely occluded, they can often be dilated through a tiny puncture wound in the groin; a catheter with an inflatable balloon on the end can sometime dilate a vessel, and sometimes stents can be placed. This procedure is called angioplasty. If angioplasty is not possible, then open surgeries have been devised to bypass the diseased segments of artery using either a vein taken from the patient, usually the leg vein called the saphenous Vein, or using a synthetic graft material such as Dacron or Gore-Tex.

Usually the smaller the vessel the greater probability of it not staying open and clotting off but, this is also influenced by what is called the run-off, namely how good the blood vessels are that are receiving the graft and the new blood supply. If they are poor, there is a greater possibility that the graft won't stay open. What do I mean by this? Whenever we repair arteries or replace them with veins or artificial grafts, one of the main complications is occlusion of the graft. When a graft occludes then the patient's symptoms return immediately and the patient may be taken back to surgery to attempt to declot the graft. Sometimes a special clot dissolving liquid can be injected into the graft and this may successfully open the blockage. Other causes of graft blockage may relate to technical problems at the connection sites or other concurrent disease in the body. Infection is a major problem after vascular surgery and requires high dose antibiotic therapy. If a synthetic graft is used and it becomes infected, it may need to be removed if the antibiotics fail to sterilize the wound.

The worst complication of this type of vascular surgery is failure of the graft and this may result in loss of tissue, loss of toes or even a leg, either below or above the knee. Diabetes mellitus, continued smoking, obesity, high blood pressure and severe arteriosclerosis are usually involved when amputation becomes a necessity. But even after amputation of a leg, there are many prostheses, artificial legs, which can be used and there are many individuals who lead near normal lives with single or even bilateral amputations if they are relatively healthy and motivated.

There are many medications your physician may use to help keep flow in the vessels when there is significant vascular occlusive disease, and these may vary from just using aspirin to anti-thrombogenic agents which prevent clotting, medications that make the blood more slippery and even anticoagulants like coumadin and heparin. The patient with vascular occlusive disease needs to explore the medical, surgical, dietary, physical therapy, and addictive, (i.e. smoking or overeating) modalities to help improve his/her physical condition and lifestyle.

Chapter 56
RENAL ARTERY SURGERY FOR HIGH BLOOD PRESSURE

*Ninety Percent of high blood pressure's Essential
Which means that we don't know the cause or potential,
It can damage the heart, liver, kidneys and brain
And the exact etiology we just can't explain.*

*But for ten percent of hypertension we have the exact cause,
And for this certain doctors deserve our applause.
By improving the flow to the kidney, their contention
Is that this will stop kidney-caused hypertension.*

We know that obesity, smoking, heart disease, pregnancy and birth control pills may cause increased blood pressure; the real cause for 90% of hypertension remains unknown or "essential". Although it seems like a small number, there are about 5-7% of people with hypertension where their elevated blood pressure is due predominantly to a narrowing of the arteries to the kidney called renovascular hypertension. Whereas with essential hypertension we can only treat the signs, namely the elevated blood pressure, by giving complex mixtures of medicine, namely antihypertensives, and diuretics, with renovascular hypertension we can often cure the disease by eliminating the cause. For this reason it is important that your doctor perform the minimal studies which can lead to this diagnosis.

Renovascular hypertension is caused by narrowing of the renal or kidney arteries by arteriosclerosis or a disease called fibromuscular hyperplasia, an abnormality of the tiny muscles in an artery wall which cause constriction of the artery. When the blood flow to the kidney is decreased by this narrowing, the kidney responds by releasing a hormone called renin which in turn causes the release of a substance called angiotensin which in turn causes the blood pressure to rise. In the course of working up a patient with high blood pressure, a serum renin revel is done and if this is elevated then a renal scan and renal angiogram may be indicated.

If the diagnosis is made then there are four choices of therapy. The most radical is done when the kidney has been severely damaged by the renal artery narrowing, and that consists of removing the kidney. This sometimes cures the hypertension. The other methods are angioplasty, opening the narrowed segment of the artery with a balloon dilation and placing a stent via the groin artery, or by open surgery where the renal artery is dissected out and operated upon. Sometimes, with arteriosclerosis, the artery can be endarterectomized, opened, cleaned out and closed, and sometimes the artery can be bypassed by a graft, and the exact connections are up to the surgeon to chose. The open surgery is fairly complex and we are moving more towards endovascular approaches over the next ten years.

Chapter 57
TRAUMA

I always marveled in the movies when the cowboy hero was shot,
That he got right up, bandaged the wound, and hurried off at a trot.
It wasn't so much the internal organs, that they were worried about
Just whether or not that frontier surgeon "got that bullet out".

And the dying man would come to life with energy left to give,
The minute Doc held up his hand and said "I got it out, he'll live!"
Now I hope you're not so very naive to believe this romantic fluff,
In real life we don't care about bullets, we concentrate on "the real
stuff"!

There is basically only one true surgical emergency and that is hemorrhage. Oh sure, absence of respiration and heart beat are emergencies, but I characterize them as medical emergencies. Hemorrhage is the only situation, strictly for the surgeon, when something must be done NOW to stop life threatening bleeding.

I present this chapter on trauma in the vascular section to emphasize that the rapid evaluation of trauma from a surgeon's point of view is to quickly recognize, locate and stem the continued hemorrhage before the patient bleeds to death. The emergency patient usually has the airway secured immediately by the ER physician or paramedic and attention to the heart must be done at the same time. The next area is the surgeon's determining the location of the trauma and how it impacts the arteries and veins in the area.

Venous bleeding is low pressure and unless a very major vein is opened and exposed, the pressure from surrounding tissue and structures will temporarily tamponade the bleeding. Slight pressure over the bleeding site will usually control venous bleeding, even if the vena cava is injured or the jugular vein lacerated. Venous blood is very dark whereas arterial blood is bright red.

Arterial bleeding is much more difficult to stop whether inside or on the surface of the body. Frequently it is almost impossible to hold enough pressure for a long enough time to control the blood loss, and if the bleeding is inside the head, chest or abdomen, time is of the essence. Bleeding in the brain will be discussed in Chapter 78. Bleeding in the chest or abdomen can be evaluated quickly by physical exam and by chest x-ray and CAT scan. With penetrating injuries to the abdomen, as with a knife or gun, or severe blunt trauma as with high falls, and auto accidents, it is important that the ER physician or surgeon evaluate the patient for possible surgical intervention.

When arteries are only partially lacerated, they bleed immediately and usually do stop. However, when an artery is completely transected, cut through and through, the body's normal mechanism for defense takes over and the artery may spasm or close, and the bleeding may stop for a while; this even occurs in major arteries in the arms and legs. In some cases the artery will stay closed long enough for a firm clot to occur which will keep the vessel from rebleeding. But more often with larger vessels, after a few minutes or even an hour the vasoconstriction or spasm of the artery will release and the vessel will open and hemorrhaging start again. After acute trauma there may be transection of a major artery with minimal bleeding initially. This may be deceptive to all but the trained physician; with severe injuries, therefore, evaluation of the blood vessels, sometimes by CAT scan or angiography, is necessary. When the injury is seen, then it can be repaired. The urgency of treatment is part of the art or medicine, where the surgeon must use his experience and judgment to evaluate whether a given injury needs surgical exploration or can just be observed. It is perhaps better to err on the side of exploration than to wait too long and have resultant severe complications. Trauma can also be caused by surgery and a surgeon must always be wary of the potential for catastrophic problems during even the simplest of cases. I recall a case where a surgeon was doing a straight forward laparoscopic appendectomy. Part of the procedure is placing a trocar or sharpened tip tube into the abdomen and then placing a camera through this opening to visualize the abdomen. Inadvertently he placed the tube too far and it went into the retroperitoneum in the back of the abdomen where it transected the right iliac artery. The artery went into spasm and there was no significant bleeding and the injury went unrecognized while he completed the appendectomy uneventfully. Twenty minutes after surgery in the recovery room, the patient showed signs of impending shock with falling blood pressure, rising pulse and pallor. I happened to be there at the time and took him right back to surgery where the transected vessel was now easy to see because it had started to hemorrhage. It was repaired but the patient had many post-operative problems, only recovering completely after months of problems. I only relate this case to you to emphasize that the simplest surgery has the potential for great injury and that each case must be done carefully and never casually. Could this complication and trauma have been avoided? I don't know. It's always easy to criticize through the retro-spectoscope which means looking back after the thing has been done, but the recognition of the injury in the recovery room and its immediate treatment are the most important lesson to learn.

The patient with a gunshot or stab wound to the thigh may seem stable but if a vascular evaluation is not done, a severe injury could be missed which could cost the individual his leg a few hours or days "down the road".

The whole field of trauma medicine and the management of vascular injuries is way beyond the scope of this chapter, but I just wanted to emphasize that it's easy to recognize the injury when blood is spurting or the patient is going into shock with falling blood pressure, rising pulse, increasing respiratory rate, decreasing urine output, and progressive confusion, but it is difficult to identify the arterial or venous injury in the apparently stable patient. If the skin and muscle wounds are closed and the broken bones repaired, but the vascular injury goes unrecognized, the overall prognosis may be very poor.

The vascular surgeon has had extensive training in trauma and knows all the techniques of repairing blood vessels, bypasses and grafting, and most of all, he has a high index of suspicion for injuries to your arteries and veins.

Chapter 58
ENDOVASCULAR SURGERY

Endovascular surgery may be the end of vascular surgery,
All that may be left is a few memories and some liturgy.
Pretty soon the surgeons will have a new but familiar toy,
Which goes beep when you hold it against the skin, like Star Trek's
Dr. McCoy.

No fields have had so many radical recent advances as vascular and cardiovascular surgery. The progress has been shifting from open surgical procedures for the correction of partially or totally blocked arteries to procedures which accomplish essentially the same results without major open operations. This new area is called endovascular surgery and is being done by vascular surgeons and invasive cardiologists and radiologists. In most major centers these procedures are being taught or learned by physicians to make the correction of patient's pathology much simpler for the patient and the doctor.

Invasive, open procedures such as peripheral vascular repair, carotid artery repair, open heart surgery and aortic aneurysm repair involve major operations with significant potential complications and several day hospital stays. The new procedures appear to offer less morbidity and shorter hospitalization and for those patients where the procedure cannot be done or where it is unsuccessful, the old tried and true open procedures are still available.

Why aren't these procedures done routinely? Basically many of these procedures are still in the investigative stage with certain centers participating in the studies. Although the early results look promising, most of us like to see long-term results comparing the old methods with the new.

In some areas, such as coronary artery dilation and stenting and peripheral vascular stenting, the clinical trials have been completed whereas with other types of endovascular procedures, the data is still being collected. Another area of advancement is in the mechanical equipment which is being produced for this type of surgery; it changes from month to month getting better and better with each new improvement. Some physicians want to wait until the technical advances are better before trying the new procedures.

What exactly is endovascular surgery? It is a way of getting to a blood vessel without a large incision, open operation. Usually a small incision is made in the femoral artery (groin) and a wire is placed into the artery. Under fluoroscopy the wire can be placed in just about any small, medium or large artery in the body. Over this wire many different apparatuses can be passed. Some are special catheters with inflatable balloons on the end which can be used to dilate partially occluded vessels; this is called percutaneous balloon angioplasty, or PTA, percutaneous transluminal angioplasty. There are also special lasers and roto-rooter type instruments to clean out vessels and when the vessel is dilated and cleaned, rigid tubes can be placed in the vessel to assure that it stays open. This is routinely being done in coronary arteries, and as I have mentioned, in my primary hospital it has been done in a long term clinical trial on carotid artery disease for a long time.

Aneurysms are being excluded by an endovascular technique which passes a wire through the diseased segment followed by a tube graft. When the graft is deployed and put in place it is secured by special stapling devices at both ends.

For previously complex procedures such as renal artery stenosis or mesenteric artery stenosis where a vessel to the intestine is narrowed and can cause severe cramping pain after eating, the endovascular surgeon dilates the narrowed segment and sometimes places a stent to keep it open. There are vascular endoscopes, little cameras which can be placed inside a blood vessel to evaluate its condition, which can monitor the success of these new procedures. The complications include bleeding, damage to the artery during the procedure, embolism from the artery or knocking off material and plaques which may block smaller arteries downstream, and inability to do the procedure for anatomical or technical reasons. As more procedures are done, the complication rate will fall, as with any new procedure.

I am sure that in the next few years, as the long term results are accumulated, more physicians will be switching to the endovascular approaches, and I know that the patients will appreciate this much more than the old open procedures.

Chapter 59
VEINS - VARICOSE VEINS, ULCERS, PHLEBITIS

You ever see the muscle-bound guys,
With veins in their arms to pop your eyes?
Well, some got veins in other places
And are looked at with less than smiling faces!

To those of you with aches and pains,
With painful sores and varicose veins,
We offer a cure for all these "goblins",
By stripping your veins, and solving the problems.

For this discussion we shall focus on the veins in the lower extremities. As we have mentioned in a previous chapter, the venous system is the low pressure system which brings poorly oxygenated blood back to the heart and to the lungs to be re-oxygenated. Because the blood flows towards the lungs, debris or clots in the veins can be swept into the lungs causing a pulmonary embolism. We will describe the anatomy of the veins and some of the more common and serious diseases and how they are treated.

The leg veins are classified as the deep, the superficial and the perforators as shown in the diagram. The deep system is the largest, draining the major portion of blood from the leg. These veins are very large and if blood clots occur in these veins and then get loose and travel to the lungs, the effect can be serious to catastrophic. The superficial veins, primarily called the greater saphenous vein on the inner side of the leg and the lesser saphenous on the outer side of the leg are much smaller and although they may be subject to phlebitis or inflammation, it is rare that the clots are large enough to cause major embolic problems, but they do cause pain and aching. The perforating veins connect the superficial system with the deep system. The veins have V-shaped valves which allow blood to flow upward, but not back down the leg, and to flow from

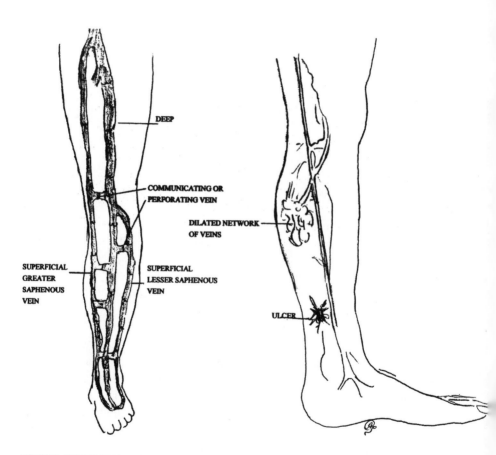

NORMAL ANATOMY OF LEG VEINS · PATHOLOGY IN LEG VEINS

NORMAL AND PATHOLOGIC ANATOMY OF LEG VEINS

DIAGRAM 32

the superficial to the deep system. Without getting more complicated, I will mention that there are several named perforators, Cockett's, Boyd's, and Hunterian, which should keep blood flowing in the correct direction.

When the valves are damaged from too much back pressure or infection, then the superficial veins dilate and you see the serpentine, large, ropy varicose veins that are so unsightly and often cause an aching and tired feeling in the lower extremities. These veins are often found to be familial with a genetic propensity in certain families, influenced by increased back pressure on the veins caused by a pregnancy or obesity, estrogen or certain other medications and several more obscure causes we need not elucidate. To prevent these occurrences, many physicians recommend wearing support hose during pregnancy and in overweight individuals.

The diagnosis of venous insufficiency or valve trouble, is made with several clinical examination tests which your surgeon may perform, called the Perthes and Trendelenburg tests, and the exact nature and cause of the varicose veins can be determined. Doppler sound studies and venograms of the legs can also be done to clarify the situation. Frequently these can be managed by conservative care such as wrapping and support hose or sometimes by injection of small veins with a sclerosing solution, a liquid which makes the veins collapse. For the larger veins and the incompetent perforating veins, the surgery is more major. The perforators are located and tied off and the greater and lesser saphenous veins may be stripped out, a somewhat barbaric appearing procedure where a small incision is made near the ankle and by the knee or the groin to find the veins. A plastic or metal tube is then passed up the vein and tied at both ends. The vein is cut and then pulled or stripped out of the leg while the leg is being tightly wrapped so that the torn branches will not bleed and will eventually seal off. It's a procedure better suited for the Spanish Inquisition than the operating room, but the results are usually excellent. If a patient delays having serious varicose veins treated, there may develop skin inflammation and infection, purplish discoloration and eventual skin breakdown and ulcerations which are often chronic and difficult to treat. They often respond to surgical removal of the offending veins but frequently get worse after the surgery before they get better. A relatively good non-surgical approach is the use of a special medicated wrap called an Unna Boot which will heal the ulcer in anticipation of definitive surgery or for those patients who are too sick to have surgery.

In patients with several areas of enlarged veins, tiny punctures can be made and the veins pulled out, literally avulsed; the incisions are only 1-2 millimeters and leave minimal scarring.

Varicose vein injections can be done in the office, but ligations and stripping are done as an outpatient procedure in the operating room. The postoperative patient has some discomfort and usually cannot return to work for several days depending on the severity of the disease.

In patients with severe ulcerations secondary to varicose vein disease and venous insufficiency, it is sometimes necessary to do skin grafting to the area of the ulcer after the offending veins have been removed.

Let us now move on to the deep system of veins. There are two major problems, the first being chronic venous insufficiency or chronic backflow into the big veins because of destroyed valves in the largest veins and this may cause a chronic swelling of the legs that is very difficult to manage. Elevation, bedrest and treatment of the skin problems and ulcerations are necessary and often the perforating veins have to be ligated to prevent the skin from breaking down. When ulcers occur they are very difficult to manage and surgery on the incompetent valves in the large veins is not very successful. Fortunately, deep venous insufficiency is not too common and most of what the surgeon sees today are superficial venous insufficiencies.

The second and most major complication with the deep venous system is deep vein thrombosis. Blood clots may occur in the leg veins or even in the large veins in the abdomen, the iliac veins and vena cava, and may be associated with coagulation or clotting problems, malignancy, pregnancy and oral contraceptives and conditions where there is slow flow in the veins or where the blood is thicker and more prone to clotting.

The signs of thrombosis are swelling and aching of the foot and leg, and the severity of the symptoms may relate to the level and severity of the thrombosis. Clots low in the leg may cause swelling at the ankle and foot; clots in the thigh veins will cause more swelling and pain and tenderness of the entire leg. The diagnosis once suspected must be confirmed by Doppler sound studies and/or venography and treatment started immediately to prevent pulmonary embolism and possible death. This consists of anticoagulation, elevation of the leg and bedrest for several days. The usual anticoagulant is heparin which is converted to the pill coumadin when patients are ready to go home. They stay on coumadin for several months.

In anticipation of this severe problem, most surgeons provide some prophylaxis for their patients to prevent thrombus formation in high risk situations. This includes special compression stockings, special cuffs and booties with sequential pressure to be sure that blood flow is good in the legs; in many situations, low dose anticoagulation is used. Patients with high risk are individuals with a history of thrombophlebitis, obesity, malignancy, orthopedic procedures on the legs and knees, multiple trauma patients, and the elderly.

Treatment of deep vein thrombosis may become surgical if the occlusion is so severe that there is risk of losing the leg. In these cases surgery is done to remove clots. In some cases where anticoagulation is unsuccessful in preventing pulmonary emboli or where anticoagulation is contraindicated such as multiple trauma or brain injury where anticoagulation would cause fatal bleeding, treatment measures are focused upon preventing the clot from getting to the lungs. To prevent pulmonary embolism, surgeons or interventional radiologists or cardiologists will place a filter in the vena cava in the abdomen to catch any blood clots that break loose and head for the lungs. These blood clots, once trapped by the filter, will be dissolved in time by the body's own anticoagulation system. Some filters are placed through open operations (The Adams--DeWeese and Miles vena cava filters) and one, called the Greenfield Filter can be put in place by a radiologist or cardiologist through a small incision in the neck.

The thing is to be aware of the signs and symptoms of phlebitis, whether superficial or deep, and to let your doctor know immediately before you develop a pulmonary embolism. To reiterate, the signs are pain and aching in the leg, especially the calf, swelling or redness of the leg, and the most serious sign being that of pulmonary embolism: chest pain, shortness or breath, and occasionally coughing up blood.

Of note is that in certain severe cases of massive pulmonary embolism unresponsive to blood thinners, a heart surgeon may actually do an open heart procedure and remove the blood clots from the vessels in the lung. It is a very dangerous and infrequently successful last ditch type procedure.

I think that the greatest hope we have to saving many patients from pulmonary embolism is education. If the patient is alert and can notice the signs and symptoms and relay these to the nurse or physician, then appropriate therapy can be started and lives saved.

C

UROLOGIC SURGERY

Chapter 60
CATHETERS - FOLEY, URETERAL, SUPRAPUBIC, NEPHROSTOMY TUBES

Whether it's kidneys or your bladder,
These docs know just what's the matter.
They will probe your private-most parts
While doing their urological arts.

With no urine, yer in trouble,
Needing their help on the double.
I've never seen a fella sadder,
Than after rupturing his bladder!

In this section we will look into the specialty called Urology, giving a basic introduction to the field and the major problems encountered and managed by these specialists. It is best to start by giving you a brief course in urological anatomy. As seen in the diagram, the blood flows through the renal arteries to the kidneys where waste products are filtered through a complex system of tubes, the glomeruli and collecting systems, excreting urine into the kidney pelvis. From there it flows down the ureters to the bladder where it is collected until the individual urinates through the urethra. In the male the testicles contain seminiferous tubules that produce sperm cells which migrate to the epididymis for storage. They then pass through the ductus deferens through the prostate to the urethra where they exit during ejaculation. Each structure we have mentioned is an organ in its own right and can have a complexity of pathology. After discussing various "tubes" in this chapter, we will have separate chapters to cover the problems found with the kidneys, ureters, bladder, prostate, penis and testicles.

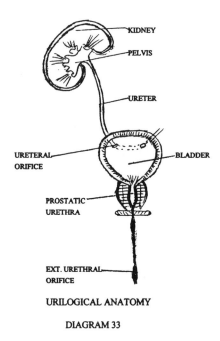

URILOGICAL ANATOMY

DIAGRAM 33

Most of you have some familiarity with the Foley catheter. This is a hollow rubber tube with an inflatable balloon on the end which can be placed through the male or female urethra into the bladder. The balloon is then insufflated with water and the catheter acts to drain urine from the bladder into a bag. This is used in patients who are unable to urinate who are in acute urinary retention because of trauma, recent anesthesia and surgery, diminished conscious states, and prostate enlargement or infection. There may be what is called a neurogenic bladder which is a malfunction of the bladder muscles because of nerve malfunction, and this may indicate spinal cord disease. Other causes of retention include spinal anesthesia, certain drugs effecting the bladder nerves, and even cancer. Often after pelvic or even inguinal hernia surgeries a patient may need to have a Foley catheter inserted for a few days until there is return of normal bladder function. Sometimes, an individual with incontinence which means involuntary loss of urine, may have an indwelling catheter for hygienic or social reasons, or may have what is called a condom catheter which is placed over the penis as a condom rather than inserted into the bladder. It must be remembered that anything inserted into a body cavity, no matter how sterilely it is inserted, always carries the risk of infection and this is true with Foley catheters if they are left in too long; there is always the risk of urinary tract infection, so the physician tries to get that catheter out as soon as possible. In cases of prostate enlargement or tumor, the underlying problem must be alleviated before the catheter can be removed.

Ureteral catheters are placed in the ureters. They are tiny wire-like hollow tubes that are placed in the ureters through the urethra and bladder while a patient is asleep. They are used to help surgeons identify the ureters during surgery or to act as a stent or a firm rod to maintain stability when a ureter is repaired after injury. When the ureter is partially or totally blocked by an infectious process or a tumor, a catheter may be able to be passed through the obstruction as a temporizing measure until the obstruction is relieved. These catheters exit the body through the urethra and are connected to their own special bag. Removing them is simple - the physician or nurse just painlessly pulls them out!

A suprapubic catheter is placed into the bladder during surgery by passing a tube through the skin and deeper tissues in the midline just above the pubic region. This tube is placed when a Foley catheter cannot be passed through the urethra either because of prostate enlargement, trauma or tumor. It too is usually a temporary tube until the causative problem is alleviated, but for some very sick people, a permanent indwelling suprapubic tube is left in place. To prevent infection, patients with tubes need to be on antibiotic coverage.

Finally, let's discuss the nephrostomy tube. It is placed when the patient is asleep or under a local anesthetic in the operating room, and is inserted through an incision in the flank or occasionally percutaneously by a radiologist, directly into the kidney pelvis to drain off urine. It is usually done for severe infection or tumor where the ureter or bladder is not functioning or obstructed. In some cases of extensive stone formation in the kidney with obstruction of the ureter, the nephrostomy tube is placed so that the stones or a large stag horn calculus, can be broken up by ultrasound and removed through the nephrostomy tube. Most urologists rarely use the nephrostomy tube, but it is available, if needed, in ureteral injuries where an immediate repair is not possible and where the surgeon feels that in several weeks the ureter may heal or be more amenable to direct repair.

Chapter 61
THE PROSTATE

The prostate is why men over fifty,
Stand at urinals looking quite shifty,
While younger men just come and go,
Their urine trickles...oh so slow.

If you're a beer or soft drink guzzler,
Or a wizened crossword puzzler,
You could have the urinal blues,
And leave some dribbles on your shoes.

The prostate gland is always described in texts and the encyclopedias as a chestnut-shaped reproductive organ. This organ in the adult male wraps around the proximal or first part of the urethra and is richly supplied by nerves, arteries and veins. It is responsible for much of the secretions added to the sperm during ejaculation; semen equals secretions plus sperm. The gland is examined by the physician with the patient bending over a table while the examiner does a gentle rectal exam. Although the size of the prostate is difficult to evaluate this way (ultrasound is much more accurate), the consistency of the gland can be evaluated. A normal prostate is firm but not hard, as is the enlarged but non-cancerous gland. The gland with cancer is usually very hard and nodular. However, small cancers of the prostate can be missed on exam.

The semen can be examined after a man has been abstinent for 48 hours and is obtained and evaluated. There is usually about 3-5 cc of fluid and more than 20 million spermatozoa in each cc. More than half should be moving and appear normal in shape. This study and many others are performed in the course of an infertility workup. Inflammation of the prostate, prostatitis, is usually bacterial and not a surgical problem. It presents with pain on urination called dysuria, bloody urine called hematuria, urgency, perineal pain, located behind the scrotum and can progress to fever, chills and severe systemic infection. It responds to appropriate antibiotic treatment.

Now let's move on to what we discussed in the poem. Many men over fifty begin to have what is called hyperplastic growth of the prostate gland. This is a benign process called benign prostatic hypertrophy. More than 90% of men have this disease by age eighty. When the prostate enlarges it may grow in a way that doesn't block the urinary flow or it may cause obstructive symptoms very early. The patient will notice a weaker urinary stream, a need to urinate more frequently which is known as frequency, a feeling of not emptying the bladder, and urgency which is a sense that you need to go right now, usually due to an increase in bladder pressure from urinary backup; incomplete urination may be due to partial obstruction, nocturia or urinating several times at night (although this can occur with excess fluid intake), slow starting and hesitancy at starting urination. Chronic partial obstruction can lead to bladder distention, stone formation in the bladder and eventual kidney failure.

The workup for this disease, aside from the digital rectal exam and the history, includes studies to rule out cancer, infection, or stones. The urologist has to be aware that the patient can have more than one problem going on; he may have benign prostatic hypertrophy, BPH, as well as infection, cancer, etc. The laboratory test PSA is routinely performed since high levels may indicate prostate cancer.

The treatment depends on the extent of the disease and the symptomatology. There is a scoring index put out by the American Urological Association, the AUA, which rates the various symptoms from 0-5. They are a measure of the amount of flow reduction, urgency, nocturia, straining and hesitancy. The treatment of asymptomatic or minimally symptomatic BPH is just observation. Moderate to severely symptomatic patients may initially be treated medically and if unsuccessful will need some surgical intervention.

The medical management is basically twofold, the first by a medication that relaxes the muscle in the prostate, partially relieving the obstruction, such as the alpha adrenergic blocker drugs terazosin and doxazosin, and another medication which actually shrinks the prostate up to 20 or 25% over several months, a 5 alpha reductase inhibitor called finasteride.

For those patients unresponsive to medical management or with such severe BPH that kidney function is threatened or impaired, there are several options. The most common is the transurethral resection of the prostate, TURP, done under general or regional anesthesia. The urologist places a special lighted tube in the bladder, a modified cystoscope or resectoscope and removes prostate tissue with a cautery loop device. The morbidity is very low and some of the complications include bleeding, infection and retention. Over several months a few patients may become impotent with loss of the ability to have an erection, incontinent or develop more narrowing requiring repeat surgery.

Another procedure is the transurethral incision of the prostate, TUIP, where incisions are made in the capsule of the prostate to allow it to expand posteriorly and reduce the obstructive symptoms and with fewer complications. For patients with huge prostates, an open prostatectomy is required which is performed through a low mid abdominal incision and prostatic tissue is removed from an incision in the prostate or an incision through the bladder coming right down on the prostate. The complications are about the same as for TURP, but remember that in the last few years new drugs have been developed such as Viagra which help to lessen the significance and incidence of impotence after treatment for BPH.

Other procedures include balloon dilation of the urethra at the prostate site, transurethral needle ablation, TUNA, and transurethral microwave thermal therapy, TUMT, all of which are minimally invasive but of questionable long term effectiveness.

Let us now turn to cancer of the prostate, which accounts for almost 10% of cancer deaths in men. We don't know the cause for this cancer but the incidence increases with age. About 30% have it at age 60 and upwards of 75% in 90 year old men - a common disease! The tests include digital rectal exam and the serum blood test PSA. Ultrasound of the prostate in suspicious cases can lead to needle biopsy by the urologist which will confirm the diagnosis. Elevation of the blood test acid phosphatase suggests prostate cancer, and elevated alkaline phosphatase suggests bony metastases.

For cancer contained to the gland itself, radical prostatectomy is often the best mode of treatment. Whereas in the past all patients would have impotence, urologists have now developed nerve sparing procedures which leave most patients continent and two thirds potent. Some physicians may recommend radiation therapy or medical therapy in patients who cannot or will not have surgery. This consists of estrogen or other therapy to reduce the male hormone androgen levels. In some cases the testicles are removed in a procedure called an orchiectomy. PSA blood levels are often followed and elevation after they have been down after surgery may indicate recurrent disease.

In advanced prostate cancer, patients may have large cancers fixed in the pelvis as well as metastatic spread to bone and lungs. In most cases their PSA levels are elevated as are the acid and alkaline phosphatase. The treatment is to reduce or eliminate the male hormone, androgen, with drugs and/or orchiectomy. Treatment of symptomatic metastases with radiation therapy is often successful. Several different medical centers are experimenting with other modes of therapy which may become available in the next few years including gene therapy and new chemotherapeutic agents. Surgery is only indicated when obstructive symptoms cannot be relieved in any other way.

Chapter 62
THE BLADDER

Micturition is the word that defines the excretion of fluid called urine.
And it is not the thing you discuss with your boss or in columns by
Abby Van Buren.
To empty your bladder you need nerves and muscles, the latter is
called the detrusor,
And if you attempt to explain this to mom, you're probably going to
confuse her.

The bladder is only a muscular sac that fills up and stores urine
gradually,
And if you have problems, like blockage or bleeding, you need a
urologist quite badually.
This can be a sign of a prostatic problem but that is not always the
answer,
'Cause sometimes the bleeding is caused by infection, a stone or even
a cancer.

The bladder is a muscular sac designed for the storage of urine. It has many arteries, veins and nerves, the latter of which cause its muscle, the detrusor, to constrict when the bladder is full in a complex series of messages between the brain and the bladder which may be partially conscious and partially unconscious. In individuals with neurological deficits such as brain or spinal cord disease or intrinsic bladder injuries, the coordinated contractions of the bladder, along with relaxation of the urethral muscle will not occur and incontinence and poor bladder control will result.

The anatomy of the bladder is shown to help you understand the pathology and surgery of the organ.

Incontinence is the involuntary loss of urine from the bladder and is associated with the above mentioned neurogenic problems and may result in men after prostate surgery or in women who are post menopausal or post partum because of relaxation of the pelvic floor; this is called stress

MALE FRONTAL SECTION

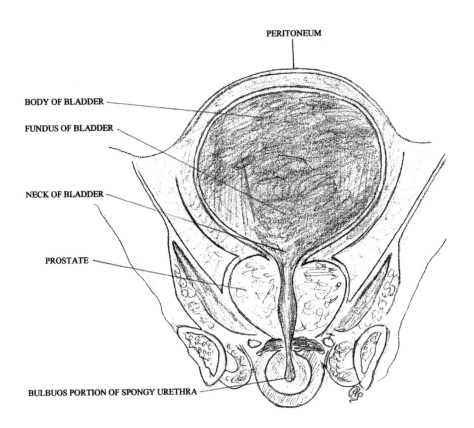

PERITONEUM

BODY OF BLADDER

FUNDUS OF BLADDER

NECK OF BLADDER

PROSTATE

BULBUOS PORTION OF SPONGY URETHRA

ANATOMY OF THE BLADDER

DIAGRAM 34

incontinence where coughing or lifting will cause leakage of urine. Infection and cancer may also cause urge incontinence which causes leakage with the first sensation of need to urinate. Incontinence is a whole field in itself and I just want to describe it to you briefly. It is managed by treatment of the underlying cause, catheter insertion, an external garment such as Depends or sometimes can be surgically corrected if the problem is related to the pelvic floor. The urologist or gynecologist can perform what is called an anterior repair which strengthens the floor and helps correct the incontinence.

Inflammation of the bladder, cystitis, is diagnosed by urinalysis and is treated with antibiotics; however, the etiology for the infection must be established and causes such as prostatitis, obstruction, tumor and kidney infection must be ruled out or treated.

Cancer of the bladder accounts for about 2-3% of cancer deaths and has been related to cigarette smoking, stones in the bladder and exposure to certain industrial chemicals. Most patients present with microscopic hematuria where there is blood in the urine which can't be seen but is detected on urine studies and can be diagnosed by examining cells in the urine and by a bladder x-ray called an excretory urogram or cystogram, and by a cystoscopic exam using a lighted tube placed through the urethra. A biopsy can also be done at this time. Further studies such as MRI, CAT scans, and chest x-rays are done to stage the cancer and help determine the best course of therapy. The depth of invasion into the bladder wall determines the staging along with the predicted long term survival, with Dr. Donald Skinner, one of the world experts in urological disease at USC having some of the best survival rates. The diagrams shows the staging of the disease (*see* Diagram 35 next page).

The superficial bladder cancers can be resected by the urologist using a cystoscope and special instruments that remove and cauterize the area of the tumor. Anti-cancer agents such as thiotepa, Adriamycin and mitomycin are placed in the bladder to prevent recurrence; however, these patients have to be watched carefully for recurrence of disease.

The treatment of more advanced bladder cancer is cystectomy which means removal of the bladder, and reconstruction can be accomplished in several ways, depending on the location and extent of the tumor. Some cancers require such extensive surgery that a bladder reconstruction using a loop of intestine, either colon or small intestine, is not possible. These patients have their ureters attached to a pouch made out of intestine which is attached to the skin as an ostomy, and drained at intervals or with a continuous bag attached to the ostomy.

In patients with advanced bladder cancer, a diverting tube such as a suprapubic cystostomy or nephrostomy are rarely needed.

The important message is to have a regular checkup including urinalysis so that any malignancy in the bladder can be found early when simple transurethral resection is possible.

REGION OF BLADDER WALL AFFECTED

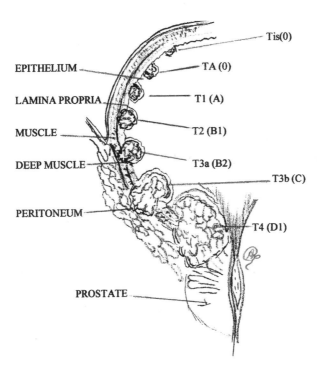

STAGING FOR BLADDER CANCER

DIAGRAM 35

Chapter 63
KIDNEY AND STONES

Why in the world are some organs double?
Twice the advantages but twice the trouble.
We don't have two hearts, to ache and attack us,
And only one brain (could we use two to wrack us?)

But certain things come in plural, namely two
The first one for us and the second for who?
The couplets are ovary, testes and kidney,
It's quite esoteric. (Are you still staying wid me?)

There's eyes and ears, arms, legs to be seen...
But only one nose and liver and spleen.
It would be much better if all organs paired,
Then if you lost one we'd act like----who cared?

If I'm ever asked by the Old Guy, (you know who),
I'll tell him that hearts and brains should be two.
But till then we're stuck with our double friend kidney.
God did what He wanted and didn't tell, didney.

The kidneys are kidney bean shaped! The two kidneys are retroperitoneal, lying in the abdomen behind the peritoneum, surrounded by fat and then by a strong tissue called Gerota's fascia. They lie on each side of the back of the abdomen partially under the rib cage under the diaphragm and near the colon. On top of the glands are the suprarenal glands or adrenal glands.

There are variable numbers of arteries and veins and many nerves. As in the diagram, there is a cortex, a medulla and a pelvis, the latter narrowing into the upper end of the ureter. We have discussed renal hypertension due to renal arterial stenosis. The right kidney is near the liver and the left kidney is near the spleen, stomach and pancreas.

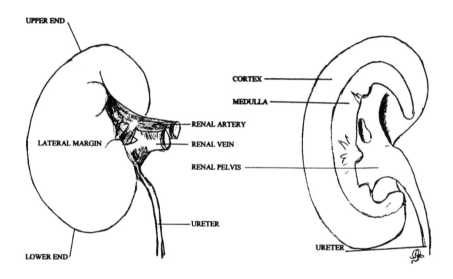

ANATOMY OF THE KIDNEYS

DIAGRAM 36

The examination of the kidneys is by observation, to see if one flank is larger than the other and by palpation, examining with the fingers, just below the rib cage on both side posteriorly and laterally. Gentle or firm tapping on the lower ribs may elicit pain if there are stones, inflammation or a tumor in the kidneys. The best studies for evaluation are urinalysis, blood urea nitrogen, BUN, and creatinine, and a several hour study called the glomerular filtration rate, GFR, which measures kidney function. X-rays of the kidneys include an intravenous pyelogram or IVP which is an intravenous dye study showing the kidney function; the dye travels through the blood and is concentrated in and excreted by the kidneys. Other studies are ultrasound, nuclear scans of the kidney to determine function, and CAT or MRI scans of the abdomen focusing on the kidney. When tumors are suspected, arteriograms may be helpful prior to surgery. As you can see there are many studies from which the urologist can choose in making his diagnosis. When trauma is present a CAT scan will delineate the degree of injury and determine whether operative intervention is indicated.

Infections of the kidney, pyelonephritis, can vary from very mild to severe, and surgery is not indicated unless an abscess develops in or around the kidney, a perinephric abscess, which needs to be drained. In severe infections where the kidney is destroyed or with extreme destruction as from tuberculosis the kidney may even need to be removed.

When a patient has a urinary tract infection in the bladder, the bacteria may travel up the ureters into the kidney and the most common organism is one called E. Coli. This can cause shaking chills, high fever and even a shock-like syndrome with falling blood pressure and increasing pulse. This is not a surgical condition and usually responds to vigorous broad spectrum antibiotic treatment.

One condition I will just mention is called papillary necrosis or destruction of part of the kidney; it has many causes including diabetes mellitus, certain drugs, and sickle cell disease. Sometimes the patient has renal failure and must be kept alive using the artificial kidney or dialysis machine, but in time the renal papillae will regrow and the patient will recover from the kidney failure.

Next let us discuss one of the most common urologic disorders: Nephrolithiasis or kidney stones. They form when calcium compounds or some other stone causing substances such as cystine or uric acid accumulate in the kidney. These may drop down into the ureter causing obstruction. The common characteristic is intermittent severe pain lasting several minutes called renal colic. The location of the pain may be in the flank or the abdomen depending where the stone is lodged.

Diagnosis of kidney stones can be made on simple abdominal x-ray or on an IVP. If the stones are small they may pass down the ureter into the bladder and then be excreted into the urine. Primary treatment consists of pain management and antibiotics, and the patient's response to these measures will determine whether hospital admission is indicated. Most stones will pass; if not, then the stones can be broken up by shock wave treatment called lithotripsy, after which they may pass. Large stones may have to be extracted from below by the urologist using a cystoscope and special baskets-like instruments. In severe cases percutaneous nephrostoli-thotomy is performed, which consists of placing a large tube through the skin into the kidney pelvis under anesthesia and introducing lasers or shock waves to break up large stones and extract them through the nephrostomy opening.

After stones have passed or been removed or after the acute episode has passed, the patient is instructed on the appropriate diet to help prevent future kidney stones. This can be a very complex process involving a careful dietary history and recommendations along with medications that help prevent stone formation. Some diets make the urine more acid, some more alkaline depending on the underlying cause of the stones. The causes are multiple and beyond the scope of this chapter but must be evaluated by the urologist and the dietician in each case individually.

Cancer of the kidney accounts for about 2-3% of cancer deaths in the United States, and is more frequent in men. There are three types, one predominately found in children, the Wilms' tumor and two in adults; renal cell carcinoma accounts for most of the malignancies and sarcomas account for only a small percent.

There is a classic triad of symptoms for cancer of the kidney: hematuria or bloody urine, pain and the presence of a mass. Although these are commonly present, a significant number of renal cancers are found when a CAT scan of the abdomen is done for some other reason and this finding is incidental. Once there is suggestion of a tumor, further workup may include an MRI and even an x-ray of the vena cava which may show whether the tumor has invaded this structure. Because of these diagnostic methods, only a few renal cancers have already spread beyond the kidney at the time of diagnosis.

The preoperative workup is standard as in Chapter 9. For some small kidney cancers or when there is only one kidney, sometimes a partial nephrectomy is acceptable. However, for most renal cancers, the preferred surgery is the radical nephrectomy which means the removal of the kidney and adrenal together; they are intimately attached and couldn't be separated without compromising the extent of the cancer operation. In addition, the surgeon also removes the lymph nodes, perinephric fat and Gerota's fascia. If the vena cava is involved a wider resection including the vein will be done with the assistance of a vascular surgeon. The kidney for these operations can be approached through the abdomen to have better access to the great vessels or through a flank incision. For large tumors a surgeon can use a thoraco-abdominal incision which means cutting into the abdomen and chest to have a good approach to the cancer and its surrounding tissues. With kidney tumors, there is a TNM staging system as in other malignancies which will guide the urologist in knowing the prognosis, and with kidney tumors the staging is based on the anatomical location of the spread. Because of the early incidental diagnosis of almost 75% of kidney tumors, the survival rate is almost 70% and with low grade the cure rate is almost 100%. Even with distant metastases in kidney cancer, some surgeons feel that after the removal of the primary tumor, the metastases sometimes get smaller or don't grow as fast as usual. The medical oncologists feel that chemotherapy has little to add to the treatment.

We will discuss cancers of the renal pelvis along with the ureter in the next chapter.

Chapter 64
URETERS AND STONES

When papa starts his moans and groans
He isn't dying, it's kidney stones.
They've lodged in the ureter causing pain
So he'll have to go to the ER again.

The stones are collected in the john in a sieve
With an agony very few patients forgive.
So watch your diet that I hope you have learned,
Cause your body will never leave one stone unturned.

The ureters are muscular tubes that go from the kidney pelvis to the bladder. Surgeons have to know their exact location in the retroperitoneum so that they are not injured during major abdominal surgical procedures such as colon resections, hysterectomies and aneurysm surgery. In cases where there is danger of injury because of severe inflammation, abscess or tumor, the urologist can place catheters in the ureter to help the surgeon identify and avoid them.

Most people hear about the ureter in relationship to stones which pass from the kidney into the ureter where they cause severe pain while passing down into the bladder. If they get stuck, and do not respond to "tincture of time" they may need shock wave lithotripsy to break up the stones. If this fails, they may need to be removed in the operating room under anesthesia by a urologist using a special instrument called the ureteroscope; a balloon or basket is placed up the ureter. A surgical procedure for stone removal is rarely needed. The pain, from ureteral stone causing blockage, is called ureteral colic and may be in the mid back down to the labia or scrotum depending on the location of the stone in the ureter. The stones can usually be seen on an abdomen x-ray, IVP or CT scan. If stones obstructing the ureter are left too long, there may be permanent kidney damage.

The ureter, like the bladder and the kidney pelvis, has an inner lining called transitional epithelium. Cancers that develop in the kidney pelvis and ureter are similar to those that form in the bladder. Treatment consists of removing a portion of, or the entire ureter. Many surgeons remove the kidney and ureter on that side to assure a better prognosis. If the ureter is obstructed by tumor, then a nephrostomy tube may be needed although in some cases the urologists can place a rigid stent through the obstruction as a palliative measure. If the kidney is left and there is not enough ureter to "rehookup" the urinary tract, then a segment of bowel may be prepared and used as an ersatz ureter.

Chapter 65
PENIS AND TESTICLES

There was a young man from St. Paul,
Whose urethra was terribly small,
He went to a doctor who said with acumen
He wasn't a man, just a strange looking woman.

The male reproductive tract is intimately connected to the urinary tract and together they function for excretion, copulation, reproduction and production of hormones. We have already discussed the prostate and will focus in this chapter on the penis and the scrotum which contains the testis, epididymis, vas deferens and the vessels and nerves to these organs (*see* Diagram 37 next page).

As seen above, the penis consists of two outer tube-like structures, the corpora cavernosa, which are responsible for the erection when they are engorged with blood, and a central area, the corpus spongiosum urethra, through which the urethra passes. The many nerves that innervate this area are important for sexual function and the nervi erigentes are of key importance in developing and maintaining an erection. These nerves pass close to and behind the prostate and in recent years surgeons have made a point to spare these nerves during surgical procedures to help prevent impotence. We have briefly described the testes in Chapter 59, and I want to explain some of the pathology of the scrotum and testes in this chapter.

The penis is such an important sexual and psychological organ that it is fortunate that anomalies are very rare. The most common problems are associated with incomplete development of the urethra resulting in hypospadias and epispadias. In hypospadias, the urethra is incompletely developed and the opening exits under the shaft of the penis and not through the tip or glans. Epispadias is just the opposite with the urethral opening on the upper surface and is much rarer than hypospadias. These abnormalities can be repaired surgically but since they can occur with some genetic sexual abnormalities, the patient has to be evaluated for this prior to any surgery. The openings may be in different locations and each requires a slightly different surgical approach, sometimes sitating staged

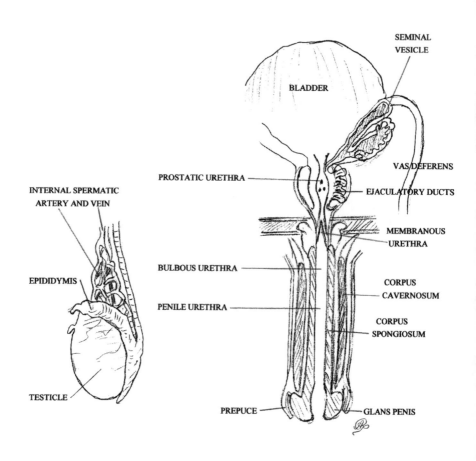

MALE GENITOURINARY ANATOMY

DIAGRAM 37

procedures which may be done weeks or months apart. Hypospadias may present with a band of tissue called a chordee bending the penis downward which must also be repaired.

The penis has a foreskin or prepuce which covers the glans and which is retracted for urination. If the foreskin cannot be properly retracted, severe constriction, phimosis, can occur causing inflammation, swelling and occasional urinary obstruction. It is surgically corrected by a dorsal slit operation freeing up the foreskin, followed then or later by a circumcision or removing of the foreskin. Another situation arises when the retracted foreskin is not replaced over the glans and this can result in a condition called paraphimosis, with severe swelling and inflammation of the penis. In the past, many male children were routinely circumcised, but there is not universal agreement on the need for this now. Religious and social customs still follow the older recommendations. The surgery on an adult requires general anesthesia and is a relatively straightforward procedure with moderate postoperative discomfort.

Trauma to the penis can occur in many ways including the classical "zipper" injuries or injuries sustained during intercourse or masturbation. These are usually managed by simple suturing under local anesthetic. However, as we know from a recent nationally publicized episode, when the penis is amputated, it can be reconnected by surgeons using microscopic surgical techniques, connecting the urethra, nerves, arteries, veins and muscles, with fairly good results.

Malignancies of the penis are rare in the United States and higher in other countries where circumcision is rarely done and where hygiene is poor. Partial or complete amputation of the penis may be needed and several plastic reconstructions are available.

Urologists can treat impotence, the inability to have an erection, surgically, with a procedure that places an inflatable implant in the penis that has a valve for inflating and deflating, before and after intercourse. Two other problems I will mention briefly are Peyronie's disease and priapism. The first is a slowly developing fibrous tissue plaque or band of tissue in the penis that causes it to bend abnormally and is more accentuated during erection. This condition often responds to medicines, radiation therapy or steroid injections, but occasionally, when severe, may require excision of the tissue and even skin grafting. Priapism, named after Priapus, the Greek God of sexuality, is prolonged often painful erection frequently unassociated with sexual arousal and is treated medically, rarely requiring a surgical procedure. The specific cause is not known but it is sometimes seen with malignancies.

Lastly, impotence may be caused by certain medications called adrenergic blockers. It may be a postoperative occurrence after bladder or prostate surgery, or may be a sign of spinal cord disease or diminished blood supply. If the spinal cord disease is reversed, the impotence may be reversed and similarly, when the iliac arteries are blocked by disease, some vascular reconstructive procedures may return potency.

Let us now move on to the scrotum and testicles. This is a very complex area with many different types of pathology. Lesions in the scrotum can be evaluated using the following diagram:

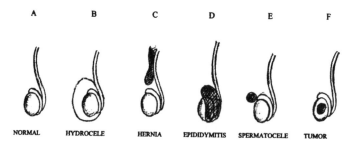

A   B   C   D   E   F

NORMAL   HYDROCELE   HERNIA   EPIDIDYMITIS   SPERMATOCELE   TUMOR

DIAGRAM OF SCROTAL CONDITIONS

DIAGRAM 38

The hydrocele is fluid in the scrotum that may or may not communicate with the peritoneal cavity. Sometimes simple aspiration will make it go away; otherwise a small surgery to tie off the peritoneal connection and remove the fluid is needed. Varicocele is essentially like varicose veins of the scrotum and is corrected by surgery to tie off the veins. Whereas most surgeons do this through the same incision as for an inguinal hernia, some surgeons are doing the procedure laparoscopically with equal success.

Hernias have been described in Chapter 29. Epididymitis is a medical condition which responds to antibiotics and does not normally require surgery. Spermatocele is a cyst which develops at the top of the testes at the epididymis and is usually small and of no consequence unless it becomes large or symptomatic, in which case it can be aspirated or surgically removed.

Before I move on to tumors of the testes, I want to describe the procedure of vasectomy, which is the sterilization of the male by tying off and dividing the vas deferens which carries the sperm. This proce- dure, while it may create some anxiety, is very simple and is done under a local anesthetic with some general sedation, after appropriate counseling with both husband and wife. A small incision is made in the upper scrotum and the vas deferens is grasped with a clamp, tied on both sides and a small center segment removed and sent to pathology as proof that the vas deferens has been divided. This is repeated on the opposite side. The patient will have minimal discomfort and is sent home with pain medication and ice compresses. However, it takes about six to eight weeks before there is no more sperm in the ejaculate and the patient must have a negative sperm test before assuming he is completely sterile. It is important to note that some men have more than one vas deferens on each side and if sperm is still present after the waiting period, a re-exploration of each side must be undertaken and the extra vas deferens found, tied and cut!

Torsion or twisting of the spermatic cord may shut off the blood supply to the testicle. Occasionally, this is a difficult diagnosis to differentiate from epididymitis, with sudden onset of pain, and swelling of the cord and scrotum. A Doppler ultrasound will help make the diagnosis. From this point it is urgent for the urologist to operate and "detorse" the cord and testicle. Torsion of more than three or four hours may lead to death of the testicle and the need for removal of testis called orchiectomy. If it occurs on one side, the surgeon may have to do a preventative procedure on the opposite side because of a tendency towards bilaterality.

Cancer of the testis is usually firm and can be determined on physical exam and by ultrasound examination. I can recall the first autopsy I saw in medical school. I had gone to grade school in the same city and discovered that the person on the autopsy table was a former classmate of mine who had died of a malignant testicular cancer called seminoma, at the age of twenty-two. I recall this vividly because today the cure rate for the disease approaches ninety to ninety five percent because of the advances in surgery and chemotherapy. My childhood friend would probably still be alive today!

There are basically three types of malignancies of the testis, the largest percentage being the seminoma, followed by embryonal cell carcinoma and then the much rarer but more serious and more malignant choriocar- cinoma. These cancers require radical orchiectomy which means removal of the testicle, the spermatic cord and the related lymph nodes through a groin incision similar to that used for inguinal hernia repairs. The seminomas are highly curable even when there are local lymph node metastases because they are very sensitive to chemotherapy and even radiation therapy. The embryonal cell carcinomas are more malignant with a more rapid spread to other locations such as lymphatics and lungs, and they are not as responsive to chemotherapy. The last tumor, the choriocarcinoma, is very rare and the prognosis is usually not good because it is diagnosed late when it has spread extensively.

Suffice it to say that the most common tumors are now very treatable with excellent prognosis, and as with most malignancies, the earlier the diagnosis, the better the prognosis. After many decades we have finally gotten women to examine their breasts for lumps. Men - it's time to start examining your testicles for abnormalities, and if something abnormal is felt, seek out medical examination and advice.

D

Orthopedic Surgery

Chapter 66
FRACTURES

Sticks and stones may break your bones, but orthopedists mend them,
Whether elbows, arms or legs, whatever you can send them.
Open, closed, asleep, awake, with staples, nails or plaster,
They're doing Humpty Dumpty today, he's had a bad disaster.

Mrs. Dumpty's little boy would never pay attention,
And over and over was told to avoid that wall of great contention.
So when Humpty sat on that wall, I was underneath to see...
And when he fell, unfortunately, the whole yolk was on me.

This is the beginning section on orthopedics and I want to start out by emphasizing that this is just a general review for the layman. We will discuss the anatomy of bones and then talk about the nature of fractures and healing, describing simple, comminuted, open and closed fractures and reductions. It should be emphasized that when fractures occur, it means that excess pressure has been exerted on a bone or that the bone itself is weaker than normal. Accompanying this trauma there may be other bodily injuries which must be assessed before the fracture is repaired. Also, it is important to evaluate the nerves, arteries and veins in the vicinity of the fracture, as there may be sharp or blunt injury causing immediate or delayed injury to these tissues. Fractures of the large bones of the pelvis and legs usually require tremendous force and concomitant injuries to the major arteries. Or, nerves to the leg must be identified, evaluated and repaired in conjunction with the fractures.

What is bone, anyway? It's the rigid framework supporting the body and allows for movement by connections with muscles, tendons and joints. It is composed of a matrix or frame made of organic living material, collagen, which is a fibrous tissue, inorganic, non living components, calcium, phosphate, and carbonate compounds which form mineral crystals. Bone protects the softer tissues of the body such as the brain, heart and spinal cord, and bone may have a central core containing marrow which has cells that produce blood cells. Only about 5% of bone is living tissue and it contains several types of tissues which I will name but not expand upon. These are osteoblasts that make new bone, osteoclasts that destroy bone, osteocytes that promote living bone tissue growth and mesenchymal cells that cause growth of the covering of the bone called periosteum. The shaft of a bone is called the diaphysis and the end is called the epiphysis; the outer part is called the cortex and the inner part contains the marrow. The bone grows lengthwise at the epiphyses and fractures in this area may affect the growth in children. Bones need blood supply to repair and to stay alive. If trauma injures the blood supply or if the bone is affected by infection, diabetes mellitus, steroids, tumors or weakness of the bone called osteoporosis, healing will be affected and bones may break more readily and heal more slowly. There are many systemic diseases that effect bone healing and growth such as vitamin D deficiency, arthritis, mineral deficiency, and other metabolic diseases. So when we talk about fractures, remember that the orthopedic surgeon is keeping all these variables in mind.

A simple fracture is when the bone is broken in a single line. When there are many fracture lines and many pieces, it is called a comminuted fracture. If the injury and the fracture cause the bone to protrude through the skin or if the wound is so large that it exposes a broken bone to the outside, it is called an open fracture and when the overlying skin is intact it is called a closed fracture. Open fractures must be cleansed and repaired urgently to prevent infection.

Fractures that occur in weakened bones as with cancer or osteoporosis are called pathologic fractures and sometimes violent muscle action may cause avulsion fractures at the insertion site of the muscle.

Enough for definitions. X-rays are taken to confirm and define the nature of the fracture and then the objective is to repair the bone as best possible to achieve appropriate length and good healing. The bone fragments don't necessarily have to be perfectly aligned and sometimes because of severe comminuted fractures, only partial alignment is possible. The process of getting the bones back into position is called reduction and this can sometimes be done with local anesthesia and sedation with manual manipulation, strong pulling and pushing!. If good reduction is not possible this way, the patient may require complete anesthesia and either closed or open reduction, repairing the fracture with the skin closed or with the skin open. Some fractures require fixation with wires, rods, screws and other stuff that look like they were purchased at your local hardware store, in order to keep the bone fragments in place. After the reduction and possible fixation, some type of immobilization is needed to prevent the bone from moving out of position, to give stability and to help healing. This is where the cast is used and the types and positions of the cast are something you can discuss with the orthopedist since it varies from fracture to fracture. The general principle used, however, is that a fracture should have a cast which immobilizes the joint proximal and distal to the fracture to achieve stabilization.

Complications of fractures were mentioned above, but complications after repair may include compartment syndrome where there is bleeding and swelling at the repair site or too tight a cast, both of which may lead to severe muscle injury and must be attended to immediately. Infection must be carefully watched for with open fractures. With extensive fractures, fat globules may be released from the fracture site into the blood causing fat embolism, a serious problem similar to pulmonary embolism which may cause acute shortness of breath, rapid pulse and even death. It's treated with steroids and oxygen and general medical support.

When a fracture heals, the bone healing cells, the osteogenic cells, cause an early healing site called a fracture callus; however, if the bone ends are too far apart or if there is intervening tissue such as muscle, non-healing or nonunion will occur. And remember for good healing you need good tissue and good blood supply. Chronically sick people or very elderly people heal very slowly.

Fractures of the spine can be painful and dangerous because of potential injury to the spinal cord. That is why we don't move patients until the spinal cord has been protected by stabilizing the spine fracture. The fractures in the neck have various names including the Hangman's fracture (for obvious reasons) and are treated with immobilization, occasionally requiring open procedures and bone grafts, placing extra pieces of bone to assure good healing. The fractures of the spine, cervical, thoracic, lumbar, sacral, and coccygeal, require differing degrees and types of immobilization and differing periods of rest before activity. If there is evidence of neurological deficit such as weakness, paralysis or pain shooting into an arm or leg, exploration of the spinal canal may be indicated to relieve the problem thereby reverse the deficit.

The bones of the arm, legs and pelvis are shown below, and you can refer to this diagram when we are describing the more common fracture sites. It is only important for you to have a general impression of the bony anatomy so you can understand where the injury is and how the orthopedist will be immobilizing it once it is reduced (*see* Diagram 39 next page).

The humerus is the large bone in the upper arm. Fracture can cause injury to the radial nerve which supplies sensory function, sensation on the back of the arm and the top of the hand and motor function, movement of the triceps muscle on the back of the upper arm and the extensors of the elbow, hand and fingers. Extension is what opens your hand when in a fist or cocks-up your wrist. Closed fractures of the humerus require varying treatment from splinting to casting, or slings and other immobilizations with minimal activity for two weeks followed by progressive activity until healing occurs, usually by ten weeks. Open fractures have to be surgically treated, closed, maintained on antibiotics, and are then subjected to the same time frames for healing.

Fractures of the clavicle are usually managed with a figure of eight device that pulls the shoulders back; this is kept in place four to six weeks.

The elbow fractures are numerous and can be complex, but in general any fracture about the elbow is treated with the elbow at a ninety degree angle, like an "L". Care has to be taken in regard to checking for the brachial artery, main artery to the arm, and the median nerve which supplies motor branches, for muscles that cause flexion of the hand and sensory branches that supply areas of the hand. The treatment of the many different fractures sites is beyond what you need to understand now. "Nursemaid's elbow" is a term given to the partial dislocation of a bone at the elbow in children under 5 caused by pulling on the arm too vigorously (darn old nursemaid). It is easily reduced and needs to be splinted for a couple of weeks.

With the forearm bones, the radius and ulna, many individual names are given to specific fractures such as Colles', Monteggia, Galeazzi's, and Smith. After reduction, the patient wears a cast for up to six weeks. Sometimes only one side of the bone appears fractured, one cortex; these are called greenstick fracture and usually occur in children. The bones of the wrist like other areas of human anatomy are often memorized by the

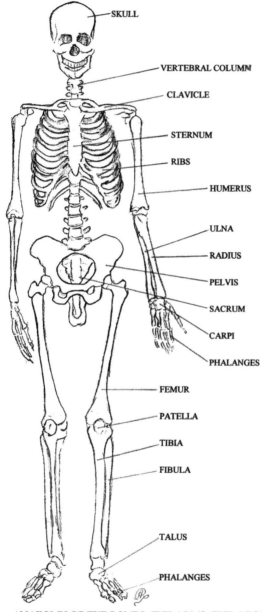

SKULL

VERTEBRAL COLUMN

CLAVICLE

STERNUM

RIBS

HUMERUS

ULNA

RADIUS

PELVIS

SACRUM

CARPI

PHALANGES

FEMUR

PATELLA

TIBIA

FIBULA

TALUS

PHALANGES

ANATOMY OF THE BONES, THE ARMS, THE LEGS AND PELVIS

DIAGRAM 39

medical student using mnemonics, making up poems or jingles using the first letter of each bone. Many of the poems are too gross to mention, but I learned the bones of the wrist using the following: "Never Lower Tillie's Pants // GrandMa Might Come Home"; the bones being the Navicular, also known as scaphoid, Lunate, Triquetrum, Pisiform, Greater Multangular now called trapezium, Lesser Multangular known as trapezoid, Cuneiform, and Hamate. These bones, when fractured, require casts for six weeks or longer.

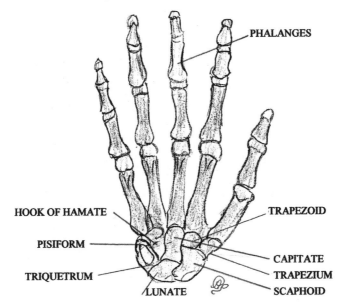

ANATOMY OF THE WRIST AND HAND BONES

DIAGRAM 40

The fractures of the finger bones may need stabilization by special pins for up to six weeks. Tendons may have to be repaired if the fracture has injured them, and of course the nerves and major vessels need to be repaired also.

We are obviously covering a lot of ground rapidly, but let us move on to the pelvis. The pelvic bone consists of three different bones, the ilium, the ischium and the pubis. The amount of force needed for fracture is often quite extensive and is often called high energy trauma and may be life threatening, because of associated injuries. When the pelvic ring (imagine the central portion of the pelvis as a circular ring) is intact after fracture, treatment is mostly limitation of activity and pain management. However, if the ring is disrupted by separation of the bones, then the complexity increases tremendously with associated complications such as massive hemorrhage, intra-abdominal organ injury, urinary tract injury, lung problems and nerve injury. These fractures usually require open operative reduction with all kinds of "hardware" such as metal plates, and screws and will need many weeks for healing and a long recovery with physical therapy and possible post fracture permanent limitations as to athletics and activity.

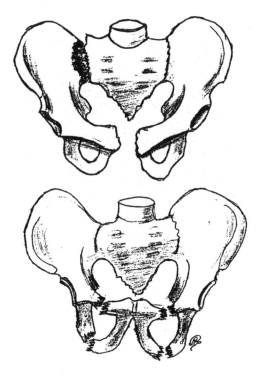

ANATOMY OF PELVIC FRACTURES

DIAGRM 41

As you can see in the diagrams, a part of the pelvis called the acetabulum is where the large upper leg bone, the femur, articulates to the pelvis. Dislocations of the hip and fractures of the acetabulum occur which often need surgical intervention. Reduction of the dislocation may occasionally be accomplished through closed manipulation, but frequently involves very complex, open surgeries requiring great skill and expertise to achieve good results. There are multiple types of surgery.

When we speak of the hip we are actually including the upper part of the femur, the femoral head and neck, and a relationship to the acetabulum. We will now discuss the problems of hip fracture and long bone femoral fractures. The diagram below shows the different types of femoral head and neck fractures. Hip fracture is a common problem in the very elderly and with all its associated complications may be the medical problem that leads to death in many very old people. The correction of femoral head and neck fractures is operative and may vary by the position, age and health of the patient from complete artificial replacement of the femoral head and neck with a prosthesis to various types of pinning and placement of large screws.

Fractures of the femur are basically four in nature depending on their position on the bone: Subtrochanteric, diaphyseal or midshaft, supracondylar and condylar, and each area has a different treatment. And, remember, there are very powerful muscles attached to the femur. When fracture occurs, these muscles often pull the different fragments out of alignment making repair very difficult. Healing may take weeks or months and physical therapy is often required to regain near-normal function. The complications are the same as we have previously discussed.

Fractures of the kneecap can be stabilized by a padded cylindrical cast if the parts are not separated, but will require open surgery and wiring if the fragments are comminuted or separated.

Now on to the lower leg. The two long bones are the outer, lateral, more delicate fibula and the inner, medial, stronger tibia or shinbone. The bones are often both fractured during the same injury and attention is focused on the larger tibia. Its repair is basically the same as any long bone trying to achieve proper length, appearance and stability. The treatments vary tremendously from upper to lower ends and may require open repairs with an intramedullary nail, a large long metal rod put down the center of the bone, metal plates, screws and everything the orthopedist can think of to get a good reduction! Open fractures are even more complex with increased complications of poor healing, infection, poor position or malunion and when the fracture and soft tissue injury is severe, amputation of the extremity may be indicated. To complicate matters orthopedists have all sorts of external fixation devices. The orthopedist's skills are certainly challenged with ankle injuries where a small deviation can impact on good function; and, if this cannot be accomplished with closed reduction, then open procedures are performed.

Fractures of the foot and phalanges or toes are usually handled by closed reduction and casting; however, if good reduction cannot be accomplished, an open repair and pinning is necessary.

Tremendous advances in instrumentation and fracture immobilization, such as the Ilizarov method, have been accomplished in the last few years with greater patient comfort, faster healing and shorter hospitalizations.

Chapter 67
TUMORS
MUSCULOSKELETAL SYSTEM

In bone and cartilage tumors, everything ends with the small word
oma,
Whether it's fibroma, osteoma, enchondroma, or the malignant
osteosarcoma.
There's fibrous histiocytoma, lymphoma and myeloma.
It seems that whether it's cancer or not, you use the same misnoma.

Fortunately tumors in cartilage and bone are rare as rare can be,
And the tumors are based on where they come from, by their histology.
Drugs today are better than before when all we had was streptomycin.
With methotrexate, cis-platinum, ifosfamide and the effective
adriamycin.

Years ago the only surgery was radical amputation,
But now more salvage procedures are earning a viable reputation.
So even though it's never good to develop malignant bone cancers.
We're rapidly learning to save the lives and limbs with better answers.

Fortunately primary tumors of cartilage and bone are not very common. The bone tumors grow at the growth plates such as the giant cell tumor, and the metaphysis, the osteosarcoma, since this is where much of the living tissue in bone resides. Tumors are basically derived from one of the four tissue types, namely cartilage, bone, marrow and fibrous tissue as the names imply. The most common benign tumors are the osteochondroma and enchondroma from cartilage, the fibroma from fibrous tissue, osteoid osteoma and osteoblastoma from bony elements, the giant cell tumor and the rarer neurilemoma from nervous tissue, lipoma from fatty tissue, and hemangioma, from vascular tissue. The major cancers malignant tumors are myeloma and lymphoma from the bone marrow cells, osteosarcomas, several types from the bony elements, chondrosarcoma from the cartilage, chordoma, Ewing sarcoma and the rarer fibrosarcoma, and malignant giant cell tumor. The staging is according to a system devised by Dr. Enneking: Intra-and extra-compartmental defines whether or not the tumor is confined to its own tissue place of origin or compartment. High and low grade are definitions of how active or malignant the tissue looks under the microscope.

Benign	Malignant
1. Latent	I A Low Grade Intra-compartmental
2. Active	I B Low Grade Extra-compartmental
3. Aggressive	II A High Grade Intra-compartmental
	II B High Grade Extra-compartmental
	III Low or High Grade and Intra or Extra Compartmental With Metastases

STAGING OF MUSCOLOSKELETAL TUMORS
DIAGRAM 42

Tumors may present as a mass, pain with rest or with motion, joint discomfort or swelling of surrounding tissue. If the tumor impinges on nerves the pain may be severe and if near a joint there may be fluid accumulation.

Although we don't know the etiology of tumors, many are associated with changes in the genes and chromosomes which can be detected. Why and when cancers spread usually depends on the grade and staging. The higher the grading the poorer the prognosis. When there is metastasis, the prognosis is poor.

Tumors, both benign and malignant, have characteristic appearances on x-ray, but sometimes, severe infections of bone called osteomyelitis can mimic changes seen with cancer. MRI scans are excellent for diagnosis and further workup for evidence of metastasis is needed including CAT scans of other bone and chest x-rays. Final diagnosis can be made with needle biopsy or open biopsy, being sure to take appropriate cultures, studying the tissue for bacteria, TB, and fungus.

Obviously the treatment of tumors is the complete eradication of the disease, if possible and secondarily, the preservation of function of the involved extremity. Whereas years ago amputation was the main surgery for malignancy, today orthopedists base their surgical planning on the staging, often doing partial resections and placing all types of modern internal prostheses to fill the gaps. The prognosis depends on the staging, with cure rates over 70-80% for stage I and 40-80% for stage II cancers.

Benign tumors may also need wide excision depending on their rating. Malignant tumors are best treated, if no metastases are present, with radical resection of bone and soft tissue. Radiation is often effective for some tumors like Ewing sarcoma, but many bone cancers may not be sensitive to radiation. However, they are often sensitive to a combination chemotherapy such as the one mentioned above containing Adriamycin, cis-platinum, ifosfamide and methotrexate.

The treatment of musculoskeletal tumors is a comprehensive one involving the orthopedist in close affiliation with the general surgeon, oncologist, radiation therapist and pathologist.

Chapter 68
AMPUTATIONS

Amputations usually come to pass at the end of a long, long trail,
With hills and valleys, ups and downs, and treatments that finally fail.
Such as stopping smoking, and drugs that thin blood, and cleansing
the ulcers with care,
And long operations to bypass the arteries and try to repair what is
there.

And the stress of the loss to the patient, and the sadness of the doctors
who failed,
And the husbands, or wives, the children who sighed and the mothers
and fathers who wailed,
Make this operation a sad one for all unless hope can be nurtured
from despair,
To give patients new visions with help and prostheses, and function
with people who care.

Amputation is the complete or partial removal of a part of the body, and we will focus here upon the extremities. Except for trauma which causes irreversible damage, and the rare tumor which demands a radical approach, most amputations come at the end of a sometimes long and difficult struggle with infection or arterial vascular disease. The most common are above knee and below knee amputations of the leg, followed by partial amputations of the foot and removal of toes. Major amputations of the arm and hand, fortunately, are quite rare and will not be discussed here. For finger and hand procedures, see Chapter 70 which is about hands.

The level of amputation is determined by several factors. In general, the philosophy is to leave as much length and tissue as possible, with a few major exceptions, and the surgeon also wants to make the result as functional as possible. With cancer, the primary focus must be eradication of the disease and this will determine the length and location of amputation. With the other amputations, it is important to take enough tissue so that the wound will heal and not require multiple surgeries to accomplish a good stump. The stump should be long enough to accommodate a prosthesis successfully but not so long as to make it unwieldy. Above knee amputations with prostheses demand twice the amount of work for walking than a below the knee amputation does even when all efforts are made to preserve the knee joint. The amputations on the foot must be designed with ambulation in mind. To save a portion of the foot but have severe discomfort walking is of little value. Although most patients want as much saved as possible, the surgeon must emphasize function over cosmesis. In the case of an upper extremity amputation, a patient can do much more with a grasping hook type prosthesis than an artificial functionless hand, although the latter may look nicer. Most healthy patients with single below knee amputations will ambulate well with a prosthesis and some individuals who are motivated will walk with bilateral below knee amputations with a cane to assist them. Unilateral above knee amputees will usually be able to walk with the help of a cane, but bilateral above knee amputees cannot generate the strength to ambulate without a walker.

Another amputation available to the surgeon is the Syme procedure which leaves a long lower leg after amputating the foot, but is very difficult to fit for a prosthesis. Very high amputations such as hip disarticulations and hemipelvectomy, which means removing half the pelvis, are rarely done and require special expertise and post operative management.

Physical therapy plays a major role with orthopedic patients, helping them return to as normal a function as possible, and the therapists are used on a routine basis in the pre- and post-operative period. Frequently, with below knee amputations, the surgeon works with a prosthetist, a specially trained individual who measures the patient, and obtains and fits the artificial leg, and physical therapists, along with a psychosocial support team, in managing the amputee. On occasion the surgeon would apply a temporary immediate fitting prosthesis in the operating room at the time of amputation and this helps the patient through the initial shock of the loss of the leg. It is sometimes better to wake up and at least see an artificial leg rather than just the stump.

Amputations require careful attention to the bony stump and nerves, to prevent post-operative pain; the muscles and skin must be handled in such a way that an appropriate stump for a prosthesis can be attained.

The complications of amputations include inadequate blood supply with tissue breakdown requiring a higher amputation, infections, bleeding, pain and poor weight bearing surface. Each of these problems must be handled by the surgeon and may require revisions of the stump in the weeks or months after the initial surgery. Most patients, after amputation, experience some degree of "phantom pain" which is a sign of the brain's confusion over the loss of the body part. Patients have periods of time when they feel the presence of the amputated leg or toe, and this usually goes away in time.

In conclusion, the patient undergoing amputation must be given a positive but realistic outlook and this can be accomplished by a sensitive, understanding surgeon, a supportive clinical psychologist or social worker, a prosthetist, a physical therapist and a vocational guidance individual, all of whom will work with, and encourage the patient in the postoperative period.

Chapter 69
SPINAL SURGERY - DISCS, SCOLIOSIS AND OTHER STUFF

I had a pain in my lower back that went down to my legs,
It always got worse in the shipping yard while lifting one hundred
pound kegs.
I went to my family doctor, who prescribed bed rest and aspirin,
But the pain never got any better and it was certainly exaspirin.

He sent me to a chiropractor who twisted my back in knots,
But all that did was make it worse until I got morphine shots.
Then off I went to the orthopod who opened up my spine
Took out some discs and sewed me up and said that I was fine.

Next morning I had the same old pain except it seemed much worse
So I had a long session with my friendly shrink who analyzed me line
and verse.
I left the office relaxed and smiling, I had a new lease on life,
But the very next day the pain was back and I started to yell at my
wife.

My life got worse, I got divorced and left my job on the docks,
And pretty soon I was out on the streets with the clothes on my back,
shoes and socks.
I still had the pain and my toes were all numb, and my underwear was
dirty,
Here I was a down and out wreck and I'm just a year over thirty.

So what is the moral of this story for you, since you've read this far
already?
What is the cause of my pain in the back? I turned over and asked my
brown Teddy.

*The only response that I give to you now, and I don't mean it as a
cute joke,
My pain went away when the alarm went off and by golly I just
awoke!*

The back is made up of thirty-three vertebral bodies made up of five divisions, seven cervical bodies, twelve thoracic, five lumbar, five sacral joined together, and four coccygeal joined together. As seen in the diagram, they each have spinous and transverse processes for muscle attachments, pedicles and laminae, and the free (not joined) ones are separated by an intervertebral disc composed of an outer circular annulus fibrosus and a central nucleus pulposus. The spinal cord runs down the spinal canal and is well protected from injury by the surrounding bones. The nerve roots come out through the neural foramina. I only mention all this anatomy because you should be a little familiar with the terms when we talk about disease (*see* Diagram 43 next page).

When there is disease with the intervertebral disc protruding or herniating, it may cause compression on the nerve roots and give the patient symptoms of paraparesis or weakness in the lower extremities, or quadriparesis which means weakness in all four extremities, and pain in the back extending into the extremities called radicular pain, which may be minimal to quite incapacitating.

There are three tracts or groups of nerves that we should know about in the spinal cord. They have long names but to be complete I'll list them for you. The outer, lateral part of the cord has the corticospinal tracts going from the brain to the extremities, and these have to do with motor or movement function. These are what we call crossed fibers in that the left side of the brain controls the right side body muscles. The lateral cord also contains the spinothalamic tract which carries messages to the thalamus in the brain transmitting pain, temperature and sensation. The dorsal, top part of the spinal cord has the dorsal columns which tell the brain about touch, vibration, and sense of position. These latter two also are crossed with the left side of the brain, alert to the right side of the body.

There are many diseases which can cause upper and lower back pain and occasional nerve deficits aside from disc disease, and the orthopedist or neurologist must rule these out before commencing on any therapy. These can include other bony disorders, such as narrowing of the nerve

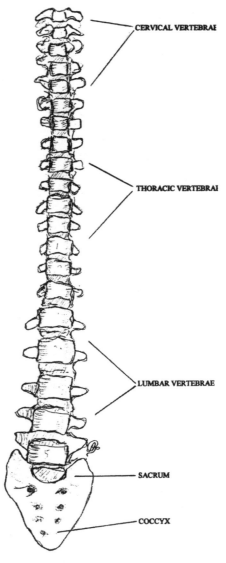

CERVICAL VERTEBRAE

THORACIC VERTEBRAE

LUMBAR VERTEBRAE

SACRUM

COCCYX

ANATOMY OF THE SPINE AND VERTEBRAE

DIAGRAM 43

root canals or spinal stenosis, spondylolisthesis--a big word for sliding of one vertebra back and forth on another because of joint instability causing nerve compression, malignancies, both primary and metastatic, rheumatoid arthritis, vascular disease, infectious problems and abscesses, spinal cord disease and many others that the neurologist or orthopedist must know about and eliminate or treat. Remember, this is a book for the public, not for physicians, so we'll just focus on the most common problems.

With degenerative joint disease as we get older, patients not only herniate or break up discs, but also form little bony projections called spurs which may impinge on the spinal cord causing symptoms. In the cervical or neck region, patients may have headaches, backaches, aching in the arms or loss of strength or sensation in the arms and hands. In the legs, the symptoms usually relate to the lumbar disc compressing the nerve roots with pain and weakness going down the legs, and weakness or loss of bladder or bowel control. Diagnosis of the disease can be made by spine x-rays, CAT scans and MRI scans. More than 65-70% of disc problems will resolve with good medical management including medications, neck or back support, avoidance of vigorous activities, physical therapy with traction and massage, and occasional steroid injection to decrease the swelling. When the medical management fails and the patient has continuing severe pain or neurological disorders, then surgery is indicated. Laminotomy or opening the lamina, and laminectomy, removing the lamina give the orthopedist the ability to remove the diseased disc.

If there is instability in the spine because of disease of the supporting structures, such as the facets and interlocking bony structures, then the surgeon may need to do a fusion. This means that he takes a piece of your own bone, usually from the hip, and inserts it into the spine in such a way that when it heals, it fuses or locks one vertebra to another vertebra above or below to assure stability.

Now you should know that there are many diseases of the spine including scoliosis, lateral or side to side curvature of the spine and kyphosis, humping deformity of the spine which requires extensive complex procedures for straightening. The list of causes for scoliosis would take up two pages and I won't bore you with all the names and etiologies. The specialists in this surgery may spend six to ten hours in a single procedure inserting all types of internal braces such as Harrington and Luque rods, Cotrel-Dubousset or Dwyer instrumentation, along with wiring and external braces and casts to correct the deformity over many months. In many cases involving the spine and spinal cord, the neurosurgeons work arm in arm with the orthopedists to accomplish the desired ends.

As for the complications, they are the same as other surgeries except for the rare problems associated with spinal cord injury with may include partial or even permanent weakness, other sensation disturbances or even paralysis.

The decision for the type of surgery needed for disc or other spinal disease may be tremendously variable. When I had a back problem, after foolishly overdoing karate with my son, I found out that I had low back disease. I cried when they used that awful word degenerative! Being like most surgeons, and petrified of any surgery, I sought out five opinions and they varied from oral medications, to physical therapy, to back injections, to simple surgery which would get me back to work in three or four days to complex surgery with spinal fusion that would lay me up for three months. So I have great reservation in recommending any procedures in this specialty without multiple second opinions! As it was, I had my back injected twice, lost some weight, gave up karate and I feel fine!

Chapter 70
JOINTS

If we didn't have joints, we'd have to have wheels
And if we couldn't bend, then we couldn't eat meals.
No walking, no grasping, no turning our heads.
We'd look pretty stiff as we lay in our beds.

Kissing would be a horrendous endeavor.
And picking our noses we couldn't do, ever.
And if we should ever attempt to try sex,
We'd end up as crumpled up soft tissue wrecks.

J oints connect one bony structure with another in the human body. The scientific names of the two major joints are diarthrosis and synarthrosis. Diarthrosis contains fluid and articulating synovium and cartilages. The ends of two bones have a smooth cartilage and synovium surface which in some ways interlocks with the other and moves against it in a fluid environment. Synarthrosis is without fluid and consists of a fibrous and cartilage containing connection. Shoulders, knees, hips and fingers are examples of diarthrodial; the three pelvic bones together, and the spine are examples of synarthrodial joints. The diagram shows an example of each (*see* Diagram 44 next page).

Diseases of the joints are among the most common causes of disability for all ages and usually have two basic causes: Inflammatory, with pain, warmth, swelling and redness, and noninflammatory. Although people over fifty years old are more prone to having joint problems, anyone at any age is susceptible. All inflammatory joint diseases are called arthritis; inflammation of the lining of a joint is called synovitis, and any inflammation of the spine is called spondylitis. Rheumatism is an older term that refers to any pain in any part of the skeletal system, tendon or ligament. Noninflammatory arthritis includes traumatic problems such as sprains, fractures, dislocations, etc.

Osteoarthritis is a degenerative condition that affects the cartilage and is most common in people over fifty, and the usual location is in the hips.

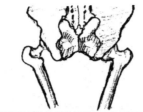

SYNARTHRODIAL JOINT-SYMPHYSIS PUBIS

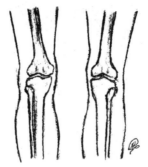

DIARTHRODIAL AND SYNARTHRODIAL JOINTS

DIAGRAM 44

There are congenital and hereditary causes and a whole host of other causes such as vitamin deficiencies such as scurvy and rickets, and other nutritional problems.

After a patient complains of joint pain or limitation of motion, a workup will include a physical examination as well as x-rays, MRI and bone scan. Serologic tests for collagen diseases, such as lupus erythematosus and rheumatoid factor, and examination of joint or synovial fluid removed with a syringe and needle, are also done. When a diagnosis of infectious arthritis is made, appropriate antibiotics are used; on some occasions the joint may be drained with a local anesthetic and small tube.

For rheumatoid arthritis, a systemic disease that affects not only the synovium of the joints but several other systems as well, including cardiac, respiratory; the first treatment is medical, with anti-inflammatory drugs such as naproxen, ibuprofen, aspirin, and corticosteroids, pain medications such as codeine, Vicodin, bufferin, and antibiotics, and splinting and muscle strengthening physical therapy. Only after medical failure will the orthopedists recommend partial or total removal of the synovium and sometimes total joint replacement. Multiple complex procedures--including arthroplasty, or repairing a joint by surgically cleaning or scraping the cartilage surface, or replacement arthroplasty, replacing the whole joint with an artificial metal joint and arthrodesis, fixing a joint by surgery with a fusion of the bones, fixing the bones together in a permanent union--are also used.

Osteoarthritis, the degenerative joint disease, affects the cartilage which is the cushion between one bony joint surface and another, and the cartilage eventually becomes so thinned and soft that the joint becomes a bone to bone interaction which leads to further bony changes and scarring and eventual partial or total loss of motion. Osteoarthritis is a slowly progressive disease which may show early changes on x-ray before the individual has any symptoms. It is often related to excessive stresses in the joint and therefore the recommendations for non-operative treatment are directed towards lessening or eliminating these stresses; walk, don't run, stop karate, take anti-inflammatory medications, just avoid stressful physical situations.

As the disease progresses, diagnosis is made by x-ray, MRI, and by diagnostic arthroscopy, by looking into a joint with a lighted scope. It may be followed by therapeutic arthroscopy where the surgeon actually removes abnormal or torn tissue and repairs the joint. When the disease becomes severe enough, the orthopedist may need to replace the joint in procedures called total hip replacement or total knee replacement. The major complication of these procedures is infection and the utmost care must be taken to prevent any contamination. This includes special air flow controlled rooms, pre and intra operative antibiotics and limiting the flow of personnel in and out of the operating room. If infections occur, they may respond to antibiotics, and if not, the hip or knee prosthesis may have to be removed and later a new one placed.

Gout is a joint disease associated with abnormal urate metabolism where urate crystals are deposited in a joint causing pain and deformity. It usually responds to medical management using Indocin, colchicine or allopurinol, and only requires surgery when severe arthritis occurs.

When disease in a joint progresses so that the nerves are damaged as in diabetes mellitus, leprosy, and syphilis, it is called a neuropathic or Charcot joint which may require braces to stabilize the joint. Severe cases may even lead to amputation.

In the foot, aside from gout which usually effects the big toe (remember King Henry VIII), the most common joint problem we hear about is a bunion or hallux valgus, outward deviation of the big toe, due to poorly fitting shoes. There are more than one hundred surgical procedures, but the one used most is called the Keller procedure where the joint is removed, leaving a shorter but painless toe.

And finally, with deference to the prince Alexei, the son of the last Czar of Russia who had the disease, hemophilia can cause bleeding into joints. This causes pain, deformity and eventual lack of function. The treatment is directed towards stabilizing the bleeding disease, preventing joint trauma and pain management. As with other arthritides, joint replacement may be needed with optimal coagulation control.

Chapter 71
HANDS

There's handball and handcuffs and Georg Friedrick Handel,
And handguns and handicaps and even a handbell.
Hands high for horses from hooves up to withers,
It's enough to go crazy like Dagwood and Dithers.

There's offhand and backhand and yes, underhanded,
Left brain is right handed, can you understand it?
"Unhand me, you villain", and hand-me-down clothes,
The list of "hand" words never ends, Heaven knows!

But just plain old "hand" is a man's grasping paw,
Which along with his brain lets him lay down the law.
We don't have to use 'em for walking like lemurs,
Because we stand upright with vertical femurs.

And since, unlike monkeys, we don't hang from branches,
Our hands are left free to write books and take chances
With playing cards, slot machines and unsundry toys,
Or gesticulate wildly while making loud noise.

So when the hand's injured we want the physician
Who can put all the hand pieces back in position.
And aside from his brain, all the patients demand
That the surgeon has a trained and a delicate hand!

Most people attribute man's development and superiority over lower species to his advanced brain and his hand with its opposable thumb. Opposable means that the thumb can move across the palm and touch the tips of all the other fingers.

The hand is a remarkable organ with the ability to perform delicate functions and yet also with the capacity for heavy work, lifting and squeezing. The ability to pick up a pin and also to grasp an object firmly is unusual for a single organ and depends on a complex arrangement of bones, muscles, tendons and pulleys as well as the nerves, arteries and veins. It is also remarkable that the hand can sustain significant injury and still perform its functions. We will discuss the anatomy briefly and then some of the more common ailments and principles needed to repair injuries and return maximum function.

We shall approach the hand for the general public in a way that will give you some insight into the ways a workup is done, the treatment of trauma and several common pathologic problems.

Evaluating the hand requires more than x-rays, CT and MRI studies because bony abnormalities may only give a small picture of what is wrong. The trained hand surgeon must know how to evaluate each muscle, tendon and nerve, along with assessing the blood supply. This physician evaluates the fingernails, and the skin and has a routine for physical examination so that minor abnormalities will not be missed. This is most important with trauma, where the patient may only focus on the overt area of injury. The physician will take in the obvious but will also be very aware of the potential for underlying injuries that could result in functional deficits. The surgical repairs of the traumatic injuries of the hand are beyond what we can explain except that hand injuries should be managed by a hand specialist. I have seen patients who have been treated by a non specialist for lacerations that were considered to be simple, where underlying minor or major injuries to the tendons or a complex pulley system and small muscles have been missed or ignored with loss of function. It is sometimes important to do a repair at the first procedure, but at other times, delayed repairs may be indicated, and only a hand specialist will be able to make those decisions. Obviously simple lacerations can be taken care of by any physician, but care must be taken to assure that the injury is indeed simple. Most physicians are able to say without losing face "I don't know" and We should call in an expert". It's taken millions of years for man to develop the hand; let's not screw it up in a few minutes of hasty misdecision!

When caring for a trauma patient's finger, we try to preserve as much length as possible and sometimes this means rotating skin from one area of the finger to another or grafting a piece of skin from a far away area to the finger. With tendon injury, surgeons may use a lesser important tendon to replace a damaged, important tendon in a procedure called tendon transfer, and nerves and vessels may need microsurgical techniques for adequate repair. In the last two decades a subspecialty of microsurgery has arisen using magnifying glasses or special magnifying scopes, which has enabled surgeons to sew back severed fingers or a hand with surprisingly good success rate and function. Remember, the brains of the matter may be in the muscles in the forearm, so that injuries of the hand or the reimplanted hand will work moderately well because the brain to muscle connection in the forearm has not been disturbed. It is when there are transections of the nerves in the upper arm that there may be terrible functional loss in the hand. Sensory nerves heal well because their specificity is less than motor nerves. The former, when healed, will deliver messages to the brain and will be reinterpreted as sensation or pain. However, the motor nerves coming from the brain heal poorly and the brain may lose the ability to connect with the exact muscle group it wants in order to perform a given function.

Infections of the hand can usually be handled with antibiotics, but abscesses or closed collections of pus must be drained. Usually this is a simple matter if only involving the fingernail called a paronychia or finger pulp, called a felon. However deep, hand infections or abscesses, usually seen in the elderly; drug abusers or immunocompromised patients, have to be handled by a specialist. Burn injuries can result in severely disfiguring scar contractures unless handled early with appropriate splinting and skin management.

Surgery for inflammation of the tendons or tendonitis is done only after failure of medical management or rest, splinting, and anti-inflammatory medications. It consists of freeing up encapsulated tendons in a delicate operation.

Let's talk about carpal tunnel syndrome. This is a condition where the median nerve is compressed in the wrist in what is known as the carpal tunnel (*see* Diagram 45 next page).

Carpal tunnel syndrome has many causes, but probably not from manual work as suspected by many patients. It is associated with diabetes mellitus, thyroid dysfunction, trauma, lipomas and obesity. The symptoms are burning or numbness is the median nerve distribution and general hand discomfort aggravated with use. Although the diagnosis may come from physical exam, it can be confirmed by MRI and nerve conduction studies measuring the nerve function and detecting injury signals.

Splints and anti-inflammatory medications are used with good success and even steroid injections may be helpful. If all fails then surgical approach is indicated with either an open procedure or endoscopy. The surgery involves dividing the transverse carpal ligament and thereby al-

CARPAL TUNNEL

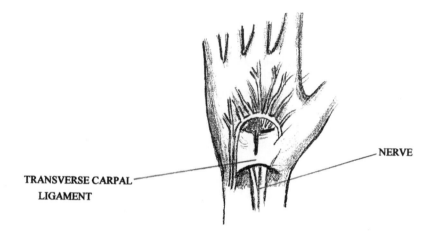

NERVE

TRANSVERSE CARPAL
LIGAMENT

CARPAL TUNNEL AFTER TRANSVERSE
CARPAL LIGAMENT DIVIDED

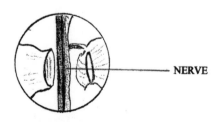

NERVE

THE CARPAL TUNNEL

DIAGRAM 45

lowing more space for the contents of the carpal tunnel. The greatest potential problem is damage to the tiny nerve that innervates the muscle in the thumb that allows opposition, and surgeons have designed their procedures to avoid this tiny structure.

Next we'll discuss Dupuytren's contracture named after French surgeon Baron Guillaume Dupuytrens, and appears in its later stages as a thickened band of tissue that causes a finger to flex toward the palm. The pathology is an abnormal proliferation of the fascia and does not respond to any nonsurgical treatments. The surgery involves an open operation with excision of the involved fascia and some type of plastic skin flap closure if the contracture has decreased the amount of local skin available. Function usually returns to normal.

Surgery for arthritis of the hand is very complex and the list of causes of the arthropathies and the repairs used occupies hundreds of pages in many books. In dealing with these various diseases, the aim is to treat the systemic disease, treat the hand in a way which will prevent severe deformity and if the deformity occurs, tailor an operation to give the best functional result.

Tumors of the hand are mostly benign and consist mainly of ganglion cysts which are mucous fluid filled spherical masses arising from a tendon sheath. At surgery, through a small incision, the ganglion cyst is removed along with the sheath base or root. This surgery can often be done under a local anesthetic with or without sedation.

Giant cell tumors of the tendon sheath of the hand are benign but need to be carefully and completely removed or they will recur. The problem with their removal is that they often occur around the nerves. Vessel bundles and the delicate pulley mechanisms and removal must be done without injury to these structures.

Malignant lesions of the hand and finger, except for skin cancers such as basal cell, squamous cell and melanoma, are rare and need not be covered in this chapter. The skin tumors are managed in the usual way with appropriate wide excisions requiring free margins.

Chapter 72
ENDOSCOPIC SURGERY

Arthroscopic surgery is used in rotten joints,
To diagnose torn menisci and to win the surgeon points.
You place a metal lighted tube inside and look around,
And take out damaged tissue by the ounce and by the pound.

It's really quite amazing that through such a tiny hole
The orthopedic surgeon can accomplish every goal.
With this small cut the orthopod now has it in his power
To reconstruct your knee or wrist, and do it in less than an hour.

Arthroscopic surgery, using a lighted tube to see and operate inside joints, is to joint surgery what laparoscopic abdominal surgery has been to gallbladder, appendix and other intraperitoneal surgeries. It's a wonderful way to perform a procedure with less pain postoperatively and minuscule scaring. Although it requires surgical expertise that many older surgeons had to pick up through post graduate course work as opposed to learning it in a residency or fellowship training course, most interested orthopedists have opted for this method of diagnosis and treatment for meniscus tears and other internal derangements of the knee. Some surgeons have also started using this technology for the shoulder, hip, ankle, elbow and wrist. Usually in the larger joints, with the patient asleep, a saline solution is injected into the joint through one opening and the scope through another. An instrument is inserted through the third port and there are all kinds of mechanical devices for cutting, sanding, and shaving for correcting the intra-joint pathology. However, many orthopedic surgeons are waiting to see the long term results of these procedures before embarking on the training.

Chapter 73
REPLANTATION OF LIMBS

In Greek mythology, seeds were planted that grew up into men
How easy the replantation of organs would be if we'd do that again.
When fingers or hands or arms are avulsed or severed or otherwise
crushed,
We wouldn't feel so urgently scared and feel so terribly rushed.

Just plant the right seed and in a few days or even a month or two,
A new hand or arm or thumb or leg could be Fed-Exed to you.
But alas the times are not so advanced and the proper seeds aren't
available,
And traumatic wounds to the hands or the arm end up on the O.R.
table.

Progress in the replantation of severed limbs made its greatest advances with the development of the operating microscope in 1960, which enabled surgeons to anastomose small vessels together. The basic theories had been present for years but the ability to actually connect the divided arteries and veins had a very poor success rate until then. Along with the ability to see smaller structures came the development of finer instrumentation and sutures so small that they wouldn't damage the minuscule arteries, veins and nerves. Replantation is the reconnecting of a body part that has been completely transected. When a small segment of skin or muscle or tendon remains attached, the procedure is called revascularization.

Today replantation is done by surgeons specially trained. Often when major replantation is needed, teams of surgeons at major medical centers are available to offer the greatest chance for success. One surgical team will be assigned to preparing the severed part and the other team will be preparing the patient to receive the severed part. An amputated finger or hand or arm survives about six hours; if it is cooled, the time can be extended to twelve hours. If there is a lot of muscle and soft tissue present, there is greater danger of severe tissue damage at shorter lengths of time. A severed limb must be cooled and kept in a saline solution until the replantation team is ready to start their work. In general, it is recommended that no work be done on the amputated part by a nonexperienced surgeon because inadvertent damage may occur from incorrect handling without magnification.

The first decision of the team is whether or not replantation is possible from a biological and mechanical point of view. If the hand, finger or arm has been terribly crushed or otherwise damaged or if the time interval between injury and replantation is very long, then it may be wiser not to attempt the procedure for fear of failure or ending up with a functionless appendage which only gets in the way. A good prosthesis may be the better choice over a very poor replantation.

Let us compare the upper with the lower extremities. The hand and arm are far more complex in their function than the legs. We have developed excellent prostheses for legs which will enable a person to function very well with minimal visible deformity. The success rate for replantation of legs is poor because of the large masses of muscle and because better stability can be achieved with a prosthesis than with a replanted leg. So, most teams do not consider the leg a suitable candidate for replantation. The opposite holds true for the upper extremity. There are no prosthetic devices any where near as good as even a partially functional hand or arm. And cosmetically, a hand shaped prosthesis is not as good as a functional hook device and this is not as psychologically and cosmetically satisfactory. Lower extremity equals good prosthesis with good function and minimal social impact; upper extremity means poor prosthesis with major visible social impact.

Because of this, replantation surgeons focus on the upper extremity. The procedures are so involved and time consuming that several criteria must be met before the surgeon will take on the case. Among the things evaluated are the severity of the injury; crush and avulsion injuries are worst, guillotine type injuries, though rare, are best. The psychological status of the individual is very important since it takes great care and cooperation to achieve replantation success. The amount of ischemic time between injury and surgery and the presence of other injuries which may be life threatening and may take priority in treatment, and the location of the injury must all be considered. Because of the complexity of the anatomy, the surgeon knows that in certain areas it may be better to complete a finger amputation than end up with a functionless digit that hinders function rather than helps it. We have discussed the motor function of the hand briefly in Chapter 70 and I want to emphasize that the flexor function, making a fist and moving the hand in that direction, and extensor function, extending the fingers and hand, are predominately controlled by muscles in the forearm. The nerves enter these muscles in the proximal forearm near the elbow. If an amputation or severe injury occurs beyond where the nerves enter and if the motor nerves are intact, there is better chance for a good functional result. This of course depends on many variables beyond the scope of our discussion, but it is important to define what needs to be done. The bones must be stabilized, often shortened a little bit so that when the nerves and vessels are reconnected there will be no tension on the new connections. The arteries and veins must be connected using an operating microscope and the muscles and tendons attached. The nerves must be reconnected as anatomically as possible, lining up the tiniest characteristics to attempt as close to an exact repair as possible.

These surgeries are complicated, expensive and very time consuming; even in the best of hands there may be complications of infection, loss of function and need for second and third surgeries.

Most reports give a 70-80-% success rate of replantation at major surgical centers.

E

GYNECOLOGICAL SURGERY

Chapter 74
HYSTERECTOMY
REMOVING THE UTERUS

In some sections of the country I think you'll agree.
There were two indications for a hysterectomy.
The first was the presence of a uterus intact,
The second was good insurance, in fact. (just joking!)

But fortunately, now, the art of the gynecologist,
Is more than just giving it to the pathologist.
More women in their forties have kids safe and sound,
So we have more reasons to keep the old womb around.

The humor attached to the uterus and childbearing has been the subject of bards and bawds for hundreds of years, including "there was no womb in the inn", "we were womb mates", "the waiting womb", "womb at the top" and so forth. But the truth of the matter is that for hundreds of years men and women knew almost nothing about the female reproductive tract, menstruation, labor and delivery. The whole subject was cloaked in mystery and superstition. Although a few isolated gynecological procedures were done in the mid-nineteenth century, there was little progress until after the widespread use of anesthesia and antiseptic surgery. The physiology of the female reproductive tract wasn't elucidated until the first half of the twentieth century and Dr. Papanicolaou didn't present his monograph on "Pap" smears until the 1940's. Oral contraceptives came out in the late 50's along with good chemotherapy for choriocarcinoma. With the development of ultrasound, CAT and MRI scanning came further surgical advances. Laparoscopy, laser procedures and the whole field of specialized gynecological oncology with gynecologists who specialize in cancer of the female reproductive organs provided the ability to handle all aspects of the surgery, including procedures previously left to the general surgeons, urologists and medical oncologists. They are the super-gynecologists.

So let us start with the female reproductive tract by giving you a brief anatomy lesson, both internal and external genitalia.

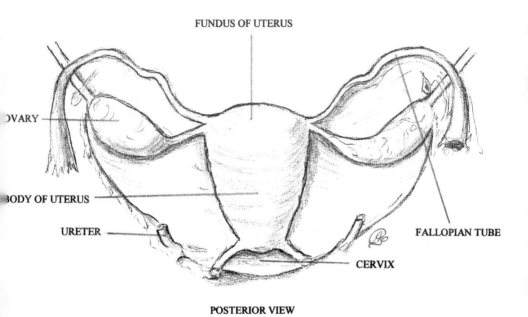

FUNDUS OF UTERUS

OVARY

BODY OF UTERUS

URETER

CERVIX

FALLOPIAN TUBE

POSTERIOR VIEW

FEMALE EXTERNAL AND INTERNAL GENITALIA

DIAGRAM 46

As you can see, the female urethra exits just in front of the vaginal opening and behind the clitoris and therefore may become intimately involved in major surgery in this area, as we shall see later. The hymen varies in extent from a very small amount of tissue to a complete closure of the vaginal opening which has to be opened surgically in a few women to allow menstruation to occur. We won't go into much discussion of the fascia and muscles supporting the perineum, the part of the body encompassing the male and female external genitalia and the anus. With many pregnancies and vaginal deliveries, the floor of the pelvis can become very stretched out leading to weakness and a prolapsing or falling out of the perivaginal tissues, among them the bladder, called a cystocele and rectum, called a rectocele, indenting into the vaginal opening. These may require surgery but only if there are symptoms of pressure, or leaking of urine or stool.

The internal anatomy consists of the vagina, cervix, uterus, fallopian tubes, and ovaries, with ample blood and nerve supply and lymphatics and with a proximity to the ureters.

Most women know the routine for their yearly gynecological checkup and aside from the usual history and physical it contains pertinent history about the age of onset of menstruation, called menarche, the time and nature of the periods, menopause, if it has occurred, abnormal bleeding, pain with intercourse, called dyspareunia, vaginal discharge, and information about pregnancies. It will include marital history, birth control and family history of any cancers or other pertinent abnormalities.

The physician asks about changes in bowel habits, pressure in the low abdomen, weight gain or loss, previous surgery and any significant medical problems. The list is even more comprehensive, but these are the major areas of interest. The woman will undergo pelvic exam where the gynecologist will examine the introitus including the perineum and vaginal opening, and will visualize the cervix; then he/she will do a bimanual two handed exam which will enable him/her to feel the uterus and the ovaries, and feel for masses or tender areas.

Any discharge will be cultured, and cells will be examined to determine the presence of yeast, Candida Albicans, gonorrhea, or Trichomonas infection, all of which will respond to appropriate antibiotic treatment. If patients have a vaginal problem that bothers them, with heavy discharge, itching or odor, they should alert their physician so that a culture may be obtained.

The "Pap" test will be done by their physician and examined by a pathologist who will look for abnormal appearing cells which may indicate cancer and might mean that further evaluation must be done.

Many patients believe that a "Pap" smear will check everything and that any exam includes a "Pap". This is not necessarily true and it's important to emphasize that a yearly exam should include a "Pap" smear which is a check for cervical cancer. You should ask your physician whether you are having a "Pap" smear. We will discuss further workup for cancer in Chapter 76. If the history suggests possible uterine abnormalities, this will include a dilatation and curettage, known as a D&C, under local or general anesthesia with possible culposcopy, looking into the cul-de sac, or hysteroscopy which is looking into the uterus. As with other areas of the body, the modality of ultrasound is frequently used to give information about the uterus and ovaries. CAT and MRI scanning is only rarely used. If the "Pap" smear shows abnormalities or "pre-cancer" cells, then a culposcopy is performed. A culposcopy is a microscopic view of the cervix and biopsies can be obtained of abnormal areas. If there is abnormal bleeding or an enlarged uterus, a biopsy of the uterus called an endometrial biopsy may be performed. Further studies might include a dilatation and curettage (D& C) or hysteroscopy (camera inside the uterus) which are done under local or general anesthesia.

In this chapter I want to discuss the benign diseases of the corpus uteri or body of the uterus and uterine cervix.

The cervix of the uterus may have the above mentioned acute infections of gonorrhea or Chlamydia with discharge and usually responds to appropriate medical regimens. Other infections such as Trichomonas and yeast are infections of the vagina.

Chronic cervicitis, a recurrent or long term disease, must be evaluated for infection and occult cancer and can be treated with antibiotics, electrocautery, laser, silver nitrate or cryosurgery (which is a cold treatment).

In the uterus itself, the usual signs of disease are abnormal vaginal bleeding, pain, and uterine enlargement and the major entities are fibroids also called leiomyomata, myomata or fibromyomata. There may also be adenomyosis, a benign condition when the lining of the uterus invades the muscle wall of the uterus, polyps which are small or large outgrowths into the center of the uterine cavity and hyperplasia which is a florid abnormal growth of the lining tissue which may be a benign or a precancerous lesion (*see* Diagram 47 next page).

Years ago most women with fibroids had hysterectomies. Today the philosophy is very different. Fibroids are only treated if they are symptomatic with pain pressure or bleeding and there is even medication, GnRH-A (gonadotrophin releasing hormone) which can be used and may shrink the fibroids in many women. GnRH-A may be used for three to six months to shrink fibroids prior to surgery or stop acute bleeding. Longer treatment leads to bone tissue loss and once the treatment is stopped, the fibroids will re-grow to their original size.

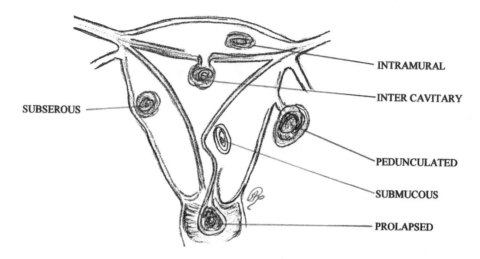

SUBSEROUS

INTRAMURAL

INTER CAVITARY

PEDUNCULATED

SUBMUCOUS

PROLAPSED

FIBROIDS OF THE UTERUS

DIAGRAM 47

Some small or asymptomatic fibroids just need to be observed on a six month to one year basis. In women who are still in the childbearing years and want more children, symptomatic fibroids can be removed surgically in a procedure called myomectomy. If the woman is past the childbearing years or wants no more children, either myomectomy or hysterectomy can be performed since fibroids usually recur.

Adenomyosis is only definitively diagnosed by the pathologist once the uterus has been removed. Because of persistent vaginal bleeding and pain, hysterectomy is often performed.

Polyps and hyperplasia can initially be treated by endometrial curettage or hormonally with progestins and if abnormal cells suggest pre-cancer and if the woman is past childbearing age, then a hysterectomy is indicated.

So let us move on to the surgeries. The usual preoperative workup is done, and checking for pregnancy should always be done in a woman of childbearing age.

The dilatation and curettage used to be a very common procedure but is now predominately used for completion of a miscarriage, termination of an unwanted pregnancy, for removal of retained placental tissue after delivery, diagnosing abnormal bleeding especially in a patient after her menopause, removal of polyps or in some cases for curetting the inner lining of the uterus for profuse hemorrhage. The patient is usually asleep and in stirrups on the operating table. The vagina is prepared and cleansed and the front of the cervical lip is held with a tenaculum, a sharp grasping instrument. Progressively larger metal rods are placed through the opening in the cervix to make the opening larger and then a curette or a metal loop shaped instrument with a sharp edge is inserted and specimens are taken of the endocervix or inner lining of the cervix if needed, and the endometrium, the inner lining of the uterus, and sent to pathology for examination. The tenaculum is removed and the site checked for bleeding. The complications include excessive bleeding and more seriously, perforation of the uterus by inadvertently putting the metal rod through the wall of the uterus into the peritoneal cavity with risk of injuring some major structure such as the intestine or causing bleeding. These are treated with watching and waiting and possibly even a laparoscopy or laparotomy if indicated. (Laparoscopy and hysteroscopy will be discussed in Chapter 77.)

The two procedures we will discuss are abdominal hysterectomy and vaginal hysterectomy and I should clarify that total hysterectomy includes removal of the uterus with the cervix, and leaves the fallopian tubes and ovaries in place. When everything is removed, it is called a total abdominal or vaginal hysterectomy and salpingo-oophorectomy.

Let me start by saying that the two most common incisions are the midline, extending from the umbilicus or bellybutton down to the symphysis pubis, the area in front of and above the mons pubis, and the Pfannenstiel, a transverse incision low in the abdomen. The Pfannenstiel is more cosmetic and many feel it is more comfortable in the post-operative period. In either case, once the skin incision is made, the muscles are separated in the midline and the abdomen entered and explored for any other pathology. Appropriate retractors are placed, and these are usually self-retaining, meaning they are held in place by mechanical arms to free the surgeon and his assistant from manually retracting. The decision to remove or leave the ovaries and tubes will have been made preoperatively although sometimes the findings at surgery may change the operative plan and the patient must be led to understand that the surgeon may have to deviate from his original plan depending on the pathology. The ureters are identified and avoided, the peritoneum is cut open and the bladder pushed away to avoid injury. The ligaments supporting the uterus and containing the great vessels to the uterus and cervix are clamped, divided and sutured and tied. The uterus and cervix are removed and the end of the vagina is sutured closed or stapled closed with absorbable staples. The peritoneum is closed posteriorly and anteriorly and the abdomen is closed in layers.

Fibroids or myomas can be removed through the same incision, leaving the uterus in place but making incisions into the uterine muscle wall and enucleating, scooping out or dissecting out the benign tumor. The muscle wall, myometrium, is carefully closed and the abdomen is closed.

The vaginal hysterectomy is performed with the patient in lithotomy position in stirrups similar to the D&C. Basically the cervix is grasped and placed on traction and the incision around the cervix is made and progressed up the side until the peritoneal cavity is entered in the appropriate place. The supporting tissues containing the blood vessels are clamped, divided and sutured until the entire uterus is brought downward with the tubes and ovaries still attached. The tubal and ovarian supporting tissues are separated from the uterus and clamped, divided and tied and the uterus is then removed through the vagina. After compete hemostasis has been confirmed with no evidence of bleeding, the wound is closed. The patient often has a urinary catheter in place for a day.

I will describe the pelvic support surgeries for cystocele, enterocele, rectocele, and incontinence surgeries when we discuss the vagina in Chapter 76.

The complications of abdominal and vaginal hysterectomies are injury to the intestine, ureter, and bladder. Most of the time these are recognized at surgery and are repaired by the gynecologists or a specialist called in to help with the repair. However, sometimes the injury is not identified until several hours or even days later and appropriate re-operation by the gynecologist in conjunction with the appropriate specialist, urologist or general surgeon, is indicated. Although the complications are not common, they do occasionally happen even in the best of hands and can usually be repaired without significant subsequent sequelae. (We will discuss laparoscopic assisted hysterectomy in Chapter 77.)

And finally just a brief note about surgery in pregnancy. On occasion patients who are pregnant may present with surgical diseases. It is felt safest to defer any elective, non-emergency, surgery until after the baby is delivered, but if this is not possible, then the surgeon tries to wait at least until after the first trimester, the first three months. The risk of losing a pregnancy to a miscarriage is very low in any case, but it is generally higher during this early period and the chances for abnormalities are of concern in the first three months. Appendectomies and gallbladder surgeries have been done on an emergency basis without any untoward problems, but the fact remains that surgery does have a remote possibility of affecting the fetus.

As far as surgery at the time of delivery, we will speak about those involving normal vaginal delivery and Cesarean section. Apparently Julius Caesar was born this way - through an abdominal incision. In the course of a vaginal delivery, an episiotomy may have to be done by the obstetrician to allow the baby's head to pass out of the vagina and prevent indiscriminate tearing of the vagina and perineum. It is basically a controlled cut made posteriorly or postero-laterally to prevent potentially harmful tissue tearing irregularly during an otherwise normal delivery. The episiotomy is then sutured closed after the baby has been delivered.

Cesarean section is done when the baby cannot be delivered vaginally either because the baby is too large, the pelvis is too small or there are complications with the mother or child that demand rapid delivery to save the child or the mother. The abdomen is opened through a Pfannenstiel incision, the uterus is opened in its lower portion and the baby is removed. One physician tends to the baby while the obstetrician closes the uterus and abdomen. The philosophy used to be "once a Cesarean section, always a Cesarean section" but many physicians have strayed away from this philosophy in an otherwise healthy woman with subsequent vaginal deliveries without complications. A trial of labor may be allowed if the previous Cesarean section was a low-transverse uterine incision and the patient understands the risks of possible uterine rupture. The obstetrician must evaluate each patient on an individual basis.

As a final note, remember, a tumor is ANY enlargement, mass or growth, and the most common tumor in the abdomen is--the Pregnant Uterus!

Chapter 75
TUBES AND TUBAL LIGATION
OVARIES

Gabriel Fallopius worked in Ferrara, Pisa and Padua, Italy and wrote
his "Observationes Anatomicae" in fifteen sixty-one.
He described the Fallopian tubes and named the vagina, the clitoris,
and the placenta
and opposed the fifteen hundred year old teachings of Galen, that son
of a gun!
He was a good friend of the famous anatomist Andreas Vesalius who
published the first great text in anatomy,
And you should always remember Fallopius every time you hear about
tubal ligation
and if I don't end this poem you're soon gonna get madatme.

This chapter is about the Fallopian tubes and the ovaries, but I want to stress that it will be about benign disease. I want to cover all the cancer of the female reproductive tract together in the Chapter 76.

The tubes and ovaries hang off either side of the uterus, with the tubes being the active conduit for the ovum or egg to reach the uterus and the sperm during the first stage of sexual reproduction.

The tubes are tied off by the obstetrician and gynecologist and a small portion cauterized and/or removed to prevent further pregnancy in the procedure called tubal ligation. It can be performed during an open procedure such as Cesarean section, or other open surgery or can be done laparoscopically through an infra-umbilical incision, in the post-partum period, after delivery of a baby. Although it is not a 100% guarantee against pregnancy, it gives about a 99.8% assurance.

The tubes are also important in that they may be the location of what is called an ectopic pregnancy, a pregnancy not in the uterus. Ectopic pregnancies in the tube cannot go to full term and the woman will have a miscarriage early in the pregnancy. The first symptoms will be pain and bleeding into the abdomen and may require an open or laparoscopic procedure which may sometimes result in the loss of the involved tube. It can also be treated medically with methotrexate in some instances. Gynecologists do all they can to preserve the Fallopian tube, but in some cases it is not possible. The tubes may also be the location of infections and abscesses, caused by organisms such as Gonorrhea and Chlamydia. These usually respond to antibiotic therapy but occasionally are so severe that an abscess forms, and open or laparoscopic surgery may be indicated and tubal removal necessary. This type of infection is usually limited to sexually active females, frequently with multiple partners. It can cause permanent scarring and may cause future problems preventing the ovum from passing down the tube and meeting the sperm. A test called a hysterosalpingogram, a study of the uterus and tubes, is done by injecting contrast dye into the uterus to see whether the tubes are open or closed, as part of an infertility test. In cases where there is severe old chronic disease in the tube, the surgeon can sometimes reconstruct the tubes and return function and fertility.

The ovaries are very complex organs, starting at menarche to produce hormones needed for the woman to develop secondary sexual characteristics. They are whitish rounded three to five centimeter organs with their own nerve, arterial and venous supply. It is an endocrine organ producing the estrogen and progestins needed for the menstrual cycle. On the surface of the ovary are microscopic follicles containing immature eggs and when a woman reaches adolescence, once about every four weeks one of the eggs matures and is extruded from the ovary eventually passing into the Fallopian tube and eventually may become fertilized. If this does not occur, it is passed from the body during menstruation.

The estrogen produced by the follicles in the ovary causes development of the breasts, growth of pubic hair, increased fat around the hips and buttocks and stimulates the growth of the lining of the uterus during the menstrual cycle. At the follicle or site of the released egg, a structure called the corpus luteum develops which produces progesterone which, among other functions, helps the fertilized egg to attach to the uterus. If the egg or ovum is not fertilized, the corpus luteum resolves and a small scar develops in the area.

So much for ovarian physiology about which hundreds of large texts have been written! What are the benign diseases? In the ovary, most masses or tumors in the woman under thirty are nonmalignant; however, after age fifty about half are cancerous, so it changes the perspective on the disease. But let us stick with the benign for now. The symptoms are usually an enlarging abdomen, pain, and tenderness. The most common are what we call functional problems, abnormal progression and regression of the corpus luteum and development of cysts, and bleeding into cysts. There may be several types of benign cysts; dermoids may contain hair, teeth, and bone and other types of tissue, endometrial cysts, simple cysts and cystadenomas.

Endometriosis is a strange benign disease where lining tissue of the uterus, the endometrium, grows in abnormal locations and may appear as tiny brownish spots on the ovaries or any other pelvic or intraperitoneal organ. It causes pain and bleeding and in the ovary may cause the development of a large cystic structure called a "chocolate cyst" because it has old blood which is brown. Other benign growths are the rarer tumors called the Brenner tumor, Leydig cell tumor, and fibroadenoma. The most important thing for the gynecologist is to make sure that it is benign and try to salvage as much normal ovary as possible. Using the diagnostic tools of ultrasound, CAT and MRI Scans and laparoscopy, the diagnosis is usually determined, but a pathological diagnosis by the pathologist is usually necessary to be absolutely certain.

Corpus luteum cysts and some other cystic masses will resolve in time and not require surgery or removal, whereas other tumors and cysts may need biopsy to confirm what they are. Occasionally cystic or solid tumors of the ovary may be found during other surgeries such as appendectomy, cholecystectomy, intestinal surgery, and the surgeon will have to use his best judgment to determine whether any partial or complete removal is indicated. In a very young woman, the tendency is to leave as much ovarian tissue as possible. In the post menopausal woman, the tendency may be to remove the ovary since the chance for malignancy is so high.

An acute problem may be torsion of the ovary, where the ovary rotates around its pedicle, the supporting tissue and blood supply, causing severe pain and occasional bleeding and must be surgically corrected by de-torsion or removal of the ovary, oophorectomy. Except in cases of huge ovarian cysts or tumors, the ovary can be evaluated and even removed through a small abdominal incision or in some cases through a laparoscope. However, I have seen ovarian cysts as large as a softball or even a football which requires a very large incision. It is important to remove the cyst or tumor intact, with its encompassing shell or capsule unbroken, so that, if it is malignant, no cancer cells will be spilled into the abdomen. (The largest ovarian cyst on record weighs 300 pounds!)

Chapter 76
VAGINA AND HYMEN

There was a young girl from Regina...
Nope - I won't even try a limerick!

In addition to describing the intrinsic problems of the vagina and hymen, I will also discuss the abnormalities of pelvic support which are apparent through vaginal examination and which can be repaired transvaginally, and the fistulas which can develop into the vagina either anteriorly, in front from the bladder, posteriorly, from behind from the rectum, or superiorly and posteriorly from the intestine. We will also describe the benign processes of the vulva.

As seen in the diagram in Chapter 73, the vulva is the term given for the external female genitalia including the labia major, labia minor, the mons veneris, the clitoris and its prepuce, the urethral opening and Bartholin's and Skene's glands.

The signs of vulvar disease may be a mass, itching or pain, burning with urination, painful intercourse called dyspareunia, and a burning sensation of the skin. With patients on antibiotics for other reasons, or diabetics or pregnant women, there may be a yeast overgrowth causing the problem which is usually Candida infection involving the vulva and vagina. It is usually very responsive to oral medication such as fluconazole, or topical vaginal creams. In young girls there may be pinworms (Enterobius vermicularis) treated with mebendazole, Trichomonas, treated with metronidazole and lice or scabies which can be treated with Kwell shampoo. Other infections due to bacteria should be appropriately cultured and treated with an antibiotic to which the organism is sensitive. Vulvitis or inflammation of the vulva may also come from irritants such as soap, vaginal lubricants, clothing and wash detergents, the latter of which would have to be eliminated from daily use. As women get beyond menopausal age, degenerative changes may occur in the vulva and vagina due to loss of estrogen support and irritation may develop; local or systemic estrogen usually resolves the situation. Then there are a whole list of other contributing causes of vulvar pathology including tumors, and dietary problems. After taking a complete history and doing a careful exam and possible biopsy, the gynecologist will have a good idea as to the cause or diagnostic workup needed and will then prescribe the appropriate therapy.

Viral infections in this area include condyloma acuminatum or warty excrescences which can be removed with cautery or lasers or sometimes by surgical excision under local or general anesthesia depending on the extent of the disease.

Another viral disease, Herpes (herpes simplex) causes painful irritation and blisters which respond to antiviral agents, such as acyclovir, but is never completely cured. The incidence of recurrence can be markedly decreased using the proper agents but infection during late pregnancy and delivery demands that the baby be delivered by Cesarean section.

A woman may be born with an imperforate hymen, meaning there is no opening at the exit of the vagina, and no fluids can exit the vagina. Usually this is not diagnosed until puberty when blood and mucous will back up into the vagina, called hematocolpos, uterus, called hematometrium, tubes, hematosalpinx or even the abdomen, hematoperitoneum. The therapy, under general anesthesia, is opening the hymen or removing it completely with rapid resolution of the problem.

Infections, cysts or abscesses of the small vulvar glands need antibiotic treatment, or incision and drainage. In severe cases of a large Bartholin cyst or abscess, surgical excision may be necessary. Small asymptomatic cysts can be left alone.

Vaginal infections have been discussed with the vulva and require appropriate culture and sensitivity or "smears" and examination under a microscope to make the correct diagnosis prior to treatment.

The uterus and vagina as well as the bladder and rectum are dependent upon the pelvic support tissue to prevent these structures from falling out through the vagina; there is a complex system of fascia and musculature. With pregnancy, the pelvic floor is stretched and may be overdistended during delivery. Often there are few symptoms until after the woman has gone through the menopause when more pelvic tissue atrophy occurs and the pelvic support is lessened. The following diagram shows where each weakness occurs and which organ will protrude into which area of the vagina, and the protrusion is into the wall of the vagina, not through the wall into the vagina itself (*See* Diagram 48 next page).

Cystocele contains bladder and urethrocele contains urethra protruding into the anterior vagina; rectocele contains rectum posteriorly and the ent-

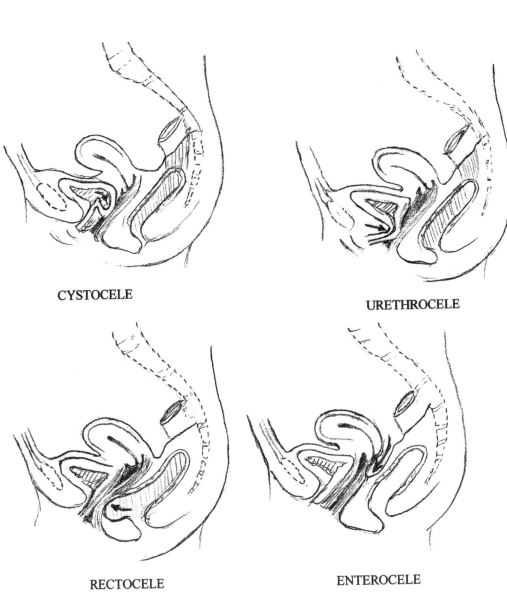

CYSTOCELE

URETHROCELE

RECTOCELE

ENTEROCELE

DIAGRAM 48

erocele contains small intestine or sigmoid colon postero-superiorly. When these problems are minimal, sometimes exercise and strengthening of the pelvic muscles will allay some of the symptoms, especially stress incontinence.

Although I can't go into a detailed description of the repairs, suffice it to say that each of these defects can be repaired through a vaginal incision. The cysto-urethrocele or bladder and urethra, needs to be repaired only when symptomatic with pelvic pressure, stress incontinence and recurrent urinary tract infections. They can be repaired in a transvaginal procedure called an anterior colporrhaphy as well as other procedures by urologists performed transabdominally called urethral sling and retropubic suspensions. They are all strengthening the pelvic floor and the angle at which the urethra exits the body so that there is no urine loss with stress.

The rectocele often accompanies the cysto-urethrocele and this along with the enterocele can be repaired transvaginally or transabdominally. Symptoms include difficulty defecating often requiring pressure to the posterior vaginal wall to force fecal material out of the invaginated rectal segment. The fascial and muscular tissue is brought together during this repair called a posterior-colpo-perineorrhaphy or posterior repair. The anterior and posterior repairs are often done in conjunction with a vaginal hysterectomy.

Prolapse of the uterus is again a failure of the pelvic floor but in this case the uterus prolapses or falls out through the vagina. In patients who are very poor operative candidates, the prolapsing uterus can be held in place with a device called a pessary, but for the active otherwise healthy woman, this is a poor substitute for definitive treatment, namely vaginal hysterectomy usually combined with an anterior and posterior repair.

Now for fistulas. What is a fistula? It is an abnormal passage or connection between one organ and another. When we use the word recto-vaginal it means a fistula from the rectum into the vagina, enterovaginal is intestine to the vagina and vesico-vaginal is from the bladder or sometimes the ureter, to the vagina.

Vesicovaginal fistulas used to occur because of traumatic vaginal deliveries with extensive vaginal tears, but are relatively uncommon from this cause today, in Western medicine. Most vesicovaginal fistulas are secondary to complex surgery, infection or radiation. The woman presents with small or large amounts of clear fluid coming from the vagina and the fistula opening may be so small that it is difficult to find. After appropriate studies including a cystogram and careful vaginal exam the size is determined and the therapy undertaken. Usually a Foley catheter is placed in the bladder to divert the urine stream from the fistula and if the opening is very small, it will close over a month or two. If it is large, then an operation is needed; it was always the custom to wait several months before attempting the removal of the fistula and repair of the bladder and vagina, to let the tissue surrounding the fistula "soften", but now many gynecologists or urologists are doing immediate repairs with great success, either trans-vaginally or trans-abdominally through the bladder.

Enterovaginal fistulas may occur secondary to injury during surgery, because of severe intra-abdominal infection or from inflammatory bowel disease, Crohn's disease, and presents with foul-smelling vaginal discharge. This type of fistula rarely closes with antibiotics or resolution of the inflammatory process, and usually requires an intra-abdominal surgery with resection of the fistula as well as the part of the intestine from which it was coming.

Colovesical fistulas occur from tissue injuries after major cancer surgeries, directly due to cancers, due to severe infections such as perforated diverticulitis or secondary to tissue weakening from pelvic radiation for rectal or pelvic cancer. This type of fistula presents with fecal material coming from the vagina and is difficult to manage. The prime treatment is diversion of the fecal stream which means bringing out a loop of colon proximal to and above the level of the fistula. In layman's terms this is a colostomy or loop of large intestine brought out to the skin; a special apparatus with a bag is placed over the opening or stoma. It takes at least a month or two for a patient to become used to living with a colostomy, after which the care becomes second nature. Colostomies for colovesical fistulas secondary to inflammation or injury after pelvic surgery may be temporary and one to two months after the procedure the fistula may close spontaneously. If the fistula does not close on its own a surgical procedure by a general surgeon is indicated. After the fistula is closed, the colostomy can also be closed in a separate surgery and normal bowel function returns. However, in the case of severe injury to the pelvis by radiation or cancer, the fistula may never close and the colostomy may have to be permanent (*see* Chapter 34).

Chapter 77
GYNECOLOGICAL ONCOLOGY
FEMALE CANCER

The woman was worried about pain and some bleeding,
And became so upset 'cause her friends were misleading.
"It's nothing, or else if it's something it's terrible",
The suggestions were foolish and all quite unbearable.

So she went to her doctor who examined her gently,
And spoke of her problem quite intelligently.
She didn't have need for a cancer apologist,
She could go to a gynecological oncologist.

Indeed she had cancer, but the news was encouraging,
Not bleak and disarming or frankly discouraging.
The tumor was treated by experts with care,
And for the next twenty Christmases - she'll be there!

I have grouped the gynecological cancers together under a single chapter because I feel strongly that they indeed belong under the care of one person...the gynecological surgical oncologist. This is a specialist who has mastered the field of obstetrics and gynecology and then gone on to have an intensive two to four year fellowship of additional training in the management of the many gynecological malignancies.

All too often this type of cancer was misdiagnosed or mistreated by the well-meaning family physician or gynecologist. And I don't mean to be overly critical; this was the way these cases were handled for one hundred years and the management met the standard of practice in the community. Now, however, the standard is changing along with new complex surgical procedures, new diagnostic tests, chemotherapy and radiation therapy that has significantly decreased the morbidity and mortality of these malignant diseases.

Several years ago when I assisted on a complex ovarian cancer operation performed by gynecological surgical oncologist, Dr. Michael Berman (no relation), I was impressed with his surgical technique in handling not only the female organs, but also his ability to operate on a cancer which had spread to the intestine, the omentum, the bladder, the liver, diaphragm and stomach. His surgical technique was excellent and he completed the complex procedure rapidly and efficiently with minimal blood loss. At a post-surgical tumor conference, he discussed the case and his comprehensive approach to the disease. This was the physician I wanted to handle gynecological cancer in my family!

I emphasize that from the preoperative workup, the case evaluation and the special diagnostic procedures, to the definitive surgery and postoperative chemotherapy or radiation, you need to have a skilled specialist who can be the captain of the ship, and this is the gynecological surgical oncologist. Let us move on to the diseases.

The vulva is an area that can be affected by a number of named premalignant diseases which I will name for you. These are: leukoplakia-- whitish patches of tissue, kraurosis vulvae, and a number of venereal diseases such as syphilis and gonorrhea. The cancer may be very limited such as carcinoma in situ, called VIN-vulvar intraepithelial neoplasia, and the treatment is surgical removal of the vulva with simple vulvectomy.

If the cancer is more extensive it is usually called a squamous cell carcinoma arising from the squamous epithelium or skin and less commonly adenocarcinoma, arising from a skin gland. These cancers are much more virulent and must be treated with a radical vulvectomy.

Many surgeons also recommend dissection of the local lymph nodes. Unfortunately cancer of the vulva is occasionally associated with other gynecological cancers and can sometimes spread widely before it is removed. This type of cancer is not sensitive to radiation therapy and the main treatment is wide excision and careful observation. Depending on the local extension of the cancer into the vagina, rectum or urethra, very radical surgery called pelvic exenteration may be indicated. This involves removal of all the pelvic organs including the bladder, rectum, and lymph nodes as well as the vulva, vagina, uterus, tubes and ovaries. Quite an undertaking, but resulting in a higher cure rate than the lesser procedures.

Cancer of the vagina is relatively rare. As opposed to vulvar cancer, it is radiosensitive and this is usually the treatment of choice. The morbidity is related to the radiation effect on the bladder and rectum with transient proctitis and cystitis. It is much more successful with less morbidity than surgical removal of the vagina.

Cancer of the cervix is a preventable disease! What a statement you may say; but it's true. With the use of the "Pap" smear, abnormal cells can be found which will show the presence of carcinoma in situ or pre-invasive cancer of the cervix. This is a 100% curable disease and if all women got regular Pap tests, the pre-invasive cancer would never progress to the stage of invasive cancer. This is important to know because pre-invasive cancer of the cervix is completely asymptomatic - no pain, no bleeding, no mass! So ladies - get your regular Pap tests.

Patients with this disease can be treated with cautery, conization of the cervix, or cutting away the outer layer of the cervix, laser vaporization or cryosurgery, which is freezing therapy. This will cure the disease in most cases but the patient needs to be rechecked on a regular basis. When there is extensive carcinoma in situ or recurrent disease, then an abdominal or vaginal hysterectomy is indicated with removal of some vagina. In cases of carcinoma in situ occurring during pregnancy, local treatment will usually suffice and the pregnancy is allowed to continue; however, if invasive cancer develops, a discussion with the gynecological oncologist will determine whether or not to terminate the pregnancy.

Carcinoma of the cervix and carcinoma in situ have been linked to cigarette smoking, herpes simplex virus type II and perhaps the human papilloma virus.

The International Federation of Gynecology and Obstetrics (FIGO) has developed a staging system for carcinoma of the cervix which I will list for you. Not that you will remember any of the details, but you can see the diagnostic expertise that is demanded of the physician, who will use the staging to determine the appropriate treatment of this disease (*See* Diagram 49 next page).

I want to give you some idea on the treatment of this disease; however, you can understand how difficult a complete dissertation on this subject would be. To be very brief, let me give you the following outline.

For Stage IA, microinvasive cervical cancer, a simple hysterectomy may be sufficient with an almost 100% cure rate. Stage IB and IIA, early invasive cervical cancer, requires a radical hysterectomy and extensive lymph node dissection or radiation therapy or combinations of both these modalities. The cure rate depends on the extent of the disease. Stage IIB to IVA, locally advanced cervical cancers, are treated primarily with radiation therapy and there are many methods and locations for delivering

FIGO Staging System for Cervical Cancer

Stage	Characteristic
0	Carcinoma in situ
I	The carcinoma is strictly confined to the cervix (extension to the corpus should be disregarded)
Ia	Preclinical carcinomas of the cervix; that is, those diagnosed only by microscopy
Ia1	Minimal microscopically evident stromal invasion
Ia2	Lesions detected microscopically that can be measured. The upper limit of the measurement should not show a depth of invasion of more than 5 mm taken from the base of the epithelium, either surface or glandular, from which it originates, and a second dimension, the horizontal spread, must not exceed 7 mm. Larger lesions should be staged as Ib
Ib	Lesions of greater dimensions than Stage Ia2 whether seen clinically or not. Preformed space involvement should not alter the staging but should be specifically recorded so as to determine whether it should affect treatment decisions in the future
II	Involvement of the vagina but not the lower third, or infiltration of the parametria but not out to the sidewall
IIa	Involvement of the vagina but no evidence of parametrial involvement
IIb	Infiltration of the parametria but not out to the sidewall
III	Involvement of the lower third of the vagina or extension to the pelvic sidewall
IIIa	Involvement of the lower third of the vagina but not out to the pelvic sidewall if the parametria are involved
IIIb	Involvement of one or both parametria out to the sidewall
III (urinary)	Obstruction of one or both ureters on intravenous pyelogram (IVP) without the other criteria for stage III disease
IV	Extension outside the reproductive tract
IVa	Involvement of the mucosa of the bladder or rectum
IVb	Distant metastasis or disease outside the true pelvis

DIAGRAM 49

the treatment. Understandably, as the stage of the disease gets higher, the cure rate gets lower. This does not mean that patients may not live for many productive years even with active disease.

Next we will discuss cancer of the endometrium of the uterus. This is the most common gynecological cancer, and is most common in the 50-70 years old age group. Although the etiology of this cancer is unknown, there appears to be some relationship between prolonged unopposed estrogen replacement, (i.e. no progestins) as well as obesity, diabetes mellitus, hypertension, early menarche, late menopause, and one or no children. Postmenopausal bleeding, or excessive premenopausal bleeding are the major symptoms and Pap smears may not show the cancer. When the symptoms suggest endometrial cancer, dilatation and curettage are indicated to evaluate and stage the disease along with ultrasound, CAT or MRI scans of the pelvis. A good pelvic exam may reveal significant abnormalities in size and shape of the uterus which may be highly suggestive of malignancy.

Similar to carcinoma of the cervix, uterine endometrial cancer is staged by the FIGO, as in Diagram 50. The treatment and survival rates are directly related to the stage, as well as the pathologist's grading of the tumor, and how abnormal the cells are and what type of cells are present.

FIGO (1988) Staging System for Endometrial Cancer

Stages	Characteristics
IA G123	Tumor limited to endometrium
IB G123	Invasion to < ½ myometrium
IC G123	Invasion to > ½ myometrium
IIA G123	Endocervical glandular involvement only
IIB G123	Cervical stromal invasion
IIIA G123	Tumor invades serosa or adnexae or positive peritoneal cytology
IIIB G123	Vaginal metastases
IIIC G123	Metastases to pelvic or para-aortic lymph nodes
IVA G123	Tumor invasion bladder and/or bowel mucosa
IVB	Distant metastases including intra-abdominal and/or inguinal lymph node

DIAGRAM 50

Stage I disease can be managed by an abdominal hysterectomy with bilateral salpingo-oophorectomy, possibly with radiation therapy added. Radical surgery is not used frequently because the success rates with standard hysterectomy, radiation and chemotherapy were found to be better. Patients with extensive or recurrent disease often respond to chemotherapeutic agents tailored to each individual case; these include Tamoxifen, Paclitaxel, Doxorubicin, Platinum and Progestins.

Ovarian cancer is predominantly of the type called epithelial; the other two are much rarer, called stromal and germ cell malignancies. A small percentage of ovarian cancers may be familial and present in individuals who have mutations or changes in the gene BRCA 1. Early diagnosis of ovarian cancer can sometimes be helped by obtaining the serum marker CA-125; however, I should emphasize that there is really no screening test for ovarian cancer. Because CA-125 can be elevated in many conditions, using it as a screening modality would lead to many surgeries for no disease or benign disease.

Ovarian cancer does not present with early symptoms and if the diagnosis is not made incidently, as during another surgery or laparoscopy, the tumor may already have reached a more advanced stage before it is identified. Early tumors have no pain or bleeding and even advanced cancer may only present as weight gain from fluid in the abdomen called ascites, vague abdominal discomfort and poor appetite. Most cancers are Grade III by the time of diagnosis, with ascites, involvement of the omentum or fatty apron in the abdomen and spread throughout the surface of the organs in the abdomen. Once again we will turn to the FIGO staging system to evaluate a cancer.

FIGO (1986) Staging System for Ovarian Cancer

Stage	Characteristic
I	Growth limited to the ovaries
IA	Growth limited to one ovary; no ascites; no tumor on the external surfaces, capsule intact
IB	Growth limited to both ovaries; no ascites; no tumor on the external surfaces, capsule intact
IC	Tumor either stage IA or stage IB but with tumor on the surface of one or both ovaries, or with capsule ruptured, or with ascites containing malignant cells or with positive peritoneal washings
II	Growth involving one or both ovaries on pelvic extension
IIA	Extension or metastases to the uterus or tubes
IIB	Extension to other pelvic tissues
IIC	Tumor either stage IIA or IIB with tumor on the surface of one or both ovaries, or with capsule(s) ruptured, or with ascites containing malignant cells or with positive peritoneal washings
III	Tumor involving one or both ovaries with peritoneal implants outside the pelvis or positive retroperitoneal or inguinal nodes; superficial liver metastases equals stage III; tumor is limited to the true pelvis but with histologically verified malignant extension to small bowel or omentum
IIIA	Tumor grossly limited to the true pelvis with negative nodes but with histologically confirmed microscopic seeding of abdominal peritoneal surfaces
IIIB	Tumor of one or both ovaries; histologically confirmed implants of abdominal peritoneal surfaces, none exceeding 2 cm in diameter; nodes negative
IIIC	Abdominal implants greater than 2 cm in diameter or positive retroperitoneal or inguinal nodes
IV	Growth involving one or both ovaries with distant metastases; if pleural effusion is present, there must be positive cytologic test results to allot a case to stage IV; parenchymal liver metastases equals stage IV

DIAGRAM 51

In the rare case of a young woman with stage IA disease, a removal of just that ovary and tube may be acceptable. In addition, the gynecological oncologist discusses the case with the pathologist to help understand not only the stage of the disease but also the grade to see how virulent or how malignant the cells look. Generally a much more vigorous approach is recommended for treatment of ovarian carcinoma, including total abdominal hysterectomy and bilateral salpingo-oophorectomy. This is often followed by systemic chemotherapy.

The term debulking is used in relationship to ovarian cancer because it has been determined that chemotherapeutic treatment is better if the surgeon can remove all areas of cancer implantation greater than 1-2 cm. In other words, there may be extensive cancer metastasis throughout the peritoneal cavity, but if the surgeon can remove most of the gross tumor so that each area is less than 1-2 cm., then the chance of the patient getting an excellent response from chemotherapy is markedly improved. This takes great surgical skill and patience in procedures that can take several hours to complete adequately. This kind of surgery, debulking, is also known as cytoreduction surgery. Small superficial tumor implants can be burned away with an argon beam coagulator which does not penetrate deeply into tissue and does a good job of destroying cancer on the surface of an organ.

The nature of the chemotherapy is beyond the scope of our discussion except to say that many of the chemotherapeutic regimens are platinum based and that paclitaxel is also used. When patients have advanced ovarian carcinoma, complications occur in the abdomen related to the tumor involvement of the intestine and patients may present with partial or complete intestinal obstruction which may be surgically corrected, by removing portions of the bowel or by bypassing the obstructed area, a decision that must be made by the surgeon at the operating table.

Chapter 78
LAPAROSCOPY

To further our skills in diagnoscopy,
We developed gynecological laparoscopy,
To look at your ovaries and tubes was the goal,
With a camera inserted through a one half inch hole.

We can now stop all thoughts about new procreation
With laparoscopic tubal ligation.
And through the small scope with a little narcosis,
You doctor will rid you of endometriosis.

We've given you an introduction to laparoscopy in Chapter 15, but I wanted to emphasize how much this procedure has become a regular part of the gynecologic armamentarium. In the past, the physician had to rely on x-ray for diagnosis and open surgery for confirmation, biopsies and even tubal ligation. Now through the laparoscope, a complete evaluation of the intraperitoneal pelvic organs can be done in a very simple procedure. Visual staging of ovarian cancer can be done, and in certain cases biopsies can be taken. Fallopian tubes can be ligated, endometriosis implants can be cauterized, and suspicious areas can be visualized and open surgery be done if needed. Large benign ovarian cysts can be evaluated and bleeding from an ovary controlled through this procedure. Laparoscopic assisted abdominal hysterectomy can be performed and when there is a question about appendicitis versus other pelvic disease, a laparoscopic "look" can be done with minimal discomfort post-operatively.

"Second look" procedures, looking into the abdomen months after an initial operation or after chemotherapy such as that for ovarian carcinoma and even for pelvic lymph node biopsies have become routine for the gynecologist and gynecologic oncologist. With better instrumentation and broader experience and training, more extensive gynecologic procedures will be done through the laparoscope.

Chapter 79
TRAUMA

I know a neurosurgeon and she's very, very smart,
She can tell a broken ankle from a pelvis or a heart
I've never seen her operate, I'm told she's very vain,
She surgerized the scarecrow so that he could have a brain!

The scarecrow hadn't said much, except golly and pshaw,
(I guess I wouldn't either if my brain was made of straw),
The surgeon used some cautery to get into his head,
Poor scarecrow's brain went up in flame and now the fellow's dead.

The Lion's very angry, and wants to chew and rip her,
Dorothy got mad and beaned her with a ruby slipper.
They're suing the neurosurgeon for all their suffering and pain,
Scarecrow never will walk upon that yellow brick road again.

I have proposed to cover all of neurosurgery in four chapters, and since you are all budding neurosurgeons, I am afraid your buds will never bloom. Well, let's get on with it anyway. I'll start by giving the most basic anatomy of the brain and spinal cord so that the explanations will make sense. The major factors we should bear in mind are that the brain cells are poor at repairing themselves in childhood and get worse as we age. Sometimes the brain compensates for a loss in one area by using another area, but in general, once there is severe injury or loss, there is no ability to transplant brain tissue - at least not at the time of this writing. We must also note that the brain is housed in a solid structure, the cranium or bony skull, and while acting to protect the brain against injury from the outside, it also prevents it from expanding when something goes wrong from the inside. When there is bleeding or infection and abscess, or a tumor in the brain, unlike in the abdomen or areas covered with "soft" tissue, it cannot be pushed to another area, it just gets pressed against the skull and the brain tissue is further damaged.

Similarly, the soft spinal cord is housed in the firm spinal canal to protect it from external injury but tumor or bleeding or bony problems cause damaging compression on the cord which may lead to irreversible neurological damage. The diagrams below show the most basic anatomy of the brain and spinal cord with some focus on the blood vessels, and nerve pathways, with the sensory nerve distributions (what levels in the spinal cord control sensation in what areas of the body). Knowing what is functioning and what is not helps the neurosurgeon and neurologist determine the exact location of the pathology, whether it be trauma, infection, disease or tumor.

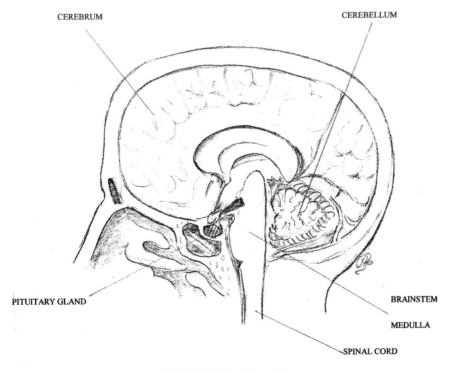

ANATOMY OF THE BRAIN

DIAGRAM 52

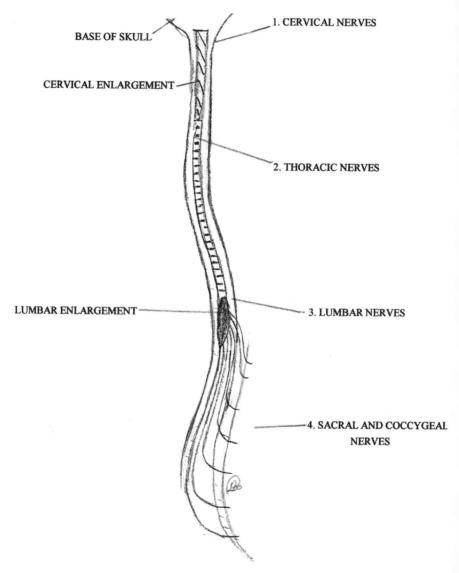

BASE OF SKULL

1. CERVICAL NERVES

CERVICAL ENLARGEMENT

2. THORACIC NERVES

LUMBAR ENLARGEMENT

3. LUMBAR NERVES

4. SACRAL AND COCCYGEAL
NERVES

ANATOMY OF THE SPINAL CORD

DIAGRAM 52

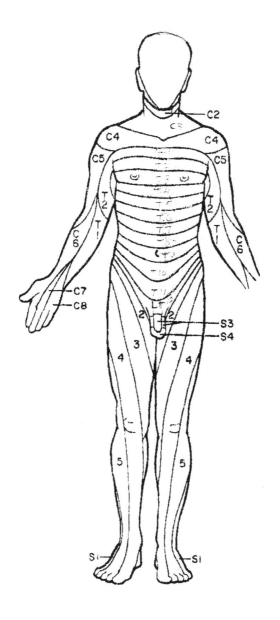

SENSORY NERVE DISTRIBUTION

DIAGRAM 53

The brain is made up of gray matter and white matter. The gray matter consists of the nerve cells, the little gray cells of Hercule Poirot - Agatha Christie's Belgian detective. The white matter is the myelinated nerves or axons with a white cover or sheath--the arms that stretch from one nerve cell to another or from a nerve cell to the end organ (muscle, skin, etc.). In the anatomy above, I have briefly outlined the areas of the brain responsible for movement, sensory, hearing, vision, balance and smell. The spinal cord has the nerve fibers which carry information from and to the brain. The motor fibers, the cortico-spinal and anterior horn tracts carry the instructions from the motor cortex to the muscles and allow movement. The sensory fibers, in the spinothalamic and dorsal column, carry stimulus information from all parts of the body to the brain for interpretation as pain, touch, vibration, heat, cold, taste, smell and etc.

The carotid and vertebral arteries supply the brain through the networks of vessels known as the Circle of Willis and these major vessels as well as the smaller arteries are well understood by the neuroradiologists, neurologists and neurosurgeons.

This chapter is entitled Trauma and we will discuss injuries to the brain and the spinal cord taking into consideration the factors which face the surgeon in his assessment of the situation.

The first consideration is the history and physical examination. The history will include the nature of the trauma, level of consciousness, nausea, vomiting, visual or hearing disturbance, weakness or paralysis, loss or change of sensation, memory problems and altered speech, to name a few. The physical examination includes checking all the above and noting changes which occur over a short period of time to assess whether there is an urgent situation which needs immediate surgical intervention. This could be a patient who comes to the emergency room alert and suddenly becomes confused or comatose, or the progressive development of a motor or sensory disorder. The Glasgow Coma Scale is used to evaluate brain function (*see* Diagram 54 next page).

After a general consideration of the acuiteness of the situation, certain diagnostic studies are indicated and these include x-rays of the head and spine for fractures, CAT and MRI scans, and several other more technical studies such as the positron emission tomography known as the PET scan, electroencephalogram called EEG, to measure brain function, and sometimes a spinal fluid analysis by spinal tap, done with a needle placed into the spinal canal to look for blood or pus.

THE GLASGOW COMA SCALE

EYE RESPONSE	None	1
	To pain	2
	To voice stimulus	3
	Spontaneously	4
SPOKEN RESPONSE	None	1
	Sounds only	2
	Inappropriate words	3
	Speaks but confused	4
	Normal speech	5
MOTION	None	1
	Minimal-unconscious extenmsion	2
	Minimal-some unconscious flextion	3
	Withdrawl response	4
	Responds locally to pain	5
	Normal	6
	Totals	3-15

DIAGRAM 54

Further studies may include an arteriogram looking for bleeding or abnormal blood vessels.

Trauma to the head, brain and spinal cord, often from motor vehicle accidents or falls, accounts for a large proportion of the morbidity and death among young people. Every family has had minor head injuries to children with lacerations from one cause or another and you know how much bleeding can come from a relatively small opening in the scalp. However, the emergency room physician must look beyond the obvious simple laceration and assume the worst until proven otherwise. A scalp wound can lose a large amount of blood and certainly can account for a lowered blood pressure, but the examiner must look for the skull fracture or the penetrating wound of the head and brain before deciding to sew up the laceration. A skull x-ray may even show what is called a "depressed skull fracture" where the bone is actually pressing in on the brain with the potential of causing brain injury. These serious types of wounds need to be evaluated, cleansed and repaired in the operating room.

Skull fractures, if small, and non depressed can usually just be observed; more complex fractures may need careful treatment in surgery.

Sometimes the appearance of bilateral black eyes, the raccoon sign, will indicate basal skull fracture. Another finding, Battle's sign, is ecchymosis or black and blue behind the ears. Since the nasal sinuses are just below the brain, separated by the base of the skull, when there is a basal skull fracture, there may be cerebrospinal fluid coming out of the nose. Most of these situations resolve without surgery, but the occasional case will need neurosurgical intervention.

When the head hits something like a dashboard, the sudden deceleration or rotational forces can cause an immediate primary injury to the brain destroying white and gray matter. After the primary injury, there may be bleeding and swelling causing secondary injury to brain tissue, further aggravated by systemic problems such as low blood pressure with poor perfusion of the brain and hypoxia with less oxygen delivered to the brain.

Whereas the initial injury may be a concussion with temporary loss of consciousness, and may be mild with no permanent injury to brain tissue, there may be moderate or severe injuries with irreversible brain damage due to the initial insult. The surgeon can't do much about that situation but it is incumbent upon him to recognize and rapidly treat the secondary problems and prevent further brain damage. Bleeding and brain swelling, called cerebral edema, will cause an increase in the pressure inside the skull. To prevent this, the surgeon may need to do a craniotomy, which means opening up the skull or cranium and remove blood clots and/or give steroids, and diuretics. High blood pressure must be controlled and the combative patient sometimes needs to be medically paralyzed or sedated to prevent motion of the head which will cause more secondary brain injury. In general, the prognosis is based on the severity of the injury, the stability of the neurological signs, the nature of the other bodily injuries and the age of the patient. Younger patients seem to have a better brain healing capacity than older individuals.

Let us talk about two types of post-traumatic bleeding. The first is called the epidural hematoma and if you refer back to the anatomy chart, it occurs between the inside of the skull called the inner table, and the dura mater. Bleeding from veins is usually not very serious in this area because of the low pressure in the venous system. However, arterial bleeding can be devastating. These injuries usually occur after a blow to the head, and the patient may have had a transient loss of consciousness. When presenting at the ER he/she may be totally alert, the so-called lucid interval; the careful physician will always do a CAT scan of the brain with this type of injury. If not, the patient may have no symptoms, be discharged home, only to be brought back to the hospital a few hours later with irreversible brain damage. Once the epidural hematoma is found or suspected, an emergency neurosurgical procedure is done to control the bleeding and evacuate the hematoma, allowing the compressed brain to re-expand. Unfortunately individuals with epidural hematomas often don't come to the ER soon enough or are so asymptomatic when seen that they are sent home only to return in a coma. The mortality rate is quite high.

The methods of opening the skull are numerous, but all consist of either using a special drill to make a small hole (trephination - like the ancient Aztecs except a little more modern) or several holes. Then, using other apparatus, the holes are joined by cutting the cranial bone and a piece of skull removed, giving access to the brain and its coverings. When the operation is done, the bone is replaced and actually sutured or glued in place with special glue.

The other bleeding condition is called the subdural hematoma, more common in the very young and very old. This type of bleeding occurs under the dura and involves veins which are a low pressure system. As opposed to the epidural hematoma, the patient may have very gradual onset of symptoms as the hematoma gets slowly larger and this can take hours, days or weeks! The signs may be changes in mental status or weakness or other neurological symptoms. The diagnosis is often made and confirmed by CAT scan and is treated by drainage of the blood clots in surgery.

Spinal cord injuries occur when the bony protection of the spine around the cord is disrupted by fracture, or the cord is injured by hyperextension, gunshot wounds, or acute herniation or protrusion of a disc into the spinal canal. You're aware of the precautions that are taken after potential neck or back injury, such as careful immobilization before movement, to prevent further injury and neurological damage. The patient needs immediate x-ray and neurological evaluation, stabilization of the condition, and correction and relief of any cord compression. This may initially involve special traction devises, such as a halo and tongs, and procedures which fuse the vertebra to prevent motion and cord injury.

With the trauma, there may be anything from no cord injury and no neurological findings to complete transection with complete paralysis and sensory loss. Injuries in the lower lumbar region may produce symptoms of loss of bladder or bowel control or changes in the reflexes when the doctor taps your knee with a rubber hammer, as well as motor and sensory changes. Often, when there is compression or partial injury, there will be return of some or all function if the primary injury is stabilized and secondary injury is prevented. Recovery from neurological injury can take days, weeks or months. When there is transection or very severe spinal cord injury, there is usually no recovery of function below the level of the injury and treatment is directed towards retraining the individual to function as well as possible with his deficits.

There is much research now in repairing spinal cord injuries, but it is still in the experimental stages. Hopefully, some day we will be able to return function in patients who now have to live with paraplegia or quadriplegia from devastating spinal cord injuries.

Chapter 80
BRAIN TUMORS
AND BRAIN ANEURYSMS

Meningioma is a benign tumor of the brain
Which used to be fatal, were it to remain,
But the deft neurosurgeon can now extirpate it,
Or in other words he can just eliminate it.

At the beginning of the twentieth century, with x-rays and anesthesia came a new breed of specialist, the neurosurgeon. With the advances in technique, instrumentation and antibiotics came the ability to successfully remove brain tumors. Although the prognosis with malignant tumors remains poor, the outlook for even large benign meningiomas, a special type of tumor arising from tissue called the arachnoid layer, changed from very poor to very good. Because of the uniformly poor results in the late eighteen hundreds, the number of individuals attempting neurosurgery decreased in the first decade of the twentieth century leaving only a handful of surgeons who specialized in this area. They became very skillful and adept at removing what were heretofore unresectable tumors. Today, the brain surgeon has at his disposal all types of diagnostic tools including CAT and MRI scan, angiography, and nuclear medicine scans and operating room microscopes, stereotactic biopsy apparatus and complex computer technology. This enables him/her to delve deep into the brain into previously unreachable areas without causing irreparable neurological dysfunction. In this chapter I want to give you a few of the names of the more common tumors and will also describe the aneurysms of the brain and how they are handled.

Brain tumors are divided into benign and malignant; however, unless they are removed, the benign tumors may be fatal because of the pressure they may exert on the brain tissue and the damage they cause to vital structures. Astrocytomas, malignant tumors arising from the supporting tissue in the brain, may present, as do many brain abnormalities, with mental changes, headaches, nausea, vomiting, and seizures. In childhood they may be low grade and after removal many children may have as high as 70-80% long term survival. If the tumor partially involves a vital structure, it may not be completely removable and can then be treated with radiation and sometimes with chemotherapy. Although there may be some long term survivals, malignant gliomas, called astrocytoma, grade 1,2 and 3, medulloblastoma, and ependymoma, are uniformly fatal in the long run, but the survival length may be tremendously variable and the patients often can lead very productive lives while undergoing therapy.

As opposed to these types of tumors, the meningioma is a relatively benign tumor although there are some malignant varieties. It causes symptoms relative to its relation to structures in the brain including visual problems, altered mentation, weakness, sensory changes, nausea, and vomiting, and often can grow very large before it is diagnosed. It was often said that meningiomas were "malignant" in their behavior; because when they couldn't be excised, they would cause death from local compression or by increasing intracranial pressure and causing the brain stem, which is responsible for many vital functions, to herniate or protrude through the base of the skull and crush itself. Complete removal of meningiomas is now attempted and often accomplished. Those that cannot be completely removed are often subjected to postoperative radiation to prevent recurrence. Radiation does destroy some non-tumor brain cells and can impact a patient's intellectual function, so, if it can be avoided, that is best. We will discuss newer procedures including radiosurgery in Chapter 83.

Tumors of the pituitary gland, in the center of the brain can now be approached through the roof of the mouth or through the nose and base of the brain with great success. Other benign tumors called Schwanno-mas, coming from cells that surround the nerve axons, are often found in the area of the nerves of hearing and are thus called acoustic neuromas. These tumors are treated surgically and are completely curable unless the tumor is very large.

Almost a fourth of all brain tumors are metastatic cancers from other areas such as lung, breast, colon. kidney and skin melanomas. They also present with symptoms of mental changes, headaches, weakness and seizures. When there is a solitary metastasis to the brain, and it is surgically accessible, it is often removed to relieve symptoms and in rare cases possibly to effect a cure. With inoperable tumors or with multiple metastatic lesions, there is often a role for radiation therapy to alleviate symptoms. Metastatic cancer to the lining of the brain, the meninges, can sometimes be palliated with chemotherapy injected directly into the ventricles of the brain. Although the prognosis is poor, there have been some long term survival. The physician, the patient and the patient's family have to discuss and agree upon the course of action, weighing the quality of the patient's life. (Tumors of the spinal cord discussed in the next chapter.)

We were first introduced to aneurysms in Chapter 54. An aneurysm is a pathologic dilatation of an artery sometimes caused by a ballooning out of a side wall. The aneurysms occur in different areas of the brain but most often in the carotid artery circulation and in the circle of Willis. Some are congenital and some are from arteriosclerosis. The symptoms of aneurysm may vary from none to visual problems and headache. If the aneurysm ruptures and bleeds, it is called a subarachnoid hemorrhage which depending on the extent of the bleeding and the location, may cause minimal symptoms of headaches and slight nuchal (neck) rigidity to deep coma and complete paralysis leading to death. The subarachnoid hemorrhage grading scale of I-V is used to evaluate the patient and then the exact location and diagnosis is made by CAT scan, spinal tap, and cerebral angiography to delineate the aneurysm, or arteriovenous malformation, another vascular abnormality which can cause bleeding into the brain. The aneurysm is treated medically by lowering the blood pressure, elevating the head with strict bed rest, with treatment directed to prevent seizures and spasm of small blood vessels which could cause a stroke. The eventual, definitive treatment for most accessible aneurysms is surgical.

The neurosurgeon, using an operating microscope, dissects out the aneurysm and places a metal clip at its base. If this is not possible, sometimes a neuroradiologist can actually cause the feeding vessels of the aneurysms to clot off, preventing a rupture. This method, as with surgery, in some cases may cause a stroke because of occlusion of a needed artery. Of course aneurysms that can be "clipped" prior to rupture have a better outcome than those that have already ruptured. I have observed the neurosurgeons doing this surgery and it is a very delicate and long operation often dissecting fractions of a millimeter at a time. In skilled hands, the outcome is usually very good.

AV malformations present half the time with hemorrhage, or with symptoms similar to that of aneurysms, especially seizure. The AV malformation may be very difficult to control and surgically difficult to remove, requiring total excision of the involved blood vessels. With inaccessible AV malformations, arterial embolization by a neuroradiologists or radiation therapy may be used.

Chapter 81
SPINAL CORD

Striking a spinal chord brings no music to anyone's ears,
Except the sound of the ambulance horn and the cries of one's family
with tears.
But fortunately most of the trauma sustained is not neurologically
harmful,
And the patient is quickly discharged from the hospital, with flowers by
the armful.

In this chapter we will discuss the spinal cord and review some anatomy and physiology. The spinal cord extends from the brain stem, the medulla oblongata, down the spinal canal to the level of the first or second lumbar vertebra where it becomes known as the conus medullaris. The nerve roots below the conus medullaris extend out like a horses tail and are called the cauda equina. If cut transversely, the spinal cord looks like a butterfly with a dorsal and ventral section on either side. At each spinal level nerve roots exit from the spinal cord from a structure called a dorsal or ventral ganglion. The nerve roots from the dorsal ganglia contain the sensory fibers, transmitting information to the brain (sensation); the ventral nerve roots transmit impulses from the brain to muscles (motor fibers) and glands. The dorsal and ventral nerve roots combine to form the spinal nerve, exiting one on each side of the spine through an opening called the intervertebral foramen. There are a total of thirty-one pairs of spinal nerves; eight cervical pairs, twelve thoracic pairs, five lumbar pairs, five sacral pairs and one coccygeal pair.

Now why should we know this anatomy? Basically, to understand why trauma, disease or tumor involving the spine or spinal cord at a certain level will partially or completely "cut off" the part of the body beyond the area of pathology. An injury to the spine or spinal cord in its dorsal area, will cause sensory deficit or loss below that level, and similarly a ventral injury will cause injury to the motor tract. This explains why a severe injury to the spinal cord can cause complete paralysis of the lower half of the body, called paraplegia, or total paralysis of the entire body from the neck down called quadriplegia from spinal cord transection by trauma, disease or tumor. We have shown the sensory nerve root distributions in Chapter 79 and have discussed the effects of trauma. The objective is to treat without causing further injury and to stabilize the spinal column, thereby stabilizing the spinal cord. Tumors of the spinal cord are classified as intradural and extradural; the dura is the thick membrane around the spinal cord and the brain.

The intradural tumors are usually central nervous system tumors and most of these are benign and can be surgically removed. They cause symptoms of weakness and sensory loss which are often completely reversed after surgery. The extradural tumors are usually metastatic cancers from breast, lung, prostate and kidney, or cancers of the bone of the vertebra, and treatment is directed at palliation of symptoms rather than cure. Abnormalities of the level called the conus medullaris may cause problems with bladder or bowel function.

The best tests for these abnormalities are MRI scan and sometimes just plain x-rays or myelograms, which are studies of the spinal canal where dye is injected into the spinal canal.

The intraspinal tumors are often surgically resectable and curable; they are the meningiomas, lipomas, ependymomas, schwannomas to name a few.

Chapter 82
PRESSURE ON THE BRAIN HYDROCEPHALUS AND INFECTIONS

Hydrocephalus means too much fluid in the ventricles of the brain;
Either too much is being produced, or not enough will drain.
So the surgeon must drain off the fluid, into the belly or into a vein,
So you won't have to worry about seizures and headaches ever
occurring again.

The poem really says it all. The cerebrospinal fluid, CSF, in the central nervous system surrounds the brain and spinal cord. Normally the fluid is produced by structures called the choroid plexus which are present in the lateral, third and fourth ventricles of the brain. This fluid circulates through the ventricular system, exits through two tiny openings called the foramina of Magendie and Luschka in the fourth ventricle and is finally absorbed into the blood stream through the arachnoid villi. When either too much is produced or too little reabsorbed, pressure builds up in the ventricles and thereby on the brain itself. There are congenital and acquired causes of hydrocephalus. The congenital can be from one of several developmental syndromes called Arnold-Chiari, Dandi-Walker or from certain cysts, and of course tumors. The acquired are usually secondary to meningitis, hemorrhages and tumors.

In infants up to age two years, where the bones of the skull have not yet fused, the increased pressure may cause the head to enlarge thereby temporarily relieving some of the pressure on the brain tissue. The cause is either congenital abnormalities meningitis or hemorrhage. The infants may present with the bulging fontanelles, that soft area between the unsealed frontal skull bones, and the hydrocephalus that must be surgically managed as soon as diagnosis is established. This is done by using a tube with a one way valve system, inserting one end into a ventricle of the brain and the other into a vein or the abdomen to drain off the fluid and lower the pressure. This is called a ventriculo-peritoneal shunt when drained into the abdomen and with these shunts the most common complication is blockage of the tube which may require partial replacement. Infections occurring in the shunt can be severe and can lead to brain damage.

Hydrocephalus in children over two years is different than in infants in that the bones of the skull are fused and the symptoms often appear rapidly causing possible seizures, headaches, nausea, vomiting, coma and even death. There may be a whole host of neurological deficits and mental changes, which can be partially reversed with surgical correction of the cause or decompression of the hydrocephalus with a shunt.

In adults the main causes are tumors, meningitis and intracranial bleeding. The symptoms will usually be gradual and include changes in mentation, urinary incontinence and changes in gait called ataxia. The treatment is either getting rid of the cause through surgery or placement of one of the shunts I have mentioned above.

This is obviously a very simplified explanation of hydrocephalus, but hopefully will give you a little insight into a complex problem.

Infections of the brain are usually labeled according to their location. If it involves the lining tissue it is called meningitis, the deep brain tissue, encephalitis, and the skull bone, osteomyelitis. The brain and spinal cord may be subject to infection by bacteria, viruses, fungus and parasites, and often occur in individuals with lowered immune resistance as with chronic disease and AIDS. Abscesses can occur in any location, epidural, subdural, or deep in the brain. Most infections respond to antibiotics with careful monitoring using CAT or MRI scans. However, surgery may be indicated in certain circumstances. A cranial bone osteomyelitis usually requires removal of the bone and later replacement with a synthetic bone replacement called methacrylate. And a subdural abscess, as with an intra-brain abscess, will need appropriate drainage in one of many ways determined by the neurosurgeon.

Meningitis usually responds to antibiotics unless there is a focus of contamination, as with the adjacent sinuses, where a defect in the lining of the brain or chronic sinusitis may need to be approached surgically. Sometimes brain infections mimic tumors and stereotactic or open biopsies may be needed to rule out malignancy. When a patient has a focal area of brain inflammation, possibly leading to abscess formation, it is called cerebritis and needs to be followed carefully by scans. Sometimes these abscesses can be repeatedly drained by needle aspirations instead of major brain surgery. They respond well to this plus antibiotics or antifungal medications depending on the causative organism. The patients are often given steroids to decrease brain swelling and are usually given anticonvulsant medications, since seizures are a common complication accompanying brain infections and abscesses.

In some infections, the neurosurgeon may be asked by the infectious disease specialist to place a catheter in the brain through which antibiotics can be given, or may need to place a ventriculo-peritoneal shunt because the infection has induced hydrocephalus. More recently over the past fifteen years there has been an increase in the number of unusual brain infections found in the population with AIDS, some of which will need biopsy by the neurosurgeon. Fungus infections usually result from long term use of antibiotics, especially for lung infections in otherwise immune compromised individuals. Surgery is occasionally required for resolution.

Although we don't see a great deal in the United States, parasitic diseases effecting the brain are much more common elsewhere in the world causing occasional abscesses which mimic tumors and often have to be biopsied, drained or excised. And, as with most CNS problems, the sooner it is taken care of, the fewer the severe residual neurological deficits.

In conclusion, I want to mention some of the techniques that are used for neurosurgical procedures. These include stereotactic tumor resection, endoscopic endonasal pituitary tumor removal, proton beam treatment, thermal surgery and most recently the Gamma knife. These methods are beyond the scope of this book and can be discussed fully with a neurosurgeon prior to their use.

Chapter 83
TRACHEOSTOMY

Farmer Brown's favorite rooster had pneumonia for a week,
And had a tracheostomy and wasn't able to speak.
So until the bird got better, all the hens had a morning spree,
And woke old farmer Brown each day with a cock-a-doodle-dee!

Before we get to the lungs and its diseases proper, I want to spend a little time with the trachea and tracheostomy. The trachea is the tube that leads from the back of the throat to the bronchi of the lungs. It is made of a membranous tissue augmented with rings of cartilage. The upper part is partially covered by the isthmus or central part of the thyroid gland which is usually seen by the surgeon during tracheostomy. Tracheostomy means the insertion of a tube into the trachea through the skin in front of it for the purpose of assisting respiratory function. The indications are either blockage of the upper airway by trauma, tumor or scarring, for control of secretions as when someone is so weak or sick that lung secretions cannot be coughed up and suctioning is continually needed, and for a method of long term assisted breathing for patients when they are not able to breathe adequately by themselves. The tracheostomy is attached by tubes to a respirator machine which breathes for the patient, and a nurse can suction the trachea and lungs through the tracheostomy. In general, the tracheostomy is more comfortable for the patient than having a tube through the nose or mouth.

Most of the time, a tracheostomy is an elective operation, done only after a patient has been intubated, meaning having a breathing tube down the nose or mouth into the lungs for a week to ten days; in some emergency situations with trauma or tumor, the procedure may need to be done at once.

Tracheostomy is often a temporary procedure, used after trauma or chronic illness and when the patient recovers sufficiently, the tube can be removed and the opening will close on its own. The tracheostomy tube has a balloon cuff near its end which is inflated when a patient is on a respirator so that air does not escape around it. Also, the cuff is inflated when there is a risk of the patient being unable to control swallowing or there is a risk of vomiting. The cuff prevents anything from getting around it into the lungs such as vomitus or other secretions. Taking vomitus or fluid into the lungs is called aspiration and can be a cause for severe lung problems and even death. In a recovering patient, the cuff can be deflated and the patient can block the tracheostomy opening, permitting air to pass through the upper trachea and larynx allowing the patient to speak. This is not possible when the cuff is inflated.

The procedure of tracheostomy can be done at a bedside in an emergency, but generally is best done in the operating room with optimal assistance, lighting, suction and surgical instruments. The patient is either fully asleep or under heavy sedation with a local anesthetic, and is placed in position with the head hyperextended to give best access to the throat. A small transverse incision is made about one to two centimeters above the manubrium and carried down through the tissue of the neck until the strap muscles in the midline are identified. These muscles are split apart and the trachea is visualized. Using any of several methods, the surgeon then opens the trachea and inserts the tracheostomy tube while the anesthesiologist removes the endotracheal tube that has been in place prior to the procedure. Appropriate connections are made to the respirator by the anesthesiologist or nurse. The entire procedure should take fifteen to thirty minutes in skilled hands.

The main complications are bleeding from irritation of the trachea by the tube, infection, and obstruction of the tube by being dislodged or by mucus plugs. A late complication after removal of the tracheostomy is narrowing of the trachea from scarring and this sometimes requires reconstructive surgery (*see* Diagram 55 next page).

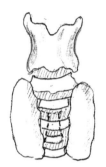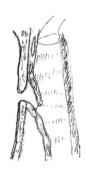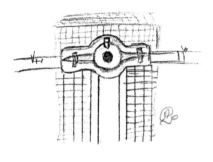

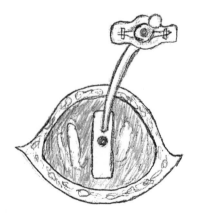

TRACHEOSTOMY

DIAGRAM 55

Chapter 84
LUNGS

If you smoke cigarettes by the pack,
Your lungs are probably turning black
And after you cough for a decade or so,
You just won't have all of your get up and go.

Twenty years later with emphysema,
You've an increased chance for an empyema.
And if you are stubborn or won't hear the answer,
You'll believe when they tell you that smoke won't cause cancer!

The lungs are two large organs of respiration or breathing located in the chest cavity. There's a right and a left lung, the right with three lobes, an upper, a middle and a lower, and ten segments or divisions, and the left with two lobes and ten segments. The lungs are encased in a thin tissue called pleura and each lung is connected to the trachea or windpipe by a mainstem bronchus; the lungs are connected to the heart by the pulmonary arteries and veins. On the inner side of the lung is an area called the hilum where the arteries, veins and main bronchi enter each lung. Each main bronchus divides into smaller bronchi and even smaller bronchioles looking like an inverted tree until they lead to tiny airsacs called alveoli where carbon dioxide (CO_2) and oxygen (O_2) are exchanged between the respiratory system and the blood stream. In addition to this respiratory function, the lungs absorb and excrete water and drugs such as those used in putting a patient to sleep. By the action of the diaphragm, abdominal muscles and motion of the rib cage, negative pressure is exerted on the lungs causing air to enter and to be expelled.

As we shall see, numerous infectious, toxic, traumatic and neoplastic processes can occur in the lungs, some of which we shall discuss in this chapter (*see* Diagram 56 next page).

The evaluation of the lungs is done with a chest x-ray. If abnormalities are found, a CAT or MRI scan, and even a pulmonary angiogram, which is a dye study of the arteries to the lung, may be performed.

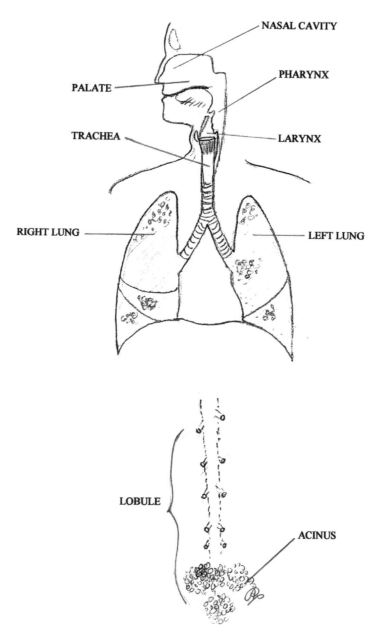

ANATOMY OF THE LUNGS-GROSS AND MICROSCOPIC

DIAGRAM 56

To measure the actual function of the lung, pulmonary function studies are done which include measurement of the capacity of the lung, the amount of air with each breath, the oxygenation of the blood; PO_2 measures how much oxygen is dissolved in the blood and PCO_2 indicates how much carbon dioxide is in the blood. These studies help determine how well someone will go through a surgical operation and also will tell the thoracic surgeon whether the patient will tolerate removal of some of the lung. Cigarette smoking, obesity, age and any anesthesia, impact the operative risk; that is why some patients need to be operated on under a regional block or local or spinal anesthesia as a safer alternative.

As an important addition to the diagnostic workup, bronchoscopy can be performed by the pulmonary physician or by the chest surgeon to look in the bronchi and do biopsies. Bronchoscopy, when properly done has very few complications although serious bleeding, respiratory and heart problems can occur and must be anticipated and able to be managed immediately.

The thoracic surgeon usually doesn't get involved with infectious processes in the lung unless the disease has not responded well to appropriate antibiotic or other medical therapy and has progressed to form an abscess which needs to be drained, or unless a segment of lung is so involved that it needs to be removed. An abscess is an area which contains pus or some other infectious process sometimes causing a cavitation or hole in that segment of the lung. The cause may be caused by aspiration of gastric contents, streptococcus, staphylococcus, E.Coli, bacteria or by fungus such as histoplasmosis, coccidiomycosis, candidiasis, or an organism called Actinomyces which causes actinomycosis or nocardiosis.

Individuals with AIDS (HIV virus) are susceptible to lung infections often not seen in the rest of the population such as Pneumocystis carinii pneumonia, as well as Candida, herpes simplex and Cryptococcus infections. For some cases, and in patients too sick to undergo an operation, a tube can be placed into the abscess cavity for drainage. However, in general, in these types of cases the surgeon has to open the chest in a procedure called a thoracotomy (thorac- meaning chest and -otomy meaning opening into) and remove a segment of lung, often by using a stapling device. After the procedure, a thoracostomy tube or chest tube, is frequently left in the chest to reexpand the lungs and to drain off infection.

Emphysema is a condition of the lungs usually associated with cigarette smoking and bronchitis, an inflammation of the bronchi. This condition has marked distention of the bronchi and smaller bronchioli down to the air sacs which also are dilated. The destruction affects the ability of the alveoli to function normally exchanging oxygen for carbon dioxide, and the lung gives the appearance of a large air filled sac, most of which is not functioning. In a condition called bullous emphysema, large groups of alveoli form an air filled sac or cysts which can rupture and cause lung collapse. The patients suffer from shortness of breath, weight loss and because of the poor oxygenation of the blood, their hands and feet sometimes appear bluish. The lungs are also deficient in a substance called antitrypsin which would normally fend off bacteria; therefore patients with emphysema have an increased incidence of severe pulmonary infections.

Until recently, there was little definitive surgical help for these patients, except for placing a thoracostomy tube to re-expand the lung after a collapse from a ruptured bulla, or actually removing a bleb. Surgeons are now doing lung reduction surgery, removing large segments of non-functioning or poorly functioning lung and thereby increasing oxygenation. When blood flows through non-functioning, non-oxygenating lung tissue, it returns to the heart poorly oxygenated; when mixed with the oxygenated blood from the good areas of the lung, the overall result is poorly oxygenated blood. By eliminating the bad areas, even though there is less total lung volume, that which is present is much more efficient overall!

Chapter 85
THORACOSCOPY

Minimally invasive is the surgeon's goal
To operate through a tiny hole.
To diagnose, biopsy, and resect;
What more can a patient ever expect?

If you're wondering why I have given over an entire new chapter to thoracoscopy, it's because thoracoscopy has opened a new chapter in thoracic surgery. Evaluation of intrathoracic problems using thoracoscopy, looking through a scope into the chest, has actually been around since the beginning of the twentieth century, but because of technical problems the procedure was not widely used until the nineteen eighties. With the development of the silicon chip and microtelevision circuitry, tiny cameras could be developed and the ability to use modern instrumentation opened the way for a new approach to thoracic surgery. Unlike laparoscopy in the abdomen, the chest is more rigid, and the lung on the side examined collapses when the chest is opened by the laparoscope. The patient is asleep during the procedure and one lung has to be selectively intubated. The scope is placed in a lower chest position and two or three small openings are made in other positions in the chest through which operating instruments can be placed. Using this technique the operating surgeon can see the inside of the chest more clearly, using the magnified video camera, than with the naked eye. This is called Video Assisted Thoracoscopic Surgery, VATS, and it is used for diagnosis and therapy.

The accepted diagnostic procedures are biopsies of the lining of the chest, the pleura and the central part of the chest containing the heart and other non-lung structures, called the mediastinum, biopsy of lymph nodes, and biopsies of certain abnormal lung findings such as thickenings and lumps. The therapeutic indications for thoracoscopy are drainage and debridement of abscesses in the chest, removal of certain benign and malignant tumors of the pleura and the lungs, bullectomy in emphysema, cutting the sympathetic nerves to increase blood flow in the arms and hands in certain conditions, and several other procedures less often performed. The more adept and skilled the surgeon is at thoracoscopy, the more able he/she is to perform more complex procedures. The objective is to do as good a job thoracoscopically as can be done with the chest open and for that reason several surgeons hesitate to do major cancer operations because they cannot do as complete a procedure as they could with the chest open. The advantages of thoracoscopy are: Less postoperative pain, fewer pulmonary problems, shorter hospital stay, and fewer overall complications and morbidity. Sometimes this procedure will be done as a less optimal choice for cancer treatment when the patient is too sick to tolerate a major, open thoracotomy and lung resection.

To aid in the surgery, as with laparoscopic procedures, there are mechanical devices that are used to staple across lungs, bronchi and blood vessels through a small opening in the chest as well as special suture devices and electrocautery, argon beam coagulation (a special apparatus that uses the energy from an argon gas beam to seal off bleeding tissue), and thoracoscopic scissors, clamps and dissecting instruments. There are several possible complications including bleeding, air leakage, wound infections and, on rare occasions, death in critically ill patients. When complications occur they can be corrected either through the thoracoscope or by opening the chest when needed. Sometimes the findings of thoracoscopy prior to an open chest surgery may cause the surgeon to abort the more major surgery as with certain cancers. Likewise, thoracoscopy may give findings which would indicate the need for further thoracoscopic surgery or for an open chest operation.

As with laparoscopy, as the years go by with better training and instrumentation, more thoracic surgeons will be doing more complex procedures with fewer problems and better results. It is certainly one of the frontiers of modern medicine.

Chapter 86
INFECTIONS AND FLUID IN THE CHEST EMPYEMA, PNEUMOTHORAX, HEMOTHORAX

The pleural cavity is in the chest,
And may have fluid which we can test.
To makes diagnoses of fact from confusion
Just insert a needle and pull out effusion.

The inside of the chest is somewhat like the inside of the abdomen in that its contents are covered with a thin layer of cells. In the abdomen it's called peritoneum and in the chest it's called pleura. The pleural tissue is very active in secreting and absorbing fluid, and more than a quart of fluid is secreted and absorbed during a twenty-four hour period. Because secretion and absorption are the same in healthy individuals, a chest x-ray will not show any fluid in the chest. However, certain pathologic processes can cause an increase in production or a decrease in absorption resulting in the appearance of fluid in the chest on an x-ray. This fluid is called pleural effusion, and taking a sample of it with a needle, using a local anesthetic and placing a needle above a rib into the fluid, can be diagnostic and is done frequently for effusions of unknown origin for aid in diagnosis.

Pleural effusion can be a sign of infection in the chest and in the abdomen. It may indicate severe infection under the diaphragm such as liver or gall bladder disease, an abscess under the diaphragm called subphrenic abscess, and certain benign and malignant tumors in the abdomen; a benign tumor of the ovary with fluid in the chest is call Meige's syndrome. There may be pathology in the chest itself such as certain infections, pneumonia, congestive heart failure, trauma, fungus and Actinomyces infections, TB (Tuberculosis), blood clots in the lung (pulmonary embolism) and cancer causing the effusion.

The nature of the effusion is important and can give a clue as to the etiology. It can be bloody which is ominous for cancer, very thin called transudate containing little protein, as seen in heart failure, or thick called exudate containing much protein as seen in malignancy, TB and infections. Examination of pleural fluid is important and will steer the physician towards more diagnostic workup or directly to a treatment modality.

Hemothorax is heme or blood in the chest. This can be secondary to trauma, tumors, or severely damaged lung from infection or pulmonary embolism. In most instances, bleeding will stop spontaneously because of the pressure of the lung against the inside of the chest wall. Small amounts of blood in the chest can just be observed and will be reab-sorbed; moderate amounts of blood will require placement of a chest tube, called a thoracostomy tube, for drainage. However, if there is continued bleeding an open thoracotomy under general anesthesia is needed and the bleeding source identified and controlled. Sometimes with massive bleeding there is need for blood transfusions and if the heart or great vessels, namely pulmonary artery and vein, aorta or vena cava are injured, the patient may succumb before the bleeding is controlled. For bleeding from cancer, removal of the tumor or other treatments may be needed. One of the diagnostic tools in hemothorax and other pleural effusions is the use of Video Assisted Thoracoscopic Surgery, VATS, and in skilled hands the definitive therapy can be accomplished through the thoracoscope.

An empyema is a collection of pus in the pleural space, and may be limited to a small area or involve the entire side of the chest cavity. It may be secondary to many things, including bacterial and aspiration pneumonia, lung abscess, a ruptured emphysema bleb, or cancer. There is often partial collapse of a lung in association with the empyema. The treatment is directed towards draining and cleaning out the empyema cavity, re-expanding the lung and treating the underlining disease process such as pneumonia, neoplasm or emphysematous bleb. Often a part of a rib may need to be removed and a large tube placed in the empyema cavity for adequate treatment, cleansing and drainage. The treatment of empyema can be very complex, but this gives you a general idea of the surgeon's approach. It may take many days or weeks for the process to resolve fully before the tubes can be removed.

Let us now turn to pneumothorax, or air in the pleural cavity. Remember that it's okay to have air in the lungs, but not in the pleural cavity. This means that there is either a leak from the lungs or from the outside and this will result in a partial or complete collapse of a lung. The causes may be an emphysematous bleb, trauma, tumor or may be iatrogenic, caused by the doctor while he is doing some procedure such as starting a central venous line or doing a lung or pleural biopsy. Diagnosis is made by chest x-ray. If a pneumothorax is small (5-15%), it is not usually treated, and just observed with repeated x-rays at six to twelve hour intervals. Small pneumothoraces will resolve spontaneously.

If the pneumothorax is increasing in size, larger than 20% or causing severe symptoms as in individuals with such severe lung disease that any loss of lung volume is serious, then it is necessary to place a thoracostomy or chest tube into the chest and hook it to a special apparatus called an underwater suction device. This is hooked to a suction machine which pulls the air out of the chest and re-expands the lung. Chest tubes can either be placed in an emergency room or at the bedside under local anesthetics and pain medication, or in the operating room, as befits the circumstances and the patient's preference. However often, when there is complete lung collapse, this is an emergency procedure and must be done where the patient is first diagnosed, usually in an emergency room or hospital bed. Most leaks causing a pneumothorax will seal off by themselves in a few days and then the chest tube can be removed. But in some circumstances a thoracoscopy or even open thoracostomy may be needed to seal off the cause of the leak.

Chapter 87
CANCER OF THE LUNG

Salem
Merit
Marlboros, Pall Mall, Chesterfield, Vantage, Misty
L&M, Lucky Strike, Virginia Slim, Philip Morris
Benson and Hedges, Parliament, Players, Satin, Now
Maverick, Belair
Dunhill, Exact
True Blue
Tarreyton
Winston,
Viceroy
Doral
Kool
Kent
True
More

There's nothing cool or true blue about lung cancer. It's the most common cause of cancer death among men and women and is directly related to cigarette smoking according to most authors, reports and studies. In this chapter we will focus on several different types of cancer in the chest including two general types of lung cancer, small cell and non-small cell, a strange entity called bronchial adenoma, and a malignancy of the pleura called mesothelioma.

The symptoms of lung cancer are varied and often may depend on the location of the cancer. Unfortunately by the time symptoms occur, the tumor has usually spread to local lymph nodes or has distant metastatic spread. Only about 5-6% of patients are asymptomatic at diagnosis which may be found on routine chest x-ray, and of course these patients often have the best prognosis. The symptoms usually consist of cough, from tumor irritating the bronchial tube, coughing up blood, wheezing, shortness of breath or chest pain. When the cancer extends to involve surrounding structures, symptoms relating to those structures may be the first indication of disease. These include voice changes with involvement of the laryngeal nerves, shoulder and arm pain with tumors of the top of the lung called a Pancoast tumor, involving nerves to these areas, pleural effusion, swelling of the veins in the neck and face, secondary to tumor pressing on the vena cava also known as vena cava syndrome.

There is Horner's syndrome with a drooping of the eyelid on one side, meiosis or constriction of the pupil of one eye, and dryness of the eye, and a group of findings called paraneoplastic syndromes. These later findings are elsewhere in the body and are usually related to substances produced by the primary tumor or by distant metastases. These include weight loss, tissue wasting, decreased appetite as well as many skin and fingernail changes, and hematologic problems of anemia, blood clots in legs and arms, diminished blood platelets and coagulation disorder; there are also endocrine problems including hyperthyroidism, abnormal calcium metabolism, increased estrogen in men causing breast enlargement, low blood sugar and many others. There may be many neurologic findings such as weakness, paralysis, breathing muscle problems (Eaton Lambert Syndrome), visual and intellectual dysfunction, and skeletal changes.

The diagnostics and staging include chest x-ray, and later the CAT scan, followed by bronchoscopy and direct or needle biopsy. To determine if the lymph nodes near the hilum are involved, a mediastinoscopy may be done which involves placing a lighted tube under the upper part of the sternum in a sleeping patient and taking biopsies. A thoracoscopy or limited thoracotomy through a tiny incision, a Chamberlain procedure, is often warranted. PET (positron emission tomography) scan and MRI scans are other modalities of more careful diagnostics for staging. Like other cancers, there is an international TNM, tumor, lymph node and metastasis staging system which can be further broken down to a Stage I-IV system to guide the physician in choosing the appropriate mode of therapy.

Before going into the specific tumors, I want to spend a moment on the Solitary Nodule. This is a single spherical nodule up to 4 cm. in diameter seen by the radiologist examining a chest x-ray and needs to be carefully evaluated. It may represent a primary cancer of the lung or a metastatic cancer from some other site in the body such as breast, colon, kidney etc. It may also be a benign granuloma, a nodule from an old infection such as TB or other benign pulmonary process. If a solitary nodule has been present for several years on old x-rays, it is almost surely noncancerous and can usually be left alone. However, aside from that situation, a diagnosis must be made, and even in cases of metastatic disease, if it is the only evidence of spread, many surgeons will remove it in an attempt to cure the patient.

TNM STAGING SYSTEM FOR LUNG CANCER

PRIMARY CANCER

Tx	Cancer Cells but no tumor seen
T1	Less than 3 centimeters in diameter
T2	More than 3 centimeters in diameter
T3	Extends to lung lining, heart lining or chest wall
T4	Extends to mediastinum or cancerous fluid in chest

LYMPH NODES

N0	No cancer in lymph nodes
N1	Cancer in lymph nodes on same side as tumor
N2	Cancer in mediastinal lymph nodes
N3	Cancer in lymph nodes on other side of chest

METASTASES (SPREAD OF CANCER BEYOND LUNG AREA)

M0	No spread
M1	Spread beyond lung

STAGING SYSTEM

STAGE	TNM TYPES	FIVE YEAR SURVIVAL
I	T1-2, N0, M0	60-75%
II	T1-2, N1, M0	25-45%
IIIA	T3, N0-1, M0	25-40%
	T1-3, N2, M0	10-30%
IIIB	T4 or N3, M0	less than 5%
IV	Any M1	less than 1%

DIAGRAM 57

Let us turn to cancer of the lung. Small cell lung cancers (SCLC) are ominous in that by the time of diagnosis most of these have already spread throughout the body, even if local lymph nodes are negative. Because of this poor prognosis, most surgeons place it in a category by itself regardless of the staging, and will not operate on the lesion because it does not add to survival. These patients, after diagnosis, are usually subjected to chemotherapy and sometimes radiation therapy, and a few are occasionally cured. In general, the objective is to give the best palliation and in some cases the patients survive up to five years.

Non small cell lung cancers (NSCLC) make up the majority of lung cancer (80%), consisting mainly of gland forming adenocarcinoma, squamous cell and large cell carcinoma. There are many other types and subtypes but we don't need to go into these in this discussion. The treatment of all the types of NSCLC is essentially the same and we will group them together in our discussion. Unlike the SCLC, these cancers have a better prognosis and are treated according to their stages. The workup has been delineated above and in general, these case are taken to a tumor board where a group of physicians at conference including thoracic surgeons, pathologists, oncologists, radiologists as well as other physicians, nurses and social workers discuss each case and decide upon a course of action. Taken into consideration is the patient's general health as well as the pulmonary status.

In general, Stage I and II non small cell lung cancers undergo exploration and surgical resection, unless the findings at surgery change the staging to the degree that surgery is no longer feasible for cure, i.e. if more areas are involved. There are many procedures available to the thoracic surgeon, named according to the amount of lung tissue which is removed. They are: Wedge resection, removing just a pie-shaped part of a lobe, segmentectomy, removing part of a lobe, lobectomy, removing one entire lobe - i.e. the right upper, middle or lower lobe and pneumonectomy, removing an entire left or right lung with all its lobes. Curative resections of any size must include clean margins uninvolved with tumor, of the bronchi and great vessels and usually hilar or adjacent lymph nodes are removed to further evaluate the staging. The long term five year survival rates for NSCLC directly relate to the clinical and pathological staging and vary from Stage I - 65%, Stage II - 55-40%, Stage III - 23-0%, Stage IV - 0%. In some advanced disease, chemotherapy and radiation therapy are used possibly in conjunction with surgical resection.

The complications of lung surgery include infection such as pneumonia and abscess, incomplete expanding of the lungs (atelectasis), pain, cardiac problems and rarely death.

Other treatments, especially in very advanced cases include endobronchial (inside the bronchus), radiation therapy, photoradiation with lasers

(Nd:YAG Laser) and immunotherapy (being experimented with at this time).

Bronchial adenoma is a name given to a less aggressive group of malignant tumors of the lung with a much better prognosis than the cancers we have just discussed. They only represent a small percentage of lung tumors, but because their curability is so high, I want to just mention their names: Bronchial carcinoid, adenoid cystic carcinoma or cylindroma and mucoepidermoid carcinoma. They usually present with cough, bleeding and partial airway obstruction and the workup involves all those procedures already mentioned. Treatment is by resection with good clear margins and if there are no positive lymph nodes and no distant spread, the cure rate can be excellent...up to 80-90% among the most common group, the carcinoid tumors.

At the other end of the survival spectrum is the mesothelioma, fortunately not a common cancer that occurs predominately in the pleura, although it has also been seen in the peritoneum, pericardium, around the heart, and elsewhere. It is a cancer directly attributable to asbestos and was one of the main reasons that asbestos was banned by the Environmental Protection Agency. The patients, between 50 and 65 years old, present with shortness of breath, weight loss, and cough, and chest x-ray shows a pleural effusion. Examination of the pleural fluid and pleural biopsy will often give the diagnosis. In rare cases the disease may be localized to a small area, but often it involves an extensive area of the pleura. Resectable tumors require extensive radical surgery which involves removing the pleura, the lung and any surrounding tissue. Lesser procedures are done when the patient will not be able to tolerate the major surgery, and chemotherapy and radiation may be indicated to give longer disease free intervals and palliation. In general it is a difficult disease to cure and often the objective is to achieve as much palliation and long term quality survival as possible.

Chapter 88
RIBS AND CHEST WALL

It must have been a genetic disaster,
To make Eve from Adam's rib, and not from plaster.
And did that cause Cain in that well known fable,
To bludgeon to death his young brother Abel?

T he bony skull and strong thoracic cage were well designed to protect the brain, heart and lungs, but somehow the abdomen and external genitalia were forgotten. That's a subject for another chapter in another book! In this chapter we will examine the congenital abnormalities of the chest, as well as the diseases caused by the position of the bones and the effects of trauma on the intrathoracic and intra-abdominal structures.

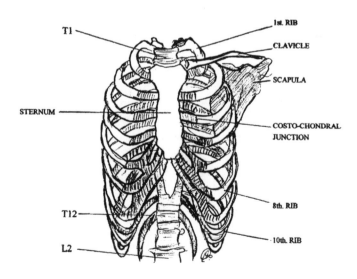

CHEST WALL ANATOMY AND BONY THORAX

DIAGRAM 58

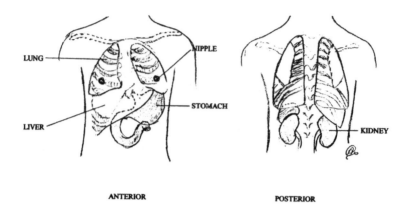

ANTERIOR   POSTERIOR

RELATIONSHIPS OF THE THORACIC CAGE TO THE ABDOMEN AND CHEST CONTENTS

DIAGRAM 59

It is important in evaluating trauma to the chest to understand that the ribs overlie the chest contents of heart, lungs, and great vessels. We are keenly aware that forces great enough to fracture ribs, sternum, clavicle or scapula, may cause internal damage to these structures and evaluation by the ER physician focuses on these areas. He/she looks for lung punctures causing pneumo- and hemo-thorax, cardiac injuries from puncture, compression, or blunt trauma and hemorrhage from great vessel injuries. However, as shown in the diagrams above, the trauma to ribs may directly affect the intra-abdominal organs. Lower right rib fractures can cause kidney damage, liver injuries and hemorrhage, and left tenth through twelfth rib fractures can cause injury to the spleen. Any abdominal tenderness or suspected injuries must be evaluated by CAT scan, and intra-abdominal bleeding or trauma may need to be evaluated by careful observation, laparoscopy or open laparotomy. Today we focus on salvaging as much spleen as possible, whereas years ago it was standard to remove a lacerated spleen. Straightforward rib fractures are painful and usually will respond to pain medication, occasional nerve blocks with local anesthetic, and splinting the chest with a firm wrap to prevent excessive motion and further injury.

The congenital abnormalities of the chest are primarily pectus excavatum, funnel or depressed sternum, and pectus carinatum, "bird chest", with protrusion of the central portion of the sternum. Pectus excavatum is present at birth and may get worse as the child grows, and depending on the severity, may cause significant cosmetic, emotional and sometimes functional physiological problems. With severe excavatum, the infant and child may have pain, EKG abnormalities from the pressure on the heart, shortness of breath and difficulty eating. It is generally recommended that severe deformity be repaired before age five to prevent postural and emotional problems, and the surgery, though complex, has a 95-98% success rate for permanent resolution of the deformity and its side effects.

The pectus carinatum deformity usually is physiologically asymptomatic, and is usually repaired for emotional and cosmetic reasons. The surgical success rate is over 98%.

Thoracic Outlet Syndrome is a name given for a group of conditions where the bony and muscular structures of the chest cause compression on nerves and blood vessels. The problem usually occurs in middle-aged women, but can occur in an individual of any age. The symptoms of nerve compression may include numbness, pain and weakness of the hands and fingers on the side of the fourth and fifth fingers, the ulnar nerve distribution, or depending on the location of the compression, symptoms may be in the neck, shoulder, face, chest and arms. Compression of the artery may cause symptoms of pain, especially with activity, weakness, and coldness and sometimes decreased sensation. Compression of the vein may cause swelling of the arm or a heavy, tired feeling.

Finding out exactly where the problem is involves physical examination, x-ray, and nerve conduction studies; a nerve will have abnormal conduction patterns when there is compression at a certain level. On physical exam, the physician will have the patient raise the arm on the involved side, bent at 90 degrees and turned outward. Then he will be asked to open and close the hand and this should reproduce the pain. Other examinations test for arterial compression by movements of the arm, but these are nonspecific and findings may be present in asymptomatic individuals. A chest, neck, and rib x-ray could show abnormal first ribs, the presence of a cervical rib which shouldn't be there, and bony scar from injuries or abnormalities of the clavicle. Arteriograms with the arm in different positions may show the site of compression, and venograms will similarly show venous compression.

These studies may confirm the diagnosis and the nerves, artery or vein or all three groups may be compressed between chest wall and a rib, clavicle, muscle or fascia. This compression is often relieved by weight loss, rest, and having the arm in a sling for several weeks. Physiotherapy and postural exercises may help. However, if the symptoms and signs persist, an appropriate operative procedure may be indicated such as removal of a cervical rib or a first rib and dividing the scalenus or other causative muscles. Unfortunately, some of the procedures have high complication rates with nerve injuries and occasional vessel injuries, and the procedures need to be performed by a surgeon fully familiar with the technique and potential complications. The approaches may be through the axilla or above the clavicle.

Finally, let us finish with a discussion of the tumors which can occur on the chest wall. The most common tumor is the lipoma, a soft fatty mass that can grow to be quite large, 10-20 cm. in diameter, is minimally symptomatic but often disfiguring. It can be easily removed with local anesthesia and sedation. Other benign tumors include bone tumors, osteochondromas, fibrous tumors, dysplasias, and cartilage tumors, chondromas. The cancers are osteogenic sarcoma, chondrosarcoma and Ewing's sarcoma, all of which present as painful masses attached to ribs or the rib-sternal junction and need wide excisions, often followed by chemotherapy and radiation therapy. Most chondrosarcomas are cured; half of Ewing's sarcomas are cured since they've often metastasized by the time of diagnosis; only about 20% of osteogenic sarcoma can be cured even with the combined regimens.

Surgery that removes part of the bony thorax presents the problem of reconstruction to maintain stability of the chest. With large defects over 4-5 cm., this requires placement of special, strong fascial tissue, artificial material, bone grafts and muscle rotation flaps to cover the defects.

Chapter 89
THYMUS

Named for the thyme leaf, which it resembles,
It's the place where the immune system T-cell assembles.
It's shaped like a pyramid, under the breastbone,
For treating myasthenia, is what it is best known.
It's responsible for development of our immune system,
It's needed in kids, but adults never missed 'em.
This organ's the thymus, bi-lobed, left and right,

That's all I can tell you, goodby and good night.

The thymus gland, until recently, was a strange bi-lobed lymphoid organ situated under the sternum in the chest and without much apparent function. The advances in immunopathology in the last twenty years have elucidated that this organ, with its central zone, the medulla, and the outer cortex layer, reaches its largest size in children and then begins to decrease in size or involute throughout the rest of adult life. It was found that animals who had their thymus removed in infancy were unable to perform certain immune functions such as rejection of foreign material and production of antibodies.

We now know that the T-cell lymphocytes responsible for this function are produced to a great extent in the thymus and are transported to the spleen, liver and bone marrow lymphoid tissue. So why the interest for the surgeon?

There is a strange disease called Myasthenia gravis which affects muscles, causing weakness, especially starting with the eye muscles but progressing throughout the body to the neck, trunk and limbs, and eventually causing difficulty breathing. Some individuals have minimal symptoms which resolve spontaneously, but others progress more seriously and if not treated can die from respiratory failure. It is apparently an autoimmune disease which means that for some reason the body's immune system interferes with the response of the muscles to neurotransmitters. The neurotransmitter acetylcholine is a substance that stimulates the muscles to contract.

The diagnosis is made through a series of fairly complex tests which measure nerve conduction and responses to certain drugs such as Tensilon. The objective is to eliminate several other diseases as the cause of the muscle weakness, such as multiple sclerosis, Lou Gehrig's disease (amyotrophic lateral sclerosis), hyperthyroidism, etc., and responses to certain drugs.

The treatment is initially medical and many patients respond well to the drug Mestinon (pyridostigmine), immunosuppressive therapy with the drug Imuran (azathioprine), and steroid therapy. Non-responders may have plasmapheresis, where blood is cycled through a machine which removes plasma and hereby removes the antibodies in the plasma that are causing the Myasthenia.

If these methods fail, removal of the thymus may be indicated, with response rates in the high ninety percent range and complete remission or complete disappearance of the disease for a long period of time in half the cases. The technique for removal of the thymus was originally through a median sternotomy which is a middle of the chest incision cutting through the sternum or breast bone. However, the transcervical technique, through the front of the neck has been used more frequently with special equipment allowing the surgeon to elevate the sternum with instruments and remove the thymus from the anterior superior mediastinum. With the advent of modern thoracoscopic instruments, the VATS procedure is being perfected for use in thymectomy in many medical centers

One other area I want to discuss for completeness is the tumors of the thymus gland. These tumors, thymomas, are 60% benign and usually the symptoms are related to large size and compression on the trachea or other adjacent organs including lung, vena cava and heart, causing cough, chest pain, venous congestion, and shortness of breath. The diagnosis is made by CAT scan, and complete removal through median sternotomy is the most common method. Patients with Myasthenia who also have a thymoma usually have a poorer prognosis. The malignant thymomas are usually diagnosed by their gross appearance and spread, and are staged according to their involvement in adjacent organs or distant spread. The therapy is complete thymectomy.

H

CARDIAC (HEART) SURGERY

Chapter 90
ANATOMY AND FUNCTION
OF THE HEART

I want to get down to the heart of the matter,
With a heart to heart talk, meant to teach, not to flatter,
After a hearty breakfast (causing heartburn galore),
You'll find it heart-warming to sit on the floor,

And study the heart, that muscular pump,
That slows when you're sleeping and speeds when you jump.
So we'll study anatomy (I'm a heartless professor,
And hardhearted man, but a fabulous dresser).

In 1628, William Harvey published a small book called De Motu Cordis et Sanguinis in Animalibus, "On the Motion of the Heart and Blood in Animals". It described the circulation of blood and the function of the heart as a pump and opened the doors to modern medicine and physiology. So simple and yet so profound it took five thousand years of medical history to arrive at that point! (*See* Diagram 60 next page.)

The heart is basically a two sided pump. Blood low in oxygen and high in carbon dioxide returns to the right atrium via the superior vena cava from the head and upper extremities and via the inferior vena cava from the lower body, and passes through the tricuspid valve into the right ventricle. From the pump action of the ventricle, the blood flows across the pulmonic valve into the pulmonary arteries and thence into the lungs where it eliminates carbon dioxide and absorbs oxygen. The oxygenated blood then flows into the pulmonary veins to the left atrium and across the mitral valve and into the left ventricle. With the pump action of the muscle of the left ventricle, the blood advances across the aortic valve into the aorta and thence to the rest of the body.

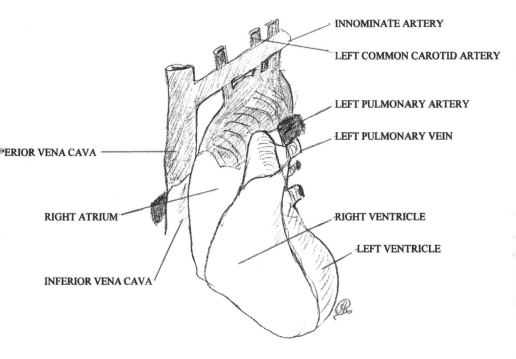

INNOMINATE ARTERY

LEFT COMMON CAROTID ARTERY

LEFT PULMONARY ARTERY

LEFT PULMONARY VEIN

ERIOR VENA CAVA

RIGHT ATRIUM

INFERIOR VENA CAVA

RIGHT VENTRICLE

LEFT VENTRICLE

ANATOMY OF THE HEART

DIAGRAM 60

Just after the oxygenated blood passes through the aortic valve, there are two small arteries, the left and right coronary arteries which supply oxygen to the heart muscle. Partial or complete blockage of these arteries or branches of these arteries causes the heart to be deprived of oxygen which results in angina or chest pain, a coronary thrombosis or heart attack, or death.

The heart is supplied by intrinsic and extrinsic nerve stimulation. The extrinsic nerves cause it to speed up or slow down, as with sleeping or exercise and the intrinsic stimulation comes from a special tissue called the sinoatrial (S-A) node, which sends a message to the atrioventricular (A-V) node and finally across an area called the Purkinje fibers so that the heart can contract approximately sixty to eighty times a minute for as long as you live!

The heart is surrounded by a sac called the pericardium, which contains a small amount of fluid. It serves to reduce any friction between the heart and its surrounding structures and hold the heart in a fairly steady position despite movements of the body. It also has a protective function shielding the heart from any infection or tumor from the lungs.

All of the structures we have mentioned are subject to abnormalities which may require surgery and which we shall discuss in this and the next three chapters. I will present the diseases of the pericardium and its surgery in this chapter. The next chapter will be diseases of the heart valves and the surgery needed to repair or replace them along with a discussion of extracorporeal circulation, the heart pump that keeps the patient alive when the heart is stopped during certain surgeries. We will then move on to coronary artery angiography, angioplasty, stenting and bypass graft surgery (CABG), to treat coronary artery problems. Lastly we will discuss the congenital abnormalities, the deformities that you are born with and discuss when and how they are repaired. Let us now move on to the pericardium.

Disease and inflammation of the pericardium, pericarditis, may occur from bacterial, viral, fungal and other infections, as well as from trauma, heart attack, tumor invasion, heart surgery itself or several other complex etiologies. The patient complains of chest pain and will have fever, chills and weakness. Aside from certain sounds heard by the physician through a stethoscope, there will be changes on the EKG and on chest x-ray. CAT scan and ultrasound, (echocardiogram) may also be diagnostic. Acute pericarditis is treated medically and often resolves without surgery, using anti-inflammatory medications either nonsteroidal like aspirin and Motrin, or steroidal such as cortisone. Sometimes a cardiologist will place a needle or small catheter into the pericardium in a procedure called pericardiocentesis to clarify the diagnosis or to remove excess pericardial fluid. When a patient has pericarditis, the lining cells may produce fluid and this can have a compression effect on the heart.

If it becomes severe, it is called cardiac tamponade which causes decrease in filling of the heart with resultant low blood pressure and weakness, and possible death. In these cases, urgent pericardiocentesis must be performed to remove as much fluid as possible. Sometimes a small catheter is left in the pericardium to drain off excessive fluid over time. If the fluid continues to reaccumulate, an opening into the pericardial sac needs to be done surgically, and sometimes complete removal of the pericardium is performed by the heart surgeon.

Another disease, constrictive pericarditis, occurs when there is thickening and inflammation of the pericardium so severe that there is a constricting effect on the heart, preventing normal filling and poor heart contraction. It sometimes responds to medical management, but often requires complete pericardiectomy.

In the case of tumors involving the pericardium, special needle biopsies can be performed to make the correct diagnosis and appropriate treatment with chemotherapy or surgery instituted.

Chapter 91
HEART VALVES

Lub dub. Lub dub, for a hundred years,
The valves in the heart is the sound that one hears.
And as long as the flow is in just one direction,
The healthy heart muscle will pump to perfection.

But if a heart valve gets diseased, or won't function
Due to a problem at the heart and valve junction,
Then you need it repaired or replaced pretty quick
And instead of lub dub, you'll hear just a loud click!

The four heart valves within the heart facilitate forward blood flow so that backflow is prevented. They are the tricuspid, the pulmonic, the mitral and the aortic valves. When a physician listens to your heart, he is listening to the sounds made by blood passing across the valves which open and close in a regular pattern. When the heart muscle contracts, expelling blood from the ventricles, the aortic and pulmonic valves leading from the ventricles open, causing a distinct sound; this is called systole or emptying of the heart and the sounds are systolic heart sounds. At the end of systole, these valves close and the blood flows into the heart through two other valves, the tricuspid and the mitral, which open just after the others close; this is called diastole and the heart sounds are called diastolic sounds. When the heart beats again, the tricuspid and mitral valves close, and the aortic and pulmonic valves open to start the cycle again.

When a valve is diseased, the openings may become smaller or stenotic, or it may not close completely, called insufficiency; however, both conditions can occur in the same valve at the same time (*see* Diagram 61 next page). When the aortic valve, leading from the left ventricle to the aorta, becomes stenotic, the heart has to work harder to push blood across the valve. Over a period of time this *wears out the heart* and can cause irreversible heart muscle damage. When there is aortic valve insufficiency, extra blood leaks back into the ventricle during

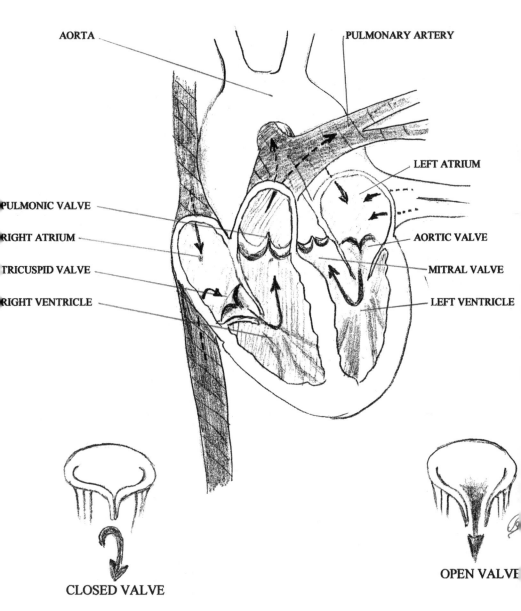

AORTA

PULMONARY ARTERY

LEFT ATRIUM

PULMONIC VALVE

RIGHT ATRIUM

TRICUSPID VALVE

RIGHT VENTRICLE

AORTIC VALVE

MITRAL VALVE

LEFT VENTRICLE

CLOSED VALVE

OPEN VALVE

ANATOMY OF HEART VALVES

DIAGRAM 61

diastole causing this chamber to get enlarged and require more work for the heart to empty. This also leads to failure of the heart if allowed to continue for a long time. Patients can have combined aortic stenosis and insufficiency which makes the problem even more severe. These types of valvular diseases can occur in the aortic, mitral, tricuspid and pulmonic valves and become progressively more symptomatic with time. I won't spent much more time on the pathophysiology except to say that the etiology of valvular heart disease can be from rheumatic disease, congenital problems, calcification of the valves and their leaflets and a host of other problems. When the physician listens to the heart of a patient with valvular disease, he will hear an altered heart sound called a murmur and the trained ear of the cardiologist can diagnose the type of valvular disease based on the type of murmur, its location on the chest wall during auscultation while listening with a stethoscope, and its timing during the cardiac cycle, during diastole or systole.

When a patient presents with the symptoms of shortness of breath, tiredness, and heart failure and signs of valvular heart disease, the cardiologist has several options for diagnostic workup including chest x-ray, EKG, echocardiography, and Doppler flow echocardiogram but the definitive study is the heart catheterization. In the latter procedure, a special catheter is passed into an artery in the groin and then into the heart to evaluate the valves and determine the extent of stenosis and/or insufficiency. In patients over 40 years of age, a concomitant study of the coronary arteries is done at the same sitting.

The indications for valvular surgery are numerous and complex and vary with each disease of each valve. The cardiologist uses his clinical judgement along with input from the cardiac surgeon and the patient to determine the timing and nature of the procedure to be done. Sometimes the patient has valvular disease as well as coronary artery disease and both entities need to be treated during the same heart operation.

Valvular surgery involves either repair of the damaged valve, or replacement with a mechanical valve or a specially preserved animal heart valve usually from a pig. The type of valve used is also determined by many factors including which valve, aortic, mitral, etc., patient age, extent of disease and irregularities of the heart. This complex surgery is performed under general anesthesia through a median sternotomy incision, and with the patient on the heart bypass machine with the heart arrested. The heart muscle is protected in the arrested state by a solution called cardioplegia. The old valve is removed and the new valve sewn into place with non-absorbing sutures.

In order to allow for complex cardiac surgery, it is necessary to stop the beating heart and develop a machine that could oxygenate blood and could pump blood through the body. The early studies were done by Alexis Carrel and surprisingly, by Charles Lindbergh, the transatlantic flier who did medical research in his later years. Eventually the complexities of oxygenating blood and pumping it correctly through the body were mastered.

The patient is put to sleep by the anesthesiologist and the chest is opened by the surgeon. Artificial tubes are placed in the patient, one in a vein to take blood from the patient, and another in an artery to pump the blood back into the body. In the heart bypass machine, the blood passes through a special chamber where carbon dioxide is released and oxygen is absorbed by the blood. As simple as it may seem, the process is fairly complex! A pump team of specially trained individuals manages the extracorporeal circulation while the surgeon stops the beating heart, and performs his procedure.

Chapter 92
CORONARY ARTERY DISEASE (CABG - CORONARY ARTERY BYPASS GRAFTING)
On and Off "The Pump"

A traveler in ancient Katmandu,
Was bothered by chest pain one day.
He figured it must be the food or ague,
And continued his adventurous stay.

But the stress and the altitude had its effect,
And his chest pain became more intense.
The cause was much more than the monks could detect,
No relief came from prayers and incense.

There were no treadmills or electric devices,
No x-rays or angiograms
No cardiac surgeons to give their advices,
And no modern cardiograms.

So our anginal traveler met with his fate,
He passed on, and what can we learn?
If you don't treat your chest pain before it's too late,
You'll end up in a funeral urn!

In the 1960's my uncle Irving, known to us as Winki, was the most athletic member of the family. An avid tennis player, muscular with no excess fat, he was the picture of health. After a vigorous tennis match, he went into the shower, collapsed, and died at the age of 49, a victim of coronary thrombosis. The family was devastated and surprised. His post mortem exam showed a single, severe area of narrowing in his left main coronary artery. If he had symptoms. he never spoke of them and in those days our ability to do screening for coronary artery disease was minimal. There was no treadmill testing, no coronary angiography, no angioplasty and no direct coronary artery bypass grafting. We will discuss these topics which have become household terms in many circles. Poor uncle Winki's heart disease came twenty years too early!

In the past, patients with signs and symptoms of coronary artery disease were treated with medicines directed at preventing blood clots from occurring in the coronary arteries and dilating the arteries. The symptoms were primarily chest pain radiating down the left arm, or into the jaw or back, called angina pectoris. With each episode of angina, the patient was treated with nitroglycerin, a powerful artery dilator, and other medications. If the patient had a heart attack, namely coronary artery blockage causing cardiac muscle death and survived, the treatment was supportive and totally medical

Then came the advent of improved diagnostics and bypass grafting, changing the whole natural history of the treatment of coronary artery disease. The diagnostics include the electrocardiogram which show changes indicating electrical abnormalities secondary to ischemia or decreased blood flow to areas of the heart. If a patient has any angina or EKG changes, the cardiologist will do a treadmill test which measures EKG changes with the stress of walking. There are also tests where radioactive liquid is injected which localizes in the heart muscle. If the blood flow to certain areas of the heart is diminished, the scan of the heart will show this abnormality. The next study is a direct angiography of the coronary arteries of the heart. The cardiologist places a catheter in the groin artery and then into the heart and injects contrast dye directly into the coronary arteries and shows all areas of narrowing and occlusion.

In many medical centers weekly conferences are held by cardiologists and cardiac surgeons to discuss elective heart problems and to decide the on courses of treatment. For many problems, the coronary disease can be corrected or improved by a procedure known as coronary angioplasty. The cardiologists can open up diseased, narrowed coronary arteries using catheters similar to the ones used for the angiogram. These catheters have balloons on the end which can be blown up in a narrowed vessel, thus dilating the vessel. This can be augmented by using lasers, drilling and reaming devices and tiny stents or hollow tubes to keep the coronary arteries open.

This procedure has resulted in outstanding successes in alleviating symptoms and correcting coronary heart problems. There are, however, complications and problems with angioplasties and among these are: Damage to vessels by the procedure, clotting off and occlusion by collapse of the vessels during the procedure, and just plain inability to correct the problem. These patients, and some with disease too severe for angioplasty, are referred for open heart surgery, or as it is called CABG, "cabbage procedures", which stands for Coronary Artery Bypass Graft surgery.

In CABG procedures, the chest is opened and the heart visualized and examined. The areas of blockage seen on the angiogram are found in the beating heart. Standard procedure for many years was to then place the patient on a cardiopulmonary bypass machine. When the machine has taken over the heart and lung function, the body is cooled to 28 degrees centigrade and cardioplegia is given into the heart and the heart muscle is protected in a flaccid state. Then the surgeon bypasses the blocked arteries using either a vein taken from the leg (or rarely the arm) or the internal mammary artery which is dissected out of the chest just behind the sternum. If a vein is used, one end is sutured to the coronary artery beyond the area of disease; the other end is sutured to the aorta. Then when the heart is restarted, the blood will flow from the aorta into the graft and thence into the distal coronary artery beyond the blocked segment. If the internal mammary artery is used, the proximal side is already in place as an artery and the distal end is sewn into the coronary artery beyond the diseased segment. The patient is rewarmed to 37 degrees, during which phase the heart may start to beat spontaneously or may need an electrical stimulation to start beating. All the tubes and connections are removed, the chest is closed using heavy wires for the bony sternum, and the patient is sent to the intensive care unit.

Complications include bleeding, heart arrhythmias, and occasional infections. In most centers doing several hundred hearts each year, the morbidity and mortality are very low because of the team effort and the experience of the surgeon and the supportive team of anesthesiologists, nurses and pump technicians. The hospital stay is usually five to ten days depending on the nature of the surgery and afterwards the patient has a strict exercise and recuperation regimen to follow for several months (*see* Diagram 62).

Over that past few years, several cardiac surgeons have been doing coronary artery bypass graft surgery off pump. This means they are able to sew the grafts in place, with the heart still beating, obviating the need for placing the patient on the heart lung machine or "pump". Special ins-

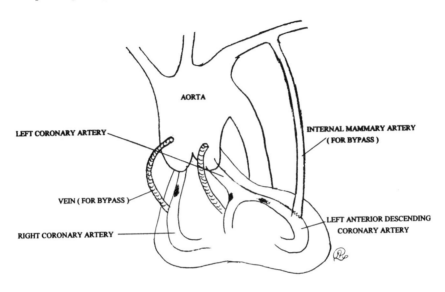

CORONARY ARTERY BYPASS GRAFTING (CABG)

DIAGRAM 62

truments and devices hold the area of heart being operated upon very still so that the fine sutures can be accurately placed in the arteries. This procedure cuts down on the morbidity and operating time. Some patients are not candidates for off pump bypass because of the nature of their heart disease, the technical difficulties and surgeon preference. The pump team is almost always standing by in case the surgeon decides he is unable to perform the surgery with the beating heart technique.

Another new procedure for coronary artery disease is called transmyo-cardial laser revascularization. It is reserved for those patients with severe heart disease where the coronary arteries are so poor that standard revascularization procedures are not possible; the vessels are so diseased or so small that they are not accessible to bypass. The patients can undergo this new laser procedure which consists of placing multiple tiny holes with a laser guided technique from the surface of the heart to the inner chamber. For some reason, not yet completely understood, new blood vessels grow within the channels thereby improving blood supply to the muscle and reducing anginal pain. The procedure is only being done at a few heart centers but if it proves very successful, it will probably become standard for all severely symptomatic otherwise inoperable coronary artery diseased patients.

With heart surgery, the more cases, the better the experience of the surgeon and the heart team, so if you have to have open heart surgery, I strongly recommend you go to a major center doing at least several hundred heart cases each year.

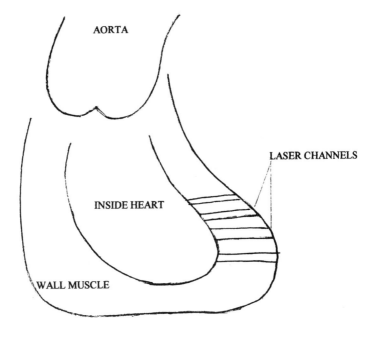

TRANSMYOCARDIAL LASER REVASCULARIZATION

DIAGRAM 63

Chapter 93
CONGENITAL DEFORMITIES, UNUSUAL SURGERY AND HEART TRANSPLANTATION

When talking of congenital deformities
It doesn't mean genital enormities.
And likewise with heart transplantations,
It's not on wife swapping relations.

So before you begin on this section,
You should know that I have predilection,
Towards things scientific, or to be quite specific,
Thoracico-cardio-congenito-transplanto-bibbidy bobbi- reflection.

There are three major areas in this chapter: Congenital abnormalities, unusual cardiac surgeries, and heart transplantation.

I remember when I was in training as a general surgeon, having a rotation through the cardiac surgery division at a major hospital where there was a renowned pediatric heart surgery program. The infants, some only a few days old, were hooked up to all types of monitoring devices, intravenous fluids, on respirators with oxygen and they seemed barely able to stand all the tubes and wires. These were the infants that somehow had some genetic defect that caused an incomplete development of the heart, which was tolerable in the uterus but intolerable in the outside world. And yet, they were the lucky ones, for most fetuses in utero with heart defects never survived long enough to be born.

These lucky babies, who never had any chance for survival one hundred years ago, now have a good chance of living to adulthood thanks to the discoveries in modern medicine which enabled physicians to make the correct diagnosis, and the surgeons to perform surgery on a heart often no bigger than a walnut. In those days, thirty five years ago, the infants were cooled almost to freezing, and the metabolism was slowed so much, that the surgeons were able to stop the heart without bypass and operate on the tiny organ without blood flow, heart beat or brain damage. The procedures were done rapidly and then the heart was restarted as the body rewarmed. I was amazed by these procedures, and by the ability to give life to an infant so close to death.

As I have mentioned, for a whole host of developmental reason, somewhere between the fourth and eighth week of gestational growth of the fetus in the uterus, the developing heart goes through tremendous changes, any one of which may result in a critical cardiac defect. By the ninth week, the heart has been fully developed, defect or not, ready to start taking over its long term function of pumping blood through the body.

There are many congenital abnormalities of the heart and great vessels and I will only describe a few important and more common ones. With more advanced pump technology, instrumentation and techniques, the pediatric cardiac surgeon can treat many of these abnormalities. I'm going to list the abnormalities and show you their appearance in diagrams and then talk about the problems they present and their surgeries. So don't cringe if the words sound foreign and unintelligible. I will go into a more detailed description as we move along.

The most common abnormalities are: Patent Ductus Arteriosus, Coarctation of the Aorta, Aortic Stenosis, Atrial Septal Defects, Ventricular Septal Defects, The Tetralogy of Fallot, Transposition of the Great Vessels, and Truncus Arteriosus. And remember, these are only the major defects; there are many more with tremendous complexity, some of which can only be repaired in several stages as the infants grow larger. Some are associated with other bodily abnormalities and are given syndrome names to describe all the accompanying abnormalities such as Ebstein's anomaly, Lutembacher's syndrome, DiGeorge's syndrome, etc.. Often the surgical correction procedure is given the name of the surgeon responsible or its development such as the original Taussig/Blalock procedure for the Tetralogy of Fallot. Now it's used very infrequently (*see* Diagram 64 next page).

Congenital heart problems are often divided into five categories according to their physiologic effects, namely what happens to circulation or blood oxygenation because of the defect. They are:

(1) Problems causing cyanosis, with bluish skin color due to decreased oxygenation where some blood is shunted away from the lungs into the

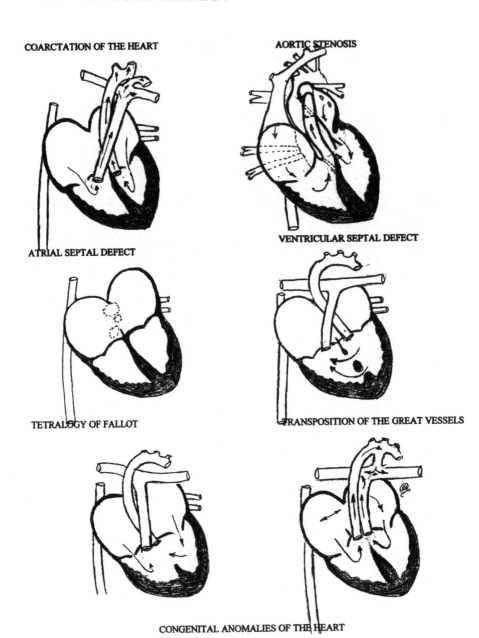

COARCTATION OF THE HEART

AORTIC STENOSIS

ATRIAL SEPTAL DEFECT

VENTRICULAR SEPTAL DEFECT

TETRALOGY OF FALLOT

TRANSPOSITION OF THE GREAT VESSELS

CONGENITAL ANOMALIES OF THE HEART

DIAGRAM 64

circulation without being oxygenated as in Tetralogy of Fallot, transposition of the great vessels, and truncus arteriosus;

(2) Left to right shunts where some oxygenated blond is moved from the left heart back to the right heart causing increased blood flow into the lungs as in patent ductus arteriosus, atrial and ventricular septal defects;

(3) Obstructive left sided abnormalities where a defect makes it harder for blood to flow out of the heart into the general circulation as in coarctation of the aorta, and aortic stenosis;

(4) Unusual origins of vessels such as coronary arteries coming from a different location causing problems; and,

(5) Other complicated abnormalities causing multiple problems, too complex to describe.

Most of these defects cause loud heart murmurs which can often be identified by the cardiologist on the basis of sound and location in conjunction with the physical diagnosis even before heart catheterization.

In the normal individual, deoxygenated blood flows into the right heart, to the lungs and gets oxygenated (it goes from being bluish to red. It then flows to the left heart from where it is pumped through the body. In defect #1, some or most of the unoxygenated blood goes back into the arterial system without being reoxygenated causing bluish appearance of these babies. If the defect is too great, the babies die rapidly, but sometimes the defect can be corrected surgically as in the cases listed above. The transposition of the great vessels is corrected by just reversing the two "confused" major vessels. The other problems have very complex curative surgeries beyond our descriptive capabilities here.

In defect #2, the problem is easier to understand. In the fetus, there is no breathing going on; the baby gets its oxygen from the mother's blood stream via the placenta so the pulmonary circulation with blood going through the lungs is not needed for oxygenation. There is a special vessel called the ductus arteriosus which is normal in the fetus, and which shunts blood from the pulmonary artery to the aorta and to the general circulation. Just after birth, when the baby takes its first breath, this ductus begins to rapidly close, forcing the blood into the lungs for the now needed oxygenation. In some babies the ductus remains open or patent and some unoxygenated blood is "shunted" away from the lungs into the general circulation having the effect of decreasing the amount of oxygen in the blood and sometimes causing problems of heart failure.

The treatment may be successful just by giving medication, indometha-cin, which stimulates the patent ductus to close or it may be closed by a radiological procedure in a cardiac catheterization laboratory with placement of a special coil into the ductus which causes it to occlude. The third method, when the above two fail or are not indicated is the surgical approach in which the cardiac surgeon or pediatric surgeon ties off the patent ductus in a procedure which often takes less than thirty minutes with essentially a 0% mortality.

The other two deformities mentioned under #2 are the atrial and ventricular septal detects. This means that there is an opening between the left and right atrium or ventricle or both. Patients with these defects have variable amounts of mixing of oxygenated and unoxygenated blood and some may have minimal symptoms for several years. The repairs are done by sewing the tissue together, if it is a small opening, or using a patch over the opening in the atrium or ventricle if the defect is too large to close proximally. The patients generally do very well. There are, however, some conditions where repair is not recommended because of other abnormalities, but these are too complex to delineate here.

The type #3 defect is what is called an obstructive left sided lesion which means that there is some partial blockage to flow into or through the aorta. In some patients there is a defect in the aortic valve where the opening is smaller than usual. This requires the left ventricle to pump harder to empty and results in eventual heart failure and permanent damage. Similarly, in coarctation or narrowing of the aorta, there is such limitation to flow that the heart must pump harder to get the blood through the narrowed segment. These are usually emergency cases and must be repaired by the cardiac surgeon as soon as diagnosed. Type #4 and #5 are more unusual and complex abnormalities which may need urgent repair but occasionally can wait until the child is older for repair in stages.

In conclusion, there are many types of congenital heart and great vessel defects which can occur during fetal development. Most of the babies will not survive and will be born dead; however, the few that do survive now have a reasonably good chance for a normal life given the innovative surgeries developed over the past fifty years and the ability to place tiny infants on heart bypass, stop the heart and perform micro-surgical procedures.

In this section I will mention the other unusual cardiac surgeries. The first is the surgical treatment of cardiac arrhythmias or the abnormal beating of the heart due to many causes. Surgery is indicated when a patient will not respond to the usual medications and has severe symptoms such as shortness of breath or stroke. The procedure, known as the "Maze" operation because it looks like a maze when completed, consists of a complex series of partial resections of the atria with incisions and closures of the heart muscle, dividing the nerve fibers of innervation from the atria of the heart and to the ventricles. In some cases, the abnormal heartbeat is due to scarring of the heart muscle from old heart attacks and this area of scar may need to be removed to prevent the arrhythmia.

Another procedure consists of excising aneurysms of the heart, usually caused by heart attack after which there has been scarring of a segment of the heart muscle.

In some patients with abnormal heart rate or too slow a heart rate, cardiac pacemakers are used. These are small devices about the size of a tiny radio, which are placed under the skin with wires coming from one end. These wires are inserted into the heart muscle, usually through a vein using fluoroscopic x-ray to place them properly. The pacemaker may give off regular impulses to keep the heart at a regular rate or may be a demand pacemaker, which means it only stimulates the heart to beat when the rate gets too slow. The pacemaker rate can be adjusted with an outside electrical instrument to go faster or slower. There are also special implantable defibrillators which will shock the heart if it stops, much the way you've seen on the television programs with external "zapping" defibrillators, which make the actor/patient bounce up three inches off the table in a dramatic fashion.

There are intra-aortic balloon pumps, which are essentially catheters with a large balloon near the end. These balloons are attached to a machine which inflates and deflates them to the beat of the heart and in patients who temporarily have poor heart function, as may occur in the first few days after a heart attack, or major heart surgery; the balloon pump acts to augment the pumping action of the heart thereby increasing the blood pressure. It is a lifesaving device in many scenarios. I have seen these inserted in patients with low blood pressure on the way to surgery for coronary artery bypass because of coronary blockages. After the bypass, when the heart is getting good blood supply, the heart muscle becomes stronger and the balloon pump can be removed.

Tumors of the heart are rare; myxoma, a benign tumor, is the most common accounting for more than half the lesions. They can actually grow quite large and have all sorts of symptoms. The diagnosis is confirmed on cardiac ultrasound and they are successfully removed in most cases (98%). Malignant tumors of the heart, primary (originating in the heart) and metastatic (coming from a distant tumor spreading to the heart), are most often not operable and there is little to be done but make the patient as comfortable as possible.

Finally, let us speak of the last words in cardiac surgery. These are heart transplantation and the artificial heart.

Heart transplantation in the experimental model on animals dates back almost a hundred years, but the first successful human heart transplant was performed by Dr. Christian Barnard at the Groote Schuur Hospital in South Africa in December 1967. This was followed by years of further experimentation with many failures until the eighties and nineties when the problems of rejection and infection were able to be overcome in most instances. Today, heart transplantation is done at many medical centers with excellent operative success rates and fairly good five year survival rates, considering that all these patients would not have survived more than a few months without the transplant. There is a long list of medications and contraindications to heart transplantation and an even longer list of the necessary studies to be done before the patient is ready for the surgery. Donors, usually "brain dead" trauma victims must be carefully screened and the donor and recipient have to be matched for blood type compatibility. There is a national registry for organ procurement which makes matching a donor and recipient easier, but there is still a long wait for a "heart" and some patients don't live long enough to receive this life saving gift.

The procedure itself is complex and requires two teams, one to "harvest" the heart, removing it carefully under sterile conditions from the deceased donor and one to prepare the recipient for the donor heart by putting the patient to sleep, opening the chest, putting the patient on the heart pump oxygenator, and at just the right moment when the new heart arrives, removing the old damaged heart and sewing in the new heart. I have watched the procedure done and it is, to say the least, very dramatic; the sadness of the death of one individual and the joy of that individual's heart living on by saving the life of another.

The solution to too few donor hearts is the artificial heart. Several have been designed and because of the multiple possible complications, few patients have survived very long. In some instances, the artificial heart has been used long enough to find a usable human donor heart, but as for a permanent artificial heart, it is still in an experimental stage, with the longest survivals in animals over 200 days. The few devices implanted (much the same technique as with heart transplantation) have been pneumatic with air pressure pumps, with the longest surviving patient living for almost two years. There are many complications including infection and strokes; newer, less bulky power packs will be needed for long term successful transplantations. Many experimental programs are underway using a battery supplied motor driven artificial heart which may be used in clinical trials in the next few years.

PLASTIC
AND
RECONSTRUCTIVE SURGERY

Chapter 94
SKIN GRAFTS AND FLAPS

The problem of covering a defect of skin,
Is a subject where skin flaps are often brought in.
Rotating from one spot to another is smart,
You can make a new ear or nose with the art.

In 1597, Tagliacozzo published a famous text in plastic surgery and wrote of the reconstruction of the nose by borrowing tissue with a "flap" from the arm. With the swordplay of the time, it was apparently not rare to cut off the nose, and nasal reconstruction was not uncommon. Plastic surgery dates way back in the history of medicine and surgery, and references to reconstruction can be found in the earliest papyri and chronicles. Whether for coverage of a wide defect of skin removed for infection or by cancer or trauma, or for reconstruction of a major defect such as an ear, nose or breast, skin grafts and skin flaps have been used for many years.

Plastic surgery is basically the field of surgery which focuses on reconstructing the appearance of the individual as well as the function. Great stress is placed on the careful handling of tissue, closing of wounds with the least possible scarring (which means less wound edge tension and anatomical approximation of edges, and fine suture). Many years ago, Dr. Langer outlined the lines of normal stress and tension on the surface of the human body and even today we use these to determine the best direction to make an incision to get the best scar. The plastic surgeon learns how to make incisions on joints and to make incisions on the face which will fall into the natural direction for lines of expression. It is not that other surgeons are not aware of, or do not keep these points in mind, it is just that the visible outer scar is often not at the top of the priority when someone is having a breast cancer or a stomach cancer removed, and the focus of each specialist is on his area of expertise. So, yes, the plastic surgeon will probably give you a better scar than the orthopedist or the brain surgeon, and if cosmesis is of utmost concern, better turn to this specialist.

Aside from this aspect, however, the plastic surgeon is the master of finding tissue and skin to cover areas of the body that need covering! When an individual has been burned and needs skin for covering the burnt area, we turn to the plastic surgeon for his expertise in taking partial thicknesses of skin from other areas of the body and placing them on the burnt area. He/she uses an instrument called a dermatome to remove very thin thicknesses of skin, and can dial in the thickness to the thousandths of an inch and arrange for the width depending on the usage.

For a skin graft to "take" to the area it is applied, there has to be a good recipient bed, which means that it needs tissue that has a decent blood supply, minimal or no infection and can be placed without tension and allowed to heal. It takes about 24 to 48 hours for new blood vessels to grow into the skin graft area and start supplying the graft, and in that critical time, oxygen diffuses through serum into the cells of the graft keeping it alive. In patients with diabetes mellitus or other vascular problems or severe infection, the graft may not "take" and other methods of wound coverage or closure may be needed. When a surgeon removes a small area of skin and cannot close the wound primarily (edge to edge because of the distance between the edges), he will take a split thickness skin graft from a donor site and place it over the defect. Split thickness means that the skin has been partially cut in its thickness. That means that the donor site (from where you take the skin) will appear like a bad sunburn or worse for several weeks, but will eventually heal, often leaving a reddish scarred site. The skin is either sewn in place, or stapled in place (the instrument looks just like a paper stapler), and often is held down in place by moistened cotton or other dressings. The surgeon tries to immobilize the recipient site so that there is no movement or shearing effect on the skin during the critical first few days.

As opposed to partial or split thickness skin grafts, there are also full thickness skin grafts. In these cases, the donor skin is removed in its entirety and the donor site must be closed much as you would a laceration. Full thickness skin grafts are used for small areas on the face, hands and fingers, but the success rate for the graft is not as good as the partial thickness graft. In some instances, when skin is not readily available, some surgeons may use porcine (pig) skin to cover a wound as a temporary coverage until the patient is ready to receive his own skin graft.

Another area of importance is the "flap". This usually means that a full thickness segment of skin and subcutaneous tissue is mobilized leaving one side (the pedicle) attached to its blood supply. Just as Tagliacozzo described almost five hundred years ago, a part of the body is brought next to another part and a flap of skin is attached where needed. Sometimes the flaps may be just adjacent to the needed area, and other times it may be from a distance. A hand needing major coverage may be temporarily "attached" to a flap of skin on the abdomen. When the attachment has healed and developed a blood supply from its attachment, the pedicle is cut and the hand and its new tissue are freed from the donor site. The donor site is then closed as best possible. Plastic surgeons spend years in training learning the ins and outs of skin coverage and flap development and I've explained it all in three minutes! I will describe TRAM and latissimus flaps in Chapter 95 when we talk about reconstruction after mastectomy.

The final area in flaps is the free tissue transfer or microvascular transfer of tissue from one site to another. With the advent of microvascular techniques for suturing using a microscope or magnifying lenses, surgeons can remove tissue from one area of the body and suture to another. This is the same technique as used in replanting a finger after amputation. Large segments of skin and subcutaneous tissue can be removed, for example, from the abdomen with the severed arteries and veins identified. These are then connected to arteries and veins in the area of a mastectomy (breast removal) and the entire tissue is sewn into place to replace the removed breast. These procedures are very successful in skilled hands but have the potential for disaster if not observed carefully by a trained team for several days.

Chapter 95
BREAST SURGERY
Augmentation, Reduction and Mammoplasty
Reconstruction After Mastectomy

For me, it would be vain, at best,
To write a poem about the breast.
With all its romance, disease and history,
It still remains a consummate mystery.

In this chapter we'll discuss the female breast from the plastic surgeon's viewpoint. The first part will be predominantly cosmetic, then a combination of cosmetic and pathologic and the third, cosmetic and reconstructive.

Living in southern California, I am convinced that every other woman has a breast augmentation or else the warm weather and sea air is good for breast development. I don't want to know the answer. Augmentation mammoplasty is a procedure where the surgeon inserts an internal mammary prosthesis under the pectoralis muscle of the chest wall (or by some surgeons just under the natural breast) to increase the projection of the breast. It is occasionally covered by insurance only in cases of significant hypomastia (absence of or very small breasts - especially when psychological problems have ensued). In general, it is a procedure which is purely cosmetic and therefore not covered by your insurance carrier. Unfortunately, because it is a "cash on the barrelhead" type of procedure, many physicians who are inadequately trained, label themselves as cosmetic surgeons, and perform the procedure in office surgery suites with less than satisfactory results. If you want plastic surgery, go to the trained specialist! If not, don't be surprised if the results are mediocre. I have seen some terrible breast augmentations!

This is usually an outpatient procedure performed in a surgeon's office operating suite or in a surgical center or hospital operating room. The main complications are bleeding, infection and occasional breakdown of the skin due to placement of too large a prosthesis. Because of the legal problems with the silicone gel, the only prostheses available for general use are the saline type, except for post mastectomy reconstruction, where the silicone is still approved. A long term complication (felt by some to be partially due to a minor Staph infection) is development of encapsulation of the implant, resulting in deformity and extreme firmness of the breast. This may require replacement of the implant and removal of the encapsulating scar tissue.

The incisions for augmentation mammoplasty can be inframammary (under the lower edge of the breast), periareolar (around the area of the nipple), or axillary (through the armpit), and when done properly, leaves an almost invisible scar. Some women, however, develop hypertrophic (raised) scars called keloids and this may impact the cosmetic result.

Reduction mammoplasty means making the breast smaller. Macromastia (large breasts) may be very painful and cause orthopedic (back pain) problems because of their size, as well as a cosmetic problem. Reduction mammoplasty can often be covered by insurance for this reason and all plastic surgeons are aware of this and will usually work with your insurance carrier to get some financial coverage. This procedure is also done for ptosis (sagging) of the breasts which occurs with aging and occasionally after pregnancy. The latter condition can sometimes be ameliorated by augmentation mammoplasty alone, but most of the times, a combination reduction and augmentation are needed to correct ptosis.

Reduction mammoplasty is much more complicated than augmentation and will leave several scars which are somewhat unsightly. The procedure involves removing skin and breast tissue and repositioning the nipple and areola in a higher position, leaving a vertical incision extending from the areola downward to an arched transverse incision under the breast (in the "inframammary fold"). The procedure is done after appropriate counseling and weight loss and the patient must understand the complications of bleeding, infection, and the rare loss of the areola and nipple if the blood supply is damaged or poor. Sensation in the nipple may be altered significantly. In some cases, a free "graft" nipple reconstruction is done by the surgeon instead of the usual procedure.

Reconstruction of the breast after a partial or modified radical mastectomy can take several forms. If the operating surgeon can leave enough skin after removing the cancer, the plastic surgeon will place a temporary expander under the pectoralis muscle after the mastectomy has been completed. Over the subsequent several months, the expander prosthesis (which is a specially designed inflatable sacs) is injected with saline and this acts to stretch the overlying skin slowly to prepare for the permanent implant. When the expansion is complete, the patient is taken back to the operating room for placement of the permanent prosthesis. There is still no areola and nipple, and the patient will have to return to the operating room a third time a few months later to have a nipple reconstruction done. Each stage has potential complications of which the patient must be made aware, and the final outcome while a significant improvement is not as aesthetically pleasing as a normal breast.

In many patients, where the implant is not desired or for medical reasons is not possible, a flap reconstruction is performed. The most common is called the TRAM flap (transverse rectus abdominus muscle flap) from the abdomen, but there is also a latissimus muscle flap from the side and back. A free flap may also be done in certain cases. What are these flap procedures?

Where there is a large defect on the chest, the flap objective is to bring up a segment of tissue with muscle, subcutaneous tissue and skin and supplied by a vascular (blood supply) pedicle. Whether by TRAM or latissimus flap, the procedure is very involved, carefully dissecting out the tissue freeing up the pedicle and then passing the entire structure under the skin of the chest where it is sutured in place. When optimally successful, this results in a more normal feeling breast; however, the complications of infection and hematoma are still possible with the major problem of complete loss of the flap tissue of the blood supply through the pedicle is not adequate. The procedure can take from two to six or more hours! The nipple reconstruction is usually done as a separate procedure several months later. Also, when the reconstruction is complete, some type of procedure is usually needed on the opposite side to make the breasts look equal in size and shape.

The free pedicle flaps are the same as the above except that the tissue is transferred to the chest and then the blood vessels are connected to new blood vessels in the chest using microsurgery. This procedure is also a very long one often taking 6-8 hours and requiring close observation of the flap to make sure it survives. The last patient I saw with this procedure had to go back for another six hours of surgery when the flap turned "gray" and the blood vessels had to be resutured. You usually don't have to worry about non-qualified individuals doing reduction mammoplasties or free grafts...it's too much work and too high risk for complications even in the best of hands!

Breast reconstruction can be started at the time of the initial mastectomy, but some surgeons prefer and recommend waiting until after the cancer surgery is completed and the wounds healed. Flap procedures and special implants are also available for patients who have undergone lumpectomy or partial mastectomy and who have poor cosmetic results. The procedure, as with all others, is fashioned to fit the patient's aesthetic needs.

Chapter 96
FACIAL PLASTIC SURGERY
Facelift, Browlift, Rhinoplasty, Cheek and Chin
Augmentation Laser and Acid Treatment

Rhytidectomy*, Rhinoplasty*, Blepharoplasty*,
You're gonna look good girl, you're gonna be classy!
Add a little cheek and a little bit of chin.
A little spray of acid and some laser, and you're "in".

You're a new woman now; there ain't no doubt about it,
Get it on, show your stuff, just move out and flout it.
You're dashing, and graceful, just cute as can be,
A plastic surgeon's dreamboat, and you're only ninety three.

*rhytidectomy = facelift
*rhinoplasty = nose reconstruction
*blepharoplasty = upper and lower eyelid surgery

With age comes aging! We develop jowls, deepened wrinkles around the mouth and eyes and forehead, bags under our eyes, and wrinkles of the neck and face. In today's world, the appearance of youth not only boosts the ego and self image, but has a positive effect in the workplace where supposedly youth equals vigor and success.

Skin loses its "tone", the nature of the underlying collagen or supportive tissue changes, there is less fat in the subcutaneous tissue, the skin becomes thinner and less elastic. Face it; growing old is the pits!

The plastic surgeon doesn't give youth; he gives the appearance of youth and it's called a facelift or rhytidectomy. With computers, the surgeon can give the patient a better idea of what to expect after a procedure so there won't be unrealistic expectations. And I emphasize, there are facelifts and there are facelifts. Some look terrific and some look pretty bad! Select your plastic surgeon very carefully.

The facelift is basically a pulling up, and back, of the fascia and skin of the face. Preoperatively the patient is advised to stop any medications which may cause increased bleeding (aspirin containing) and stop smoking if possible. The procedure may be done in an outpatient surgery center of physician's office and can be done under local or general anesthesia. The procedure may take several hours and some physicians arrange for a one or two day stay in a post-operative facility where the patient can have nursing care, medication and observation.

The essentials of the surgery are the initial incision which extends from the scalp 6 inches above the ear, along the front margin of the ear and around the earlobe and back into the hair bearing scalp. The skin is elevated from the facial fascia and dissection is carried almost to the outer edge of the nose. The underlying fascia (SMAS - superficial muscular aponeurotic system) is dissected out over a short distance, tightened and sewn to the fascia in front of the ear. Tissue from the neck is also "pulled up". Excess skin is then excised and the skin is then sutured into place, leaving an almost invisible scar line in front of the ear. There are many different additions to this procedure and it is a tedious, careful surgery taking many hours. The complications are bleeding and infection; injury to the facial nerves is extremely rare. There is usually some facial swelling for up to four weeks but patients often return to normal activity in about two weeks.

The browlift, once only done through an incision behind the hairline, can now be done endoscopically through three tiny incisions in the front of the scalp behind the hairline. The forehead muscles are cut to relax the features of the forehead and in cases of excess skin or 'winkles, this can be pulled up from above with the older incision.

Eyelid surgery is called blepharoplasty. Sometimes only fat needs to be removed, but in most instances, a small amount of skin is excised through incisions just above and just below the eyelids, which are essentially imperceptible once healed. This surgery gets rid of the "bags" under the eyes and gives a more youthful appearance; it has very few complications. Sometimes patients have a black and blue appearance for a few weeks.

Rhinoplasty is surgery on the appearance of the nose. There may be airway partial or total obstruction and in these cases the surgery will be covered by insurance. The surgery is performed through open or closed techniques, depending on surgeon preference and the extent of the procedure. The open procedure has small incision at the lower front of the nose and the closed procedure has a small opening made just inside the nose. Through these, cartilage at the tip of the nose can be refashioned and the nasal bone itself can be "trimmed" using a cutting instrument called an osteotome. Bones can be broken and reset to narrow or lower the nose as desired. The procedure is done under general or local anesthesia in an outpatient setting, and complications are unusual. During the procedure, the surgeon may also correct airway obstruction by excising overgrown tissue (in turbinates and nasal septum). Small changes in the nasal profile can make major aesthetic appearance improvements.

In the last decade great advances have been made in the use of prosthetic devices for changing the contour of the face. The high, full cheekbones of youth give way to a deflated cheek as one ages and this can be improved with cheek implants. Similarly, a small or recessed chin can be augmented by a small implant into the chin to give the face a more balanced appearance.

Finally, fine aging lines, small areas of pigment change, and superficial scarring (as from acne) can often be improved using facial "peels". Fine wrinkles and scars are usually not improved with face lift and will respond to removal of the top layer of the epidermis by one of several methods. These include dermabrasion by a spinning "sanding" wheel, or by the application of chemicals that act to burn the skin (phenol or trichloroacetic acid). The depth of the peel is dependent on the amount of chemical and length of time of the exposure. After a peel, there will be a reddening of the skin that fades in about 2-3 months. The peel is often done under mild sedation and the patient needs to avoid sun exposure for several months.

More recently, several physicians have started to use the laser (Light Amplification by Stimulated Emission of Radiation) for face peels by vaporizing the most superficial skin layers.

Chapter 97
LIPOSUCTION
AND ABDOMINOPLASTY

Jack Spratt's wife had gone to fat and Jack was getting mean,
The Missus went to a Plastic doc to see if he'd suck that fat clean.
But she canceled the surgery when she heard the cost, just in the nick
of time,
Cause you just don't make a heck of a lot, by being in a nursery
rhyme!

Liposuction is the extracting of fat through a tube hooked to a suction machine and it's the most common plastic surgical procedure performed in the United States. There may be a secret connection between the American Society of Plastic Surgeons and McDonald's restaurants. Although the procedure is not technically difficult to do, it's very difficult to do well! It had been designed for individuals who were not necessarily very overweight, but who could not get rid of the stubborn areas of fat around the thighs and hips and abdomen which don't respond easily to dieting. However, its usage has been extended to include anyone who wants it and has even become a quick weight loss regimen. This has led many surgeons to do over-extensive procedures leading to greater blood and fluid loss and complications.

Liposuction in men is usually for waist, abdomen and chin, while women go for the thighs, buttocks and hips. The procedure is usually done under local anesthesia with heavy sedation or general anesthesia and the length of the procedure depends on the extent of the surgery. Prior to beginning the surgery, many surgeons inject saline (salt solution) with epinephrine (a blood vessel constrictor to cut down on the bleeding) into the fatty areas. Small openings are then made and a blunt tipped catheter connected to a strong suction machine is inserted and literally sucks out the fat. There is usually significant bruising and the patient is required to wear some type of pressure garment for several weeks. A well planned and executed procedure results in an excellent cosmetic outcome, but often the poorly trained physician attempting liposuction will end up with a patient with uneven contours, ugly scars and occasional loss of skin from too vigorous suctioning. It is a procedure not without serious complications such as blood clots to the lung and excessive fluid and blood loss, and should not be taken casually or lightly. It should only be done by a trained surgeon under optimal safe surgical conditions.

Abdominoplasty is a plastic surgical procedure for removing skin, fat and subcutaneous tissue from the abdomen to improve the appearance. A large ellipse of skin and subcutaneous tissue is removed leaving the umbilicus in place. The upper abdomen is freed up and advanced down to connect with the area above the pubis where the segment has been removed. An opening is then made in the segment which has been brought down, and the umbilicus is brought through the opening and sutured in place.

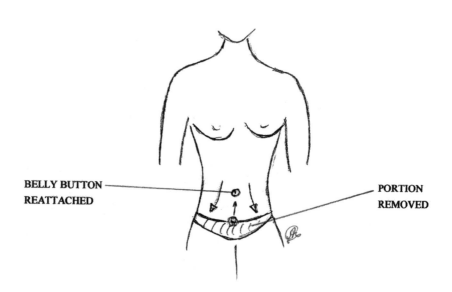

BELLY BUTTON REATTACHED

PORTION REMOVED

DIAGRAM OF ABDOMINOPLASTY

DIAGRAM 65

Chapter 98
COMMON
CONGENITAL REPAIRS

Cleft lip and cleft palate are a shock for all families,
We just don't expect to see kids with anomalies.
"Craniofacial defects" are the medical scripts,
For abnormal skull, nose, eyes, ears, mouth and lips.

One of the most devastating things I encountered in medical training were the congenital abnormalities found in newborns. The effect on the parents, nurses and physicians was greater than in most medical situations, and the expertise and team approach required for resolution of the problem is an example of comprehensive care at its best. The team approach to these severe facial anomalies involves the plastic surgeon, the pediatrician, the psychologist, the orthodontist, the otologist, and the speech and language pathologist. The pediatrician must first stabilize the infant from a physiological medical point of view before any correction of the defects can be undertaken. The focus of the caregivers must be both on the infant and on the family who require education and tremendous psychosocial support after a time of expectant joy has turned to death or to one of grave disappointment and sadness.

There are a multitude of major craniofacial developmental abnormalities and obviously I won't be discussing more than a few of them. The important thing is to recognize that today we have the ability to make major improvements in function and appearance, often resulting in appearances which the average individual will accept as a normal variant. Many of the patients lead normal lives after years of reconstruction thanks to the effectiveness of the craniofacial team approach to these serious problems.

The cleft lip and the cleft palate are the abnormalities about which most people have seen or heard. The cleft lip develops from incomplete formation of the nose in the embryo so that the left or right or both sides of the upper lip are not connected and a fissure extends up into the nostril on the involved side. Before repair, the infant will undergo some oral orthopedic procedures and have the repair done under general anesthesia at about age ten weeks, when the baby weighs about ten pounds. The nose deformity may be repaired at the same time or may have to wait until the baby is older, often just before the child enters school at age five years. Complete cosmetic repair of the cleft lip may require several surgeries and good team approach is important in long term scheduling and psychosocial support.

Cleft palate means that there is incomplete or absent closure of the roof of the mouth, separating the oral and nasal cavities. It may accompany cleft lip and has many variations. The patients without a complete palate (roof of the mouth) will be unable to breast feed and will have a nasal speech quality; they also have other abnormalities which predispose to chronic ear infections and have to be watched and treated carefully to prevent hearing loss. The repair of a cleft palate is often delayed until the child is six to eighteen months old and may require several stages over several years to accomplish the complete aesthetic result. The procedures for both cleft lip and palate are too complex to explain here, but they are done with developmental, functional and cosmetic considerations in mind.

The other areas I want to mention are the cranial or skull deformities, which lead to all types of appearance deformities and can cause brain damage and even death not treated early and appropriately. Until the 1960's many of these defects could not be safely corrected; then with advances in neonatal anesthesia and surgery and intensive care, surgeons were able to do extensive surgeries of the skull of the newborn. For example, in one deformity, some of the bones of the skull become fused too early not allowing the normal development of the skull and brain, resulting in mental retardation, and vision problems. The names applied to some of these defects are craniosynostosis (premature closing of a skull suture or separation line between the bones), hypertelorism (increased distance between the orbits [eyes]), dysostosis (bony deformities causing depression of the midportion of the face [Treacher Collins' syndrome, Crouzon's syndrome]).

Congenital deformities of the ear, microtia (absent or small ear) is usually associated with decreased hearing in the involved ear and reconstruction requires taking cartilage from a costochondral area (rib area), and in a several stage procedure, forming a new ear.

Reconstruction usually begins before the child enters school at age five, but the entire process may take several surgeries over several years. Patients with prominent ears can have otoplasty (surgery to correct this deformity) at an early age with excellent results.

The point I want to stress in this chapter is that the approach to marked facial deformity in newborns should be a comprehensive one involving the patient, the family and several specialists and putting together a time frame which the family can look to for emotional and physical resolution of the problems.

J

OPHTHALMIC SURGERY

Chapter 99
ANATOMY OF THE EYES

Lids, Lacrimal Apparatus and Conjunctiva

I'm always amazed when I study the eye,
That there's so much to learn, so I ask with a sigh,
How can an organ of such tiny size
Have so many parts? It's a major surprise.

There's optic foramen and lacrimal groove,
Optic nerve, cornea, and muscles to move,
The lens and the eyeball, there's limbus and iris
Choroid and vortex and CMV virus.

Then Bowman, Descemet and zonules of Zinn
Pars plana and Schlemm, Tenon's capsule and skin.
There's pupil and canthus and orbicularis,
Macula, fovea, and charts made by Ferris.

Abducens, oblique and small levator muscles
Puncta, canaliculus, and red cell corpuscles,
Wolfring's accessory lacrimal glands,
Axenfeld's syndrome, rods, cones, spectral bands.

This walnut-sized organ is driving me crazy,
And not 'cause I'm stupid or slow or just lazy.
So when somebody says: They'll keep an eye out for you,
By George, there's one hell of a lot they must do!

The eye is a sensory organ that relays light and object images to the brain by way of a complex system of structures. Light passes through the cornea and the anterior chamber, through the pupil,

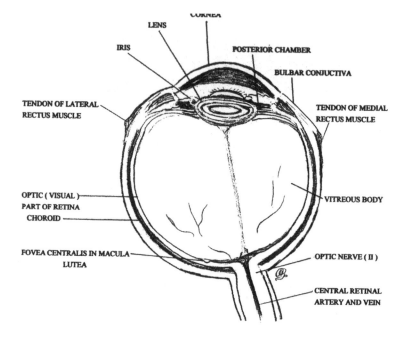

CORNEA

LENS

IRIS

POSTERIOR CHAMBER

BULBAR CONJUCTIVA

TENDON OF LATERAL
RECTUS MUSCLE

TENDON OF MEDIAL
RECTUS MUSCLE

OPTIC (VISUAL)
PART OF RETINA
CHOROID

VITREOUS BODY

FOVEA CENTRALIS IN MACULA
LUTEA

OPTIC NERVE (II)

CENTRAL RETINAL
ARTERY AND VEIN

ANATOMY OF THE EYE

DIAGRAM 66

the lens and the vitreous and the image is focused on the retina. The light image is picked up by the photoreceptor cells, the rods and cones of the retina and transmitted through the optic nerve to the optic chiasm in the middle of the brain, where the things seen by the right eye cross to the opposite side of the brain, then on through the geniculate ganglion to the back of the brain and the visual center of the cerebral cortex. But to accomplish this seemingly straightforward task, there are a myriad complex cellular and organoid activities that take place, and something can go wrong at every step of the process.

In these six chapters, I will give you an introduction to ophthalmology and describe a few of the more common procedures performed by eye doctors. As you can see from the anatomy, the eye is very complex and there are areas we will not discuss at all.

Some of the symptoms of eye problems are: Partial or complete loss of vision with many causes including optic nerve and brain injury, retinal detachment, and corneal problems, spots before the eyes from particles in the vitreous, and loss of certain fields of vision where parts of an object or print seem to disappear due to retinal detachment or vascular lesions. There is "seeing stars" or flashes of light due to trauma to the eye, migraine, or beginning retinal detachment, and there's photophobia where light bothers you, due to corneal abrasions, inflammations of eye and conjunctivitis.

Diplopia is double vision due to muscle problems; there are halos around lights possibly indicating the beginning of glaucoma or lens problems, poor night vision due to old age or myopia and color blindness with trouble differentiating green and red. There is pain in the eyes, from burning to sensation of something in the eye such as a foreign body or inflammation dryness due to aging or conjunctivitis, tearing which may be emotional or due to inflammation or lacrimal problems, and itching due to allergy or fatigue. Lids may stick together from inflammation of the lids, and bulging of the eyes may be due to inflammation, thyroid disease, or aging. And this is not even a complete list. Hopefully, you can see why our evaluation and review will be focusing on the main, surgically addressed problems.

Let us start with the eyelids. The most common abnormality is epicanthus which means the inner fold of the eyelid is prominent and appears as a web. It is normal in many Asian races and in Western population it often disappears or markedly diminishes by age five or six. Any surgery is usually deferred until then. Entropion is turning in of the eyelid and ectropion is turning out of the eyelid. Untreated, these conditions lead to irritation of the cornea called exposure keratitis so they should be corrected surgically, often by very minor procedures.

There are two common inflammatory masses of the eyelid, the chalazion which is usually sterile and a hordeolum, usually a Staphylococcal infection. Both these conditions affect the Meibomian glands and if not responsive to medical management will need excision through a small incision. A small hordeolum is called a sty. Ptosis is a drooping of the upper lid and has many causes. The treatment is surgical and requires a small incision in the eyelid and removal of a muscle causing the drooping. There are several tumors of the eyelid. Xanthelasma is a yellowish pigmented mass on the lid which can be excised for cosmetic reasons, and benign papillomas are also only removed for diagnosis or cosmetic indications.

The major cancers of the lid are squamous and basal cell carcinoma which need to be fully excised with free margins. If the tumor is large, a plastic reconstruction of the lid may be necessary. Malignant melanoma does occur in the eyelid and the same principles for melanoma anywhere else apply - wide excision with good margins.

The Lacrimal apparatus is the organ which forms tears and drains them into the nose. The only surgical problems arise when there is an abscess or tumor which needs to be opened in the operating room under anesthesia, or when the duct from the eye to the nose is blocked causing dacryocystitis and needs to be opened. Dry eye syndrome, keratoconjunctivitis sicca, is a disease of too few tears; an immune based one is known as Sjogren's syndrome. If persistent and severe, this may need temporary or permanent blockage of the lacrimal duct by surgical means, sometimes using lasers. An overflow of tears, epiphora, is only handled symptomatically and responds to medications in most cases; most other problems of the lacrimal apparatus are handled medically.

The conjunctiva is the thin mucous membrane that covers the inner side of the eyelid, palpebral conjunctiva, and extends onto the bulb of the eye to the cornea, the bulbar conjunctiva. Inflammation of the conjunctiva is called conjunctivitis, sometimes called pinkeye, the most common eye disease in the world! Most are not treated surgically. Trachoma is a disease affecting a large proportion of the world population (500 million) mostly in Africa and Asia which, if not treated with $2.00 worth of medication, can result in severe eye damage or blindness. It may cause inturning of eyelashes which will destroy the cornea and a minor surgical procedure may be needed in late chronic cases to evert the eyelashes.

Pinguecula are tiny yellow nodules that appear on the bulbar conjunctiva at the edge of the cornea at the limbus and is a normal appearance in older people. However, especially in people exposed to wind, dust and UV light, this pingueculum may enlarge and starts to cover the cornea; then it's called a pterygium and may need to be surgically excised to prevent visual problems.

Tumors of the conjunctiva are extremely rare and often require radical surgeries.

Chapter 100
UVEA, SCLERA, CORNEA, LENS (CATARACTS), RETINA

He has one blue eye and one green eye,
And women all adore him.
He's arrogant and self possessed
And you just can't ignore him.
He doesn't look his age at all,
There's not an ounce of fat.
The important thing to know, of course, is
Ernest is my cat.

In covering the many subjects of this chapter, I want to focus on the major problems and their treatments. Please refer back to the anatomy in the last chapter as needed.

The uvea refers to the iris, the ciliary body and the choroid of the eye. The iris is the pigmented, colored section of the eye surrounding the pupil, and it has muscles that make the center circle, the pupil, larger or smaller, determining how much light gets into the eye. The iris arises from the ciliary body forming this diaphragm and divides the anterior segment of the globe into anterior and posterior chambers.

Each of these chambers is host to a large number of diseases called anterior or posterior uveitis, and the causes are diverse from bacterial, viral and fungal infections, to malignancy, autoimmune disease, trauma, parasites and a whole host of unknown etiologies. Most of these processes respond to medical management, and surgery is only needed when the adjacent lens is so damaged that it needs to be replaced, or in diseases of the iris such as melanoma or a parasitic disease, like cysticercosis, where larvae have to be surgically removed. A strange disease called sympathetic ophthalmia is a bilateral inflammation of the entire uveal tract caused by a penetrating wound to this area in only one eye. The injured eye is called the "exciting" eye and the opposite eye is the "sympathizing" eye. If the disease progresses, it may be necessary to actually remove the "exciting" eye to prevent both eyes from causing complete blindness. Removing the "exciting" eye stops the process! It's a very strange phenomenon.

The choroid is the posterior, back part of the uveal tract extending to the optic nerve, and contains many vessels and three layers. The choroid itself is usually only the object of the surgeon when it has a tumor that needs to be resected.

The cornea is the transparent outer covering of the eye through which light passes on its way to the retina. It is composed of five layers; the epithelium, Bowman's membrane, stroma, Descemet's membrane and endothelium. I only mention this to let you see that even paper thin structures are much more complex than they seem! Normally there are no visible blood vessels in the cornea, and vessels are only seen when inflammation is present. Diseases of the cornea are either from the outside or exogenous such as trauma, foreign bodies and certain bacteria, or from the inside, endogenous, usually allergic or immune problems, and adjacent spread, as from conjunctivitis or uveitis spreading to the cornea. Untreated or poorly treated corneal ulcers are the major cause of blindness and decreased vision in the world today and appropriate diagnosis and treatment would prevent most of this.

The physician examines the cornea with a fluorescein stain after anesthetizing the eye, and can diagnose corneal injuries; one may use a special biomicroscope called a slit lamp for further examination of the cornea. In general, it is a very resistant structure, but repeated insults or injuries may cause chronic damage which is unable to heal. Inflammation of the cornea is called keratitis and must be treated vigorously or else it can progress to ulcers which can eventually cause perforation of the cornea and even eventual loss of the eye. The cornea has many nerve fibers and is very sensitive when irritated, as with a foreign body; inflammation causes more severe pain and may require local pain medication, as well as antibiotics.

The various types of keratitis are bacterial, viral, fungal and protozoan. Superficial and deep keratitides are generally treated medically but if they progress, clouding and opacity of the cornea may occur leading to functional blindness and corneal surgery or transplant may be necessary to retain or restore sight. Corneal transplantation has become a standard procedure in ophthalmology and when a donor cornea is obtained from a deceased individual, it is stored in special containers and fluid. The recipient has a portion of the diseased cornea removed and the donor cornea is sutured in place with line sutures using a special operating microscope. Medical advances have cut down on some of the problems of graft rejection, but it remains the most major complication. We will talk about refractive corneal surgery, correcting nearsightedness and farsightedness, in Chapter 104.

Another disease of the cornea is the asymptomatic arcus or annulus senilis which is a gray-white band around the outside of the cornea often seen in the elderly.

The lens in the eye focuses light ray images onto the retina. It has ciliary muscles and special zonular fibers which interplay to cause a change in the shape of the lens. This allows us to focus on near and far objects in a process known as accommodation. Pathology of the lens is caused by clouding, injury or abnormalities in shape which result in painless blurred vision. The examining physician can look at the lens with an ophthalmoscope, slit lamp or other light source and see the abnormalities. A cataract is an opacity, not letting light through the lens. There are many causes of cataracts: Congenital, traumatic (work related, BB shot, stone, etc.), age related (senile cataract), infectious, or toxic secondary to certain drugs. Obviously I can't explain cataract surgery in detail. The diseased lens is removed with one of three methods, phacoemulsification extracapsular or intracapsular, but today most surgeons use the phacoemulsification method and then place an artificial intraocular lens in the posterior chamber of the eye. The procedure is done under local or general anesthesia on an outpatient basis and requires wearing protective glasses and avoiding any straining for about a month. The patient will require a new glasses prescription one to two months after the surgery.

The retina is the most complex organ in the eye. The paper thin neural membrane has about twelve layers and near the innermost is a layer with photoreceptor cells called rods (for black and white) and cones (for color). In the center of the posterior retina is a round disc like area called the macula and in the center of this is the fovea; this area is mostly cones and has the highest level of visual interpretation. As you move outward there is less discrimination and more night or scotopic vision with shape identification. The retinal nerve cells receive the light and image and transmit it through the optic nerve to the brain where it is interpreted and understood.

Diseases of the macula and fovea, and the entire retina may be age related and often not treatable; however, many diseases are treatable with various types of lasers for photocoagulation of problem areas. Disease of the retina is called retinopathy. Retinal detachment means separation of the neurosensory layer of the retina from its outer pigment layer and unless corrected, leads to blindness. The retinal surgeon can use several types of instruments such as lasers and cryotherapy to "glue" a retinal tear. Retinal detachments require surgery. There are ophthalmologists who specialize only in retinal surgery, and there are a multitude of diseases which have complex delicate treatments using modern therapies with different types of lasers.

Diabetic retinopathy is a serious case of blindness in the world today and, like most tissue complications of diabetes mellitus, is related to microvascular or tiny vessel problems. This can be helped with laser treatment if done in a timely manner and photocoagulation can sometimes stem the progression of serious retinopathy.

A more severe problem is occlusion of the arteries to the retina or the main retinal artery. Depending on the location and size, resultant partial or complete blindness may occur rapidly and is usually not correctable. Similarly, retinal veins may occlude and result in partial or complete blindness. The use of lasers is becoming more common in an attempt to limit the complications of this problem. Other problems causing visual pathology are hypertension, arteriosclerosis and changes in the retinal arteries secondary to a process called toxemia of pregnancy.

Retinoblastoma is a malignant tumor occurring in childhood which may be managed by enucleation which means removal of the eye, or by radiation, chemotherapy, laser treatment and cryotherapy to preserve vision.

Chapter 101
GLAUCOMA

Hey bub, yeah you, whatcha complainin about,
You got a little ulcer or a little bit a gout?
Under some pressure at work or at home,
Wanna move from high stress LA, move up to Nome?

Well, let me tell ya, you got it real easy,
What you call dat stress is, to me, just plain sleazy,
Now me, I'm an eyeball, and I got real stress,
They call it glaucoma and it's a real mess.

My pressure is up, its affectin' my bod,
From my cornea right on down to each rod.
My old Schlemm canal is in quite a bind
If things don't improve, I'm gonna go blind!

G laucoma is a disease of the eye characterized by increased intraocular pressure. Left untreated it can lead to blindness, as is seen in almost 100,000 Americans; a totally preventable outcome to a somewhat insidious disease. A watery fluid, aqueous, is produced by the ciliary body and enters the posterior chamber; it passes through the pupil into the anterior chamber and then into the trabeculum and on into the canal of Schlemm to be reabsorbed.

We will talk about the anterior chamber, the chamber recess and the chamber angle in the subsequent discussion. Here's the anatomy (*see* Diagram 67 next page).

If the fluid in the eye is not reabsorbed, the intraocular pressure rises and the eye becomes more firm. The pressure is exerted on all the intraocular structures and over a period of time, causes damage to the photoreceptor cells of the retina leading to eventual blindness. There are two basic types of glaucoma; open angle and closed angle. Closed angle means that there is disease in the anterior chamber angle and chamber re-

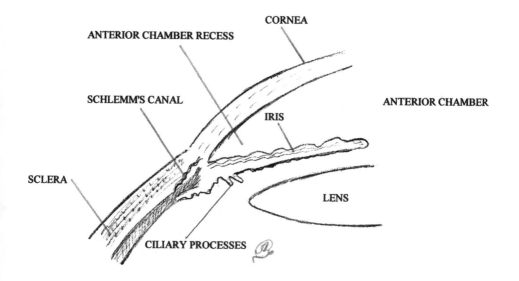

ANATOMY OF GLAUCOMA; THE FLOW OF AQUEOUS

DIAGRAM 67

cess making it so narrow that aqueous can't get into the drainage system. Open angle, the more common type, means that there is disease of the trabeculum or canal of Schlemm which prevents drainage. There are many etiologies for glaucoma, but all you basically need to know is that it causes increased pressure and that the pressure must be alleviated medically, or if that is not successful, then surgically.

Patients with acute glaucoma or closed angle glaucoma may present with headaches or pain in the eyes. Unfortunately, patients with the more common open angle glaucoma may have almost no symptoms until late in the disease when there has already been damage to the retina and the photoreceptors. Some patients have intermittent episodes of increased pressure which revert back to nominal but over many years can cause severe damage. So how does the average individual prevent the complications of glaucoma? The most important thing is regular eye exams by an ophthalmologist or a primary care physician who can do the appropriate studies.

Intraocular pressure is measured by tonometry, and there are many different types of tonometers on the market. And remember, since some individuals have intermittent elevated pressures, several readings at different times are needed to rule in or rule out glaucoma. Another measurement is the angle we have been talking about, to determine if the anterior chamber angle is normal, narrow or closed. This study is called gonioscopy and is performed by the ophthalmologist with a special light or a slit lamp. The physician will also examine the optic disc and the visual fields to assess any changes indicative of glaucoma.

As I mentioned, the primary treatment is medical, either to decrease the amount of aqueous formed (using alpha adrenergic blockers: Iopidine; beta-adrenergic blocking agents: Timoptic, Timolol, betaxolol, levobunolol, etc; carbonic anhydrase inhibitors: Diamox) or increase the outflow of aqueous (pilocarpine, Humorsol, etc.). Fluid can sometimes be "drawn out" of the eye by dehydrating the patient and forcing watery fluid into the general circulation.

If you look at the diagram, you can understand why, in the treatment of closed angle glaucoma, physicians want to keep the pupil of the eye constricted; this tends to open the anterior chamber angle. However, in other types of glaucoma, it may be better to have the pupil dilated. Only your ophthalmologist can make this determination! So you've gotten the diagnosis, gotten your medicines and still no improvement. Then it's time for the ophthalmic surgeon to do one of the many procedures available to him. These include lasers (argon, Holmium and neodymium: YAG lasers), implantation of silicone tubes for drainage, cryotherapy, ultrasound and a host of other complex yet very delicate procedures. Some of the procedures cause increased drainage while others attempt to obliterate the ciliary body production of aqueous.

My final recommendation: Get routine glaucoma evaluations and if you have early glaucoma, start treating it early to prevent visual problems.

Chapter 102
STRABISMUS
(Misalignment of the Eyes)

If your eyes don't look straight, it should give you a hint,
That you've got strabismus, or as you say, a squint.
You want to look left, but one eyeball stays straight
You want to look right but the left eye comes late.

There are multiple names and diverse kinds of squint,
Comitant, noncomitant and also divergent.
The problem, most often, is probably muscular
And it's seen during daytime and even crepuscular*.

*crepuscular - at twilight (okay, you try to find something else I can use that rhymes with muscular!)

S trabismus is an abnormality of the eyes in which they are misaligned due to a muscular problem. These are the individuals who appear to have something wrong, either when they are looking straight ahead or with movements of the eyes. The eyes should be perfectly aligned at all times to give us the best binocular vision. As with all other medical problems, let's look at the anatomy.

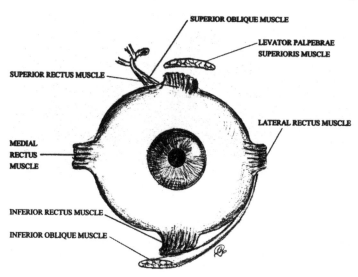

ANATOMY OF THE MUSCLES OF THE EYE

DIAGRAM 68

Under normal conditions, the muscles of the eyes all work in a complementary manner. That means that when you look up, both superior rectus muscles move the same. When you look to the right, the right lateral rectus and left medial rectus work together to pull the eyeball into the exact same position. However, to accomplish this, the antagonistic muscles, those doing the opposite, must also be relaxing at the same time as the others are contracting. If there is any difference in any aspect of these functions, the eye movements will not lock correct. It's a complex system. A few definitions: Heterotropia and esotropia means cross-eyed; exotropia means wall eyes or eyes turning outwards; hypertropia means one eye looks up; hypotropia means one eye looks down; heterophoria means there is a tendency of the eye to start turning away from the normal when looking straight ahead; esophoria is one eye turning inward; and exophoria is one eye turning outward.

Because of the different types of strabismus, there will be different brain interpretations of what is seen. The major ones are diplopia or double vision and amblyopia, a condition in young children with strabismus, one eye becomes less used and vision in that eye decreases. The diagnosis of the correct problem is through a series of eye tests by the ophthalmologist. Know, however, that strabismus does not go away without treatment! This problem occurs mostly in children and there is a significant psychological disability associated with strabismus; the "funny looking" kid on the playground gets teased!

The treatment should be started as soon as diagnosed and the success rate will often depend on the timing and vigorousness of the treatment. In many cases the strabismus can be treated medically with a patch over the good eye, for varying amounts of time depending on the pathology. Also, special glasses or medications may be prescribed.

Those patients who do not respond to medical management or with major muscle alignment problems, will be candidates for surgery. Muscles can be made shorter or removed from their insertion in the eye and resewn into a different position on the eyeball. Sound simple? It isn't. The correction of the muscles must be exact and requires superb technical skills by the ophthalmologist.

Chapter 103
TRAUMA, REFRACTIVE SURGERY, KERATOTOMY AND LASERS

Who would ever have thought or expected,
That you could now have your vision corrected,
By a Laser with star war like action within it,
And have the whole thing done in less than a minute?

In this chapter, we'll talk of two diverse subjects; First, trauma to the eye and how it is best handled, and second the whole area of lasers and their impact on ophthalmic surgery.

Trauma causes most of the loss of an eye in children due to penetrating injuries. We think of children with sticks, toxic materials such as Drano and battery fluid, sporting injuries and car accidents. When there is a question of an eye injury, determine if it is trauma or a toxic agent. If there is injury from a liquid such as acid or lye, immediate irrigation of the eye should be done with copious amounts of water using one to two quarts, at least, since timing and damage are intimately related. Get the stuff out as soon as possible! If there is trauma to the eye, protect it with an inverted paper cup bottom and get the individual to an emergency room as soon as possible.

The emergency room physician will know what to do. This will include a complete emergency eye exam and he will decide whether the injury can be handled in the ER or whether an eye specialist must be consulted. Injuries to the eyelids can be repaired carefully by the ER physician and minor bruises appropriately dressed. Sometimes the patient will feel as if something is in the eye but is only feeling the residual abrasion of the cornea. The physician will place an anesthetic in the eye and special dye to evaluate superficial corneal abrasions and treatment will usually consist of antibiotic ointment and an eye patch for a few days.

If the injury to the eye is severe, the full examination and treatment will need a general anesthetic and exploration by an ophthalmologist in the operating room. Foreign bodies embedded in the cornea will be removed, lacerations closed with suture and evaluation of bleeding in and behind the eye assessed. Blood in the anterior chamber is called hyphema. If minimal, it may be left to clear on its own, but the physician must evaluate and make this decision. There are several ways that the eye doctor will evacuate the clots, and use lasers to stop any further bleeding. Even with optimal care there is the danger of the complication of glaucoma in the future.

Burns by fire, hot water, ultraviolet radiation, snow blindness from looking at light reflections in snow, on the job exposures and sun exposures are usually treated medically. If the injury to the macula and retina are severe, there may be permanent visual loss.

When bony fractures of the orbit, bones around the eyeball, are suspected, appropriate x-ray films will be taken and the extent of the fracture determined. Depending on the nature of the injury to the orbit called a blowout fracture, there may be eye muscle injury, bleeding or optic nerve injury, the latter of which may lead to an irreversible decrease or loss of vision. Immediate surgical evaluation and repair offers the greatest chance for return of optimal function.

Let us now turn to lasers in ophthalmic surgery. Actually, this is one of the first fields that used lasers and still represents a major portion of eye surgery. We will briefly discuss radial keratotomy (RK) which is no longer an accepted treatment and then go on to the methods that are used today. These are laser in-situ keratomileusis (LASIK) and a general introduction to the use of lasers.

As we have mentioned, laser means Light Amplification by Stimulated Emission of Radiation. It can be used medically by disrupting, decomposing, coagulating, and by evaporating tissue. In other chapters, we have alluded to their use in glaucoma and retinal surgery. Here we are going to discuss the use of lasers for refractive surgery or vision correction.

Until the development of lasers, refractive errors could only be corrected with eyeglasses or contact lenses. Certain individuals are candidates for surgery on the cornea to adjust the focusing of light on the retina.

Radial keratotomy was a surgical procedure for correcting nearsightedness myopia. This was done through a carefully planned operation where small incisions are made in the outer area or periphery of the cornea. This allowed the cornea to flatten and corrected the ability of the lens to focus the image properly on the retina. The procedure was done in the ophthalmologist's office under local anesthesia. The risks were post-operative glare or starburst effect for a few months which usually cleared up; there was occasional over- or under-correction and a whole host of other complications including glaucoma, astigmatism, cataracts, hazing of vision, and the other complications of any surgery. The procedure was done for 18 years and was generally safe with good results but has now been replaced by the much superior and safer laser guided procedures that follow.

Photo refractive keratectomy (PRK) is a procedure performed with an instrument called the excimer laser, in which the surgeon vaporizes a thin layer of cornea to change the refractive index of the cornea. The corneal epithelium must be removed first. A contact lens is fitted to the cornea after the procedure for comfort.

The next major area is the LASIK procedure (laser in-situ keratomileusis). Using a microdermatome, an instrument to cut very thin slices of tissue, a hinged layer of cornea is cut called a flap. This flap is elevated and the surgeon uses an excimer laser to vaporize a portion of the cornea to change the refraction of light. There is a very minor, less than 1% risk of complications such as swelling of the eye, increased pressure, vision decrease and distortion of the cornea. The same minor often transient postoperative complications of haziness, glare, and difficulty with night vision occur, but in general it is a very safe and effective operation. Discuss these carefully and fully with your ophthalmologist before selecting a procedure; the physician who is too busy to explain everything thoroughly is not the one for you.

J

OTO-RHINO-LARYNGOLOGY
(Ear, Nose and Throat)

Chapter 104
EARS

We've heard that Marc Antony said: "Lend me your ears",
To speak to the people who had many fears.
What should have been said, to be more rhetorical,
Was something like: "Populus, lend me an auricle".

But the Bard was a dummy, and knew no anatomy,
(I know that to say that must just make a cad of me)
What I would have said to the Populus Romanum,
Was: "Give me a moment with your membrane tympanum".

And if I were Antony speaking that day
I'd pull on my toga at the Forum and say,
To my Friends, Romans, countrymen, as they await us:
"Lend me your external auditory meatus".

To the assassins of Caesar and Roman escapees
I'd yell at their malleus, incus and stapes,
And when I was done, I would take a grand bow,
For expostulating all of my otic know-how.

I n order to cover this subject clearly, we'll divide it into the External, Middle, and Inner parts of the ear. The external ear consists of the outer ear, or auricle, the external auditory canal and the eardrum or tympanic membrane; the middle ear includes the ossicles or ear bones (malleus, incus and stapes meaning hammer, anvil and stirrup), tiny muscles, the eustachian tube and the mastoid air cells. The inner ear consists of the labyrinth, divided into three parts, the vestibule, the cochlea and the endolymphatic duct. It sounds complicated, but bear with me, it's really quite simple. The cochlea changes sound energy to a form that can be passed through the organ of Corti to the auditory or hearing nerve and then to the auditory cortex of the brain; the vestibular system with its semicircular canals, utricle and saccule, is one of the three organs along with vision and feeling that helps us maintain balance and equilibrium. The endolymphatic duct plays an intimate part in the vestibular system containing fluid whose movement helps in motion and equilibrium determination.

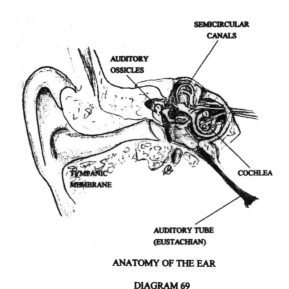

ANATOMY OF THE EAR

DIAGRAM 69

The physician uses an otoscope to look into the auditory canal and look at the eardrum. For certain problems, he/she may also use x-rays of the bony structure around the middle and inner ear, the temporal bone, including the mastoid air sinuses. CT scans are invaluable as well as MRI scans for diagnosing mastoiditis, cancers, studying the ossicles (hammer, anvil and stirrup), evaluating trauma and a disease called cholesteatoma which we shall describe later. It can identify other pathology which we will cover such as otosclerosis, labyrinthitis, and brain tumors impinging on the ear area.

For evaluation of the hearing aspect of the ear, audiology, there has been tremendous advancement in the past few years to measure the nature of the hearing deficit and to measure the presence of disease in the cochlea, the auditory nerve and even the brain. And it must be emphasized that most adults and children with hearing loss are helped without surgery and with the use of hearing aids, which have become smaller and smaller. There is now a tiny apparatus that fits deep inside the ear near the eardrum! I won't go into the specifics of testing and hearing aids because it is very complex and all you really need to know is that the testing can be done easily by a trained audiologist.

The evaluation of the vestibular system, vestibulometry, is relegated to several tests with long names, by which the expert can determine the nature of the disease and the treatment needed. These include computerized dynamic posturography, CDP, vestibular autorotation test, VAT, electronystagmography, ENG, and the rotary chair test, the Barany chair. They all measure the patient's response to motion, evaluating the movement of the eyes, and balance. All types of computerized programs have been devised in this field to help in the diagnostics.

Let us move on to the external ear or auricle. The surgeon becomes involved when there is trauma which needs suturing or for removal of benign growths such as cysts, fibromas and papillomas which are usually small and can be removed with a local anesthetic. Sometimes infections of the earlobe can develop from otitis media or internal, severe infections of the canal or eardrum which can infect the supporting structure, the cartilage of the ear, causing perichondritis which may actually cause loss of part of the earlobe and require plastic reconstruction. Fortunately such cases are rare with today's antibiotics. Squamous cell and basal cell cancers of the earlobe are not uncommon and need to be removed under a local anesthetic with clear margins. If the tumor is extensive, a plastic surgeon may be needed to reconstruct the ear using skin grafts to have a good cosmetic result. There are occasional tumors in the ear canal, ceruminoma and carcinoma, which need to be removed and may be done under a local or occasionally, a general anesthetic. Whereas the cure rate for cancer of the auricle or earlobe is 99%, carcinoma of the ear canal, though rare, has a relatively poor survival rate because it has often spread to the bone and surrounding tissues by the time it is recognized and removed. Melanomas are rare but can occur in the auricle or ear canal.

How often have we seen people with protruding ears and asked ourselves if something can be done. The answer is "yes" but the problem is that this is often considered cosmetic surgery and many insurers will balk at paying for it. Developmental abnormalities range from complete absence of the auricle to abnormal shapes and protrusions and if presented appropriately should be covered by insurance. There are several types of procedures for protruding ears, depending on the severity of the problem, which may require local or general anesthesia with removal of some cartilage and skin to reposition the ear to a more normal position. Other congenital deformities can involve extensive complex plastic procedures requiring skin flaps and occasionally, several stage procedures to arrive at a good result.

Otitis media is an acute or chronic infection of the middle ear which occurs in more than 60-70% of children at least once. It responds well to antibiotic treatment most of the time and the surgeon only becomes involved when it no longer responds to medication or progresses to complications such as hearing loss, fluid buildup in the middle ear and impending rupture of the tympanic membrane. In these eases a ventilation tube is placed in the ear drum to allow infectious material out and relieve pressure in a procedure called a myringotomy.

Chronic otitis media may remain just a nasty infection but occasionally may develop into a more severe form called cholesteatoma which contains a lining called squamous epithelium, and has the potential to cause severe infection and complete hearing loss. The following order of procedures is recommended. If the ear drum is partially destroyed a myringoplasty is performed to occasionally reconstruct the eardrum. If the mastoid air cells are not involved, then a tympanoplasty is performed which eradicates the inner ear infection and reconstructs the mechanism for hearing without need for a mastoidectomy (which means removal of the mastoid air cells along with the infection). The next stage would involve the last procedure with the addition of a limited mastoidectomy. Finally, the modified radical mastoidectomy removes extensive mastoid and middle ear disease without causing complete loss of hearing. In the past, a radical mastoidectomy involved removing the entire middle ear, a very destructive process with resultant hearing loss. For extensive tumors, radical surgery may be indicated and the nature and details of this procedure are beyond our scope.

Now you may ask, why does this chronic otitis media need such radical procedures? It's because the complications and potential complications of this infection can be life threatening causing pain, infections, meningitis, abscess in the brain, hydrocephalus, and many other severe problems. The severity of the otitis media has been markedly diminished by our armamentarium of antibiotics, but there are still deaths from its complications, which could be prevented by appropriate surgery at the appropriate time. With modern microscopes, after the infection has cleared, the ossicles can often be reconstructed and some hearing can be restored.

Infection in the inner ear can also involve the labyrinth with all types and extents of disease. Labyrinthitis can present with severe symptoms of nausea, vomiting, dizziness and inability to walk or function without losing balance, as well as bearing loss. Treatment is with bed rest and antibiotics and symptomatic medication. If infection persists or an infected area called sequestrum of bone does not improve, then surgical drainage or even removal of the labyrinth is needed. The opposite side can take over the complete functions for balance, equilibrium, etc.

Otosclerosis, sometimes apparently a familial problem, is a disease of the bony labyrinth characterized by a fixation of one of the bones needed for hearing, the stapes, and thereby causing marked decrease in hearing. The surgical procedure is stapedectomy, removal of the diseased stapes bone, and replacement with an artificial stapes made of one of several different types of metal or synthetic material, or another procedure called stapedotomy and placement of a stapes piston, which if you need, your doctor will have to explain to you. The artificial stapes is a very tiny structure and must be placed with great skill by a surgeon using a special operating microscope. It must be emphasized that this procedure can only be done when there is no concurrent ear infection and complications may occur to prevent its success in restoring good hearing.

Another interesting inner ear problem is called Meniere's disease. This strange disease is characterized by intermittent episodes of decreased hearing, ringing in the ears called tinnitus and dizziness or vertigo which can last for a few minutes to several hours and can be quite incapacitating. The disease is sometimes divided into "cochlear Meniere's" which affects mostly hearing and "vestibular Meniere's" with dizziness, but no hearing loss. The etiology is still unclear and the tests for Meniere's are mostly based on clinical findings, although there are some esoteric studies available for the ENT specialist. The pathology is in the endolymphatic duct system which is apparently engorged and indicates some type of blockage in the endolymphatic system. ENT surgeons have developed several procedures to alleviate the symptoms of Meniere's disease including those which cause increase in the drainage or resorption of endolymph, sometimes draining it into the spaces around the brain with the assistance of a neurosurgeon. There is also a medical treatment for debilitating Meniere's disease which involves a transtympanic injection of gentamicin.

The final area I want to discuss is cochlear implants, a surgical procedure used in deaf or almost deaf individuals. A part of the cochlear implant, the implant induction coil is placed in the inner ear cochlea, and then connected to a microphone and a speech processor. The patient has to have extensive training in interpretation of what he "hears" and the performance results vary from individual to individual. There is continued work on cochlear implants with new computerized implants replacing older models on a regular basis. Sound and speech perception is combined with visual and intense auditory training.

Chapter 105
NOSE AND SINUSES

"Proboscus Patty" was known though the school,
As a champion swimmer in every league pool.
She was "one of the guys", (but her face was no rose),
And at every school swim meet, she'd win by a nose.

She never went out on a date with the guys,
Her looks always lost, while her nose took first prize.
So during the summer before senior year,
She decided one evening she'd just disappear.

So she said fond farewell to the dolls Santa'd brought her,
Got into the car that her parent's had bought her,
And taking her savings and the clothes she would need,
(Left a note in the parlor for her parents to read).

She raced down the street, through the first intersection,
And was hit by a truck from the other direction.
When she woke in a hospital bed she felt fine,
Except that her head was all bandaged with twine.

Her parents were seated nearby in the room,
And the whole place was filled with emotions of gloom.
They told her, her face had been bumped here and there,
But the best plastic surgeon had done the repair.

The next day the dressings were finally excised
And Patti was more than a little surprised.
Her face was quite lovely, her nose was quite small,
This face wasn't "Proboscus Patti's" at all.

Two weeks later she returned as a senior, to school
But nobody knew who she was, or was cruel.

She was followed and whistled at and wooed by the guys,
Who had never seen more than her nose's great size.

And they all were amazed when they found out her name,
(Although deep inside she had still felt the same).
In the school paper, her picture said: Prom Queen, with a rose,
(But she lost every swim meet by exactly a nose!)

I n this chapter we'll discuss the nose and, also the eight sinuses, four on each side of the skull, the frontals, ethmoids, maxillaries and sphenoids, which are bony cavities filled with air that communicate by small passages to the nose.

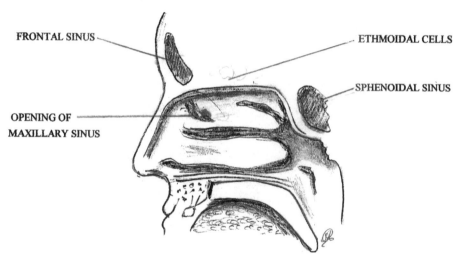

FRONTAL SINUS

ETHMOIDAL CELLS

SPHENOIDAL SINUS

OPENING OF
MAXILLARY SINUS

ANATOMY OF THE NOSE AND THE SINUSES

DIAGRAM 70

The anatomy of the nose and its relationship to the sinuses, as shown above, is important for reconstruction, and for understanding the diseases of this area. The nose may be the portal for infection into any of the sinuses and their proximity to the brain and possibility of cerebral or brain pathology is always in the back of the ENT surgeons's mind. Most of us hear about the nose in relationship to epistaxis or bleeding, rhinoplasty which is the "nose job" or aesthetic reconstruction, and fractures. Of course, we all have experience with colds and runny nose, rhinorrhea, but these are generally not needing of surgical intervention.

Let us begin with the rhinoplasty. Whether for congenital abnormalities or post-traumatic problems, this procedure, done on an outpatient basis under local or general anesthesia, is usually done for aesthetic reasons, and the ability of the surgeon to fashion an appropriate nose and nasal tip to fit the patient's face is of utmost importance. Several surgeons I have known give everyone the "same nose". While an improvement over the original, it often lacks the individualization needed. Be sure to look around before choosing a surgeon for rhinoplasty! Correction of a nasal deformity may also help clear the nasal tract and improve nasal breathing. The surgery involves many different types of incisions and good outcomes demand careful planning. The surgery can be complex with careful removal and repositioning of nasal cartilage. After the surgery, a splint is applied and left in place for about a week and the patient is advised against blowing the nose, any sports activities (where there may be nasal injury) and, in general, a period of relative inactivity. Problems with the nasal septum and the nasal tip can be corrected but extreme care has to be taken not to overdo the procedure.

Trauma or skin deficits left after removal of nasal skin tumors must often be repaired with flaps of skin artfully taken from other areas of the face and head in such a manner that they are hardly visible. This is preferable to skin grafts where the skin is too thin to adequately fit the purpose.

Epistaxis, or nasal bleeding, is usually handled at home, but on some occasions may need treatment in an emergency room. Anterior nasal bleeding is more common in children and young adults and posterior bleeding in the elderly. The bleeding in the younger group may be from superficial arteries, dryness and excessive inflammation and nose blowing and if not controlled with pressure or packing, may require cauterization with a silver nitrate stick or electrocautery after local anesthetics. Posterior bleeding may require the placement of a posterior packing, which is uncomfortable but effective. A number of diseases may lead to epistaxis and obviously patients on aspirin or blood thinners such as coumadin and heparin may be more prone to severe bleeding.

Rhinitis is inflammation of the nose and may be acute or chronic. There is a whole list of causes ranging from viral and bacterial, to allergies, systemic diseases and benign and malignant tumors. The benign polyps and papillomas can be excised; the medical syndromes are treated systematically and symptomatically, i.e. lupus, cystic fibrosis, TB, syphilis, and allergies.

The sinuses are air-filled, chambered cavities communicating with the nose and can be infected by many different bacterial, fungal or viral organisms which cause inflammation called sinusitis. In most cases this responds to appropriate medical management, but in cases of recurrent acute and chronic sinusitis, and several other problems, surgery may be indicated. The workup is performed by physical and nasal exam and confirmed by x-rays and CAT scans which may show diseased sinuses, fluid, or bony destruction. The surgery may consist of endoscopic sinus surgery under local or general anesthesia as an outpatient and is well tolerated.

As a young man, I had severe maxillary sinusitis, and the surgeon widened the natural drainage canal in a procedure called a nasal antral window. It allowed the diseased fluid to exit the sinus into the nose or throat and relieved the symptoms. Other surgeons prefer an open exploration of the maxillary sinus through the mouth, the Caldwell-Luc procedure. Surgery to drain the ethmoid, frontal and sphenoid sinuses can also be performed through hidden incisions. Trephination, making a hole in the bony skull, is performed over the frontal sinuses for drainage and obliteration. Complications of sinus surgery are unusual but may be bleeding, cranial nerve injuries, cosmetic deformities, venous hemorrhage in the brain, deviated septum, meningitis etc.

Cancer in the sinuses has a tremendously variable course. Small tumors can be removed endoscopically and large tumors may require radical sinus surgery often followed by radiation therapy and rarely chemotherapy; cure rates vary from 40-60% over five years, depending on the type, squamous cell carcinoma, melanoma, sarcoma, or lymphoma, location and clinical staging including tumor and lymph node involvement classifications.

Chapter 106
MOUTH, TONGUE, PHARYNX, AND LARYNX

If we were all docs in the late Cretaceous,
We'd know each beast as he turned round to face us.
His skull and eyes and his nose and mouth,
His pharynx and larynx to continue on south.

But I'd have to be doing a full mouth exam
On a tyrannosaurus, and I don't give a damn,
If the medical board found me slack and remiss,
If I didn't see tonsils on that toothy miss.

I had asked her politely to open up wide,
So I could look fourteen feet safely inside,
But instead she just gave me a dinosaur smile
And went back to knitting a sweater for a while.

You see, tyrannosaurus was becoming extinct
For a genetic defect made a change, quite distinct.
Instead of a vicious meat eater, teeth gritting,
She'd taken up cereals and large sweater knitting.

So whenever you see the big bones on display
Be sure that you stand firm that day and just say:
This wasn't a mean and vile beast of her day,
She was born looking vicious and there just was no way.

She could have nose, jaw and her dental work changed
For which she'd have gladly some swealers exchanged.
But no Cretaceous ENT surgeons would know,
How to change a T. Rex to T. Marilyn Monroe.

The mouth, tongue, pharynx and larynx are all part of the upper gastrointestinal and respiratory tracts. The only part we won't discuss is the teeth; but then, I have always had a "thing" about dentists and try to stay as far away from them as possible. The diagrams will help you locate the nasopharynx, hypopharynx, oropharynx, tonsils, tongue, soft and hard palate, larynx, and vocal chords.

ORAL CAVITY AND TONGUE

LARYNX

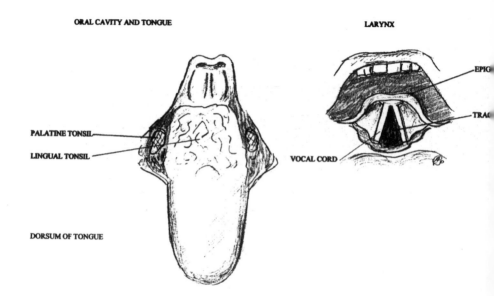

PALATINE TONSIL

LINGUAL TONSIL

DORSUM OF TONGUE

VOCAL CORD

EPIG

TRA

ORAL CAVITY, TONGUE, PHARYNX AND LARYNX

DIAGRAM 71

We will discuss the most common congenital anomalies of the head and neck in Chapter 108 including brachial clefts, cleft palate and lip, thyroglossal duct cysts.

The anatomy of the head and neck is extremely complex, and the memorization of the many muscles, nerves and vessels is the bane of all medical students. We often used mnemonics or poetic memorization to remember such things as the cranial nerves, the branches of the external carotid artery, etc., and they are all too salacious to print here. But let us move on.

There are several benign tumors of the head and neck, and they are removed surgically with local or general anesthesia; similarly, minor trauma is managed in the emergency department with simple suturing. Major injuries may be associated with other severe trauma which may need general anesthesia and may take immediate priority. We have discussed tracheostomy in Chapter 83.

The tongue, one of our five sensory organs (sight, touch, smell, hearing are the others), has several functions aside from that of taste; a complex system of nerves and muscles help us with eating, beginning to swallow, talking and expression such as kissing. There are very few indications for surgery of the tongue except for lacerations and tumors. Partial or complete removal of the tongue, as you can imagine, causes tremendous psychosocial and functional problems. The most problematic disease of the tongue is similar to the other structures we are discussing in this chapter, namely cancer.

The lining cells of the oral cavity, the lips, mouth, tongue, pharynx and larynx are all subject to developing a malignancy called squamous cell carcinoma, SCC, and this is almost universally related to tobacco, either smoking or chewing. Because the disease is basically similar in all these areas, what I say here regarding the tongue is often applicable to the other areas. Unfortunately, head and neck SCC has a mortality rate of about 50% because it has the tendency to be a systemic disease early in its development. Although the primary original tumor may be small, the tumor cells may already be in other areas of the body, and therefore, a combined, comprehensive approach to SCC has been adopted at most major cancer centers, including surgery, radiation and chemotherapy along with the psychosocial support and group decision-making.

The tumors are staged 0-IV based on the TNM classifications, and may vary from site to site. Basically T_O means there is no tumor found. T1 means 2 cm. or less in size, T2 means 2-4 cm., T3 is greater than 4 cm. and T4 means it involves adjacent structures. The status of the lymph nodes is: N_0 equals no involvement, N1 means metastasis in a single node, 3 cm. or less, on the same side as the primary tumor, N2 means a single node 3-6 cm. or multiple nodes same or both sides. N3 indicates a node or nodes greater than 6 cm.; The M stands for distant metastases. The best approach to a cancer cure is removing the SCC early and at the first sitting, and laser surgery is being used with increased frequency.

Recurrent disease is very difficult to control and therefore, the first surgery must be fairly extensive after group discussion and followed by appropriate radiation and chemotherapy. It would be easier to fight the disease if there were just one cell type, but unfortunately, this, like many cancers, has many different cell types, each responding differently to the radiation and chemotherapy. This may account for the fact that a cancer may initially respond well to chemotherapy and yet when it recurs, is very poorly responsive to the same therapy. We have selected out the nonresponsive cells, and these are the ones that grow and multiply. The cancer can spread through tissue planes, blood vessels and lymphatic channels and treatment should address all these variables. So you see that treatment of this cancer is complex and has to be individualized for each specific area, even though the cancer type may be similar (SCC).

The oropharynx, nasopharynx and hypopharynx have a ring of lymphoid tissue called Waldeyer's ring which contains the tonsils and the adenoids. These are lymphatic tissues now known to be of importance in the production of B-cell lymphocytes which may be of significance at the development of the immune system in children. Therefore, tonsillectomy and adenoidectomy, once done frequently and with impunity, are now only done for severe chronic infection, or obstruction of the eustachian tube or airway. Almost all tonsillectomies and adenoidectomies or as they're known, T&A's, are done under general anesthesia, although it is possible to do it under local and sedation in adults.

For many years a snare has been used for tonsils and an adenotome for adenoids and remaining tissue is curetted out. Recently, many physicians are doing the procedures using lasers with less blood loss and less postoperative pain. The complications are bleeding, infection and anesthetic complications and the rare fatality. We've come a long way from ether drip anesthesia and tonsillectomy on the kitchen table at home, in the early twentieth century! Abscess or Quinsy in the space near the tonsils, may be opened, needled or treated with tonsillectomy. Abscesses in other areas of the pharynx must be treated with drainage.

The human larynx has several functions: Phonation or speech and sounds, respiration, the transition from the mouth to the trachea and lungs, and protection from aspiration of material into the lungs. For the first function there are the vocal cords, for the second, the tubular larynx, and for the third, the epiglottis, a valve-like structure that sits over the top of the larynx. When you swallow, the epiglottis covers the opening into the larynx and prevents liquid and food from entering the larynx and going into the lungs. Examination of the larynx is done in two ways: indirect laryngoscopy where the doctor uses a local anesthetic spray and looks down the throat with a long handled mirror and direct laryngoscopy done under local anesthesia and sedation or general anesthesia. It consists of placing a lighted tube down the throat to look directly at the structures; biopsies can be taken and sent to pathology for evaluation.

Cancer of the larynx may present with a voice change such as hoarseness, a lump in the neck, earache, sore throat or rarely, bleeding; sometimes the patient has difficulty swallowing or a sensation of fullness in the throat. Most cancers occur in the vocal cords, but also could be above and rarely below this area. Depending on the extent of the tumor as determined by visual exam or CT study, treatment may require only a partial removal of the vocal cords or may need a complete laryngectomy. Partial procedures may result in voice changes, but the patient will still have vocal communication.

Laser surgery may be used for small cancers on the vocal cords, but whatever the procedure, it may be done in conjunction with radiation and even chemotherapy. Total laryngectomy, complete removal of the vocal cords, also necessitates placement of a tracheostomy and results in inability to communicate verbally until artificial sound generating apparatuses are used. There are many different types and they require training for effective use. The psychological effect of total laryngectomy is tremendous on the patient, affecting his family, his work and his social interactions. A strong psychosocial program and rehabilitation program is needed for full adaptation and recovery. There are laryngologists and speech therapists who specialize in this therapy and who are brought into the "loop" early in the post-operative period.

There are many surgeries now for reconstructing the ability to produce sound which involve the patient's own tissue, often in conjunction with artificial devices.

Trauma to the larynx must be evaluated immediately to assure adequate airway. The need for emergency tracheostomy is rare and in cases of severe laryngeal injury it is usually possible to place an endotracheal tube rather than going ahead with an emergency tracheostomy.

Chapter 107
SALIVARY GLANDS
AND FACIAL NERVE

The salivary glands are as "low" as ya git,
Cause all that they do is produce lots of spit.
Eating and kissing, I say with a sigh,
Would be awful hard, cause your mouth would be dry.

The salivary glands have several secretions which we need for normal mouth and throat function. They produce saliva which contains liquid to start digestion and lubrication of food liquid that protects the teeth, controls bacterial counts in the mouth and immune functions. The saliva is mostly water. The main salivary glands are the submandibular gland, producing 70% of the saliva, the parotid gland, 25%, and the sublingual and some unnamed minor glands in the lips, tongue, nose, larynx, pharynx, etc., producing the rest. The major glands have ducts or tubes through which saliva enters the oral cavity.

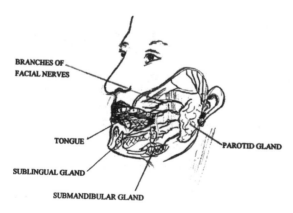

ANATOMY OF SALIVARY GLANDS

DIAGRAM 72

Sialoadenitis is inflammation of the salivary gland, most often in the parotid which is called parotitis. In some cases, a stone may form in the ducts and may have to be removed surgically under general anesthesia to return normal salivary function. Plain x-ray films can delineate these stones. Chronic inflammation of a salivary gland may result in pain, swelling and recurrent infections and if not responsive to medical management, may need surgical excision of that one gland.

When a mass is found in a salivary gland, the workup includes a complete head and neck evaluation, looking for enlargement of lymph nodes, as well as CAT and/or MRI scans of the head and neck to delineate the size and spread of the tumor.

Benign tumors occur in the salivary glands, and the most common are called pleomorphic adenomas and Warthin's tumor. While not malignant, they have a tendency to recur if not completely removed and wide excision is recommended.

The most common malignant tumors have long names: Mucoepidermoid carcinoma, adenoid cystic carcinoma, adenocarcinoma and malignant mixed tumor. They present as masses and have the staging as we have described in Chapter 106. Stage T1 and T2 tumors are completely removed surgically and higher grade tumors, in addition to surgical removal, usually have removal of certain lymph nodes in the neck as well as post-operative radiation treatment. We will discuss lymph nodes in the next chapter. Removal of the submandibular and sublingual glands is very straightforward with care taken not to disturb a branch of the facial nerve supplying movement of the lip and lower face, and the hypoglossal nerve which affects strength and motion of the tongue, unless the nerves are invaded by the tumor. The parotid gland at the side of the face is another matter. It is divided into a superficial and deep lobe and between the two lobes is the facial nerve which is responsible for the major movements of the facial muscles. For benign tumors, usually in the superficial lobe, a superficial resection is often adequate, but for cancer, the entire parotid gland must be removed and the facial nerve preserved unless involved with cancer. It is a delicate surgery requiring a skillful, well trained surgeon to dissect out the hair-sized branches of this important nerve. In some cases, when the nerve must be removed along with the tumor, nerve grafts are done in an attempt to return some of the facial nerve functions.

The facial nerve, known as the seventh cranial nerve, is responsible for facial motion but also has a tiny branch responsible for taste.

The branches of the facial nerve splay out from the outer border of the parotid gland and have been grouped into five main areas: The temporal, the zygomatic, the buccal, the mandibular and the cervical branches. Whether injured by trauma or surgically, the branches must be identified and reconnected surgically in an attempt to regain the lost function. Even in the unconscious patient, the various branches can be evaluated by a transcutaneous or direct nerve stimulator. If the nerve is intact, the muscles it supplies will twitch. During removal of the parotid gland many surgeons use a nerve stimulator to identify each branch and thereby preserve them.

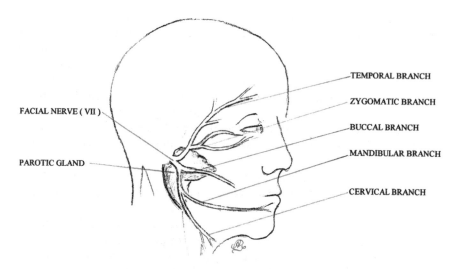

FACIAL NERVE (VII)

PAROTIC GLAND

TEMPORAL BRANCH

ZYGOMATIC BRANCH

BUCCAL BRANCH

MANDIBULAR BRANCH

CERVICAL BRANCH

FACIAL NERVE ANATOMY

DIAGRAM 73

Chapter 108
HEAD, NECK,
AND EMERGENCIES

When Alice went out with Fred one night
She was nervous and her lips were dry.
She got into his car and he held her hand,
She was happy enough to cry.
She reached in her purse for a lipstick,
a subtle shade of blue.
But by mistake she grabbed the wrong tube,
and moistened with Super Glue.

And when they kissed their lips held tight,
in a permanent lover's grip.
And this pleasant beginning all ended up,
In a local emergency room trip.
The ER doc, tried not to smile.
As he sprayed them with glue remover.
And he counseled the two not to kiss for a while,
Or else try a much different maneuver.

In this last ENT chapter, I want to cover two important areas. First, an overview of the head and neck anatomy with regard to masses in the neck and lymph nodes, and second, a look at some of the major emergencies and their management. It seems that everyone at some time or other feels their neck and finds some lump or bump and assumes the worst. It is important to know that there are many normal structures in the neck which can be felt through the skin and yet which we may not be aware of until one scary moment when we are feeling one particular area and come upon the mass. Also, the first indication of a tumor in the head and neck, or even spread from another area of the body, may be an enlarged lymph node somewhere in the neck, and we need to discuss this issue. Most enlarged lymph nodes, called swollen glands, are NOT cancer, but are due to a whole host of infectious or other diseases which will respond to medical therapy. Only in suspicious cases will biopsy, either by needle or open surgery, be indicated (*see* Diagram 74 next page).

The lymph nodes as shown above often drain the glands and tissue most adjacent to them, and tumors will spread into these regional lymph nodes. Often, the enlarged lymph node with cancer is discovered first, and only after careful ENT evaluation will the primary tumor be identified. Lymph nodes associated with infectious disease should disappear after a week on appropriate antibiotics. Enlarged nodes that do not disappear will have to have a complete head and neck and ENT evaluation. Biopsy without having this complete evaluation is usually not appropriate except when a specific diagnosis is strongly suspected, such as lymphoma which often has a characteristic appearance clinically and on CT or MRI scan. Needle aspiration for biopsy is the standard of care today to make a definitive diagnosis.

The diagram shows the areas of cervical nodal metastases from certain tumors and may be helpful to the surgeon in determining where the primary lies. Often the node enlargement may be many times larger than the primary tumor which is so small that it is missed on laryngoscopy.

What are head and neck emergencies? These are situations where immediate or urgent surgical intervention must be undertaken to save a life. As we have mentioned elsewhere, the only true surgical emergency is hemorrhage whereas the medical emergencies arc respiratory and cardiac. Neurological situations come a close third.

The head and neck hemorrhage emergencies are secondary to trauma, post-operative surgical bleeding, severe epistaxis, and rarely cancer. Trauma to the head and neck, excluding the brain which is covered in Chapter 79, may be due to injury to the jugular or other large vein, injury to the carotid artery or one of its major branches or generalized massive scalp, head and neck trauma with diffuse bleeding from many sites. In an otherwise healthy individual, most generalized venous bleeding will stop with gentle pressure until surgical management is undertaken. When the bleeding area has a steady rather than pulsatile flow, gentle to firm pressure should be applied without causing further injury to avoid exsanguination. Arterial bleeding is pulsatile and may need firm pressure to stop the hemorrhage. To prevent neurological damage and to control

LYMPH NODE LOCATIONS IN THE NECK

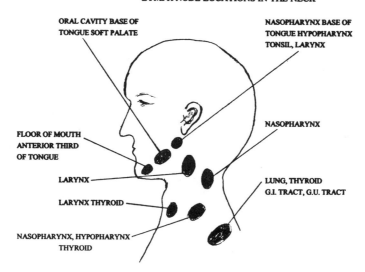

ORAL CAVITY BASE OF
TONGUE SOFT PALATE

NASOPHARYNX BASE OF
TONGUE HYPOPHARYNX
TONSIL, LARYNX

NASOPHARYNX

FLOOR OF MOUTH
ANTERIOR THIRD
OF TONGUE

LARYNX

LARYNX THYROID

NASOPHARYNX, HYPOPHARYNX
THYROID

LUNG, THYROID
G.I. TRACT, G.U. TRACT

NORMAL ANATOMICAL MASSES IN THE NECK

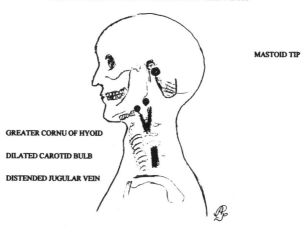

MASTOID TIP

GREATER CORNU OF HYOID

DILATED CAROTID BULB

DISTENDED JUGULAR VEIN

MASSES AND LYMPH NODES IN THE NECK

DIAGRAM 74

hemorrhage from the carotid artery may be difficult, but if the bleeding is not controlled, the individual will die of blood loss! The wounds must be explored under local or general anesthesia by one experienced with the anatomy, so as not to cause more damage with the exploration and to carefully suture the injured vessel without future negative sequelae.

One source of bleeding may be post-tonsillectomy hemorrhage which is usually self limiting but occasionally may be massive. In cases of excessive dangerous hemorrhage, the patient should be taken back to the operating room and explored under an anesthetic and the bleeding site visualized and sutured. Attempts to secure the bleeding site without the proper instruments, lighting, and personnel may result in severe complications of aspiration, further damage, airway problems and even death. In cases of postoperative bleeding after neck surgery, the surgeon must determine whether return to the operating room is necessary or whether simple drainage under local is indicated. The experienced surgeon never hesitates to take a patient back to surgery whereas sometimes a lesser surgeon may hesitate because he thinks it reflects badly upon him as a surgeon to have to "take the patient back" to the operating room.

The next area of emergency is respiratory. Some inflammations of the throat in children, and rarely in adults can be considered emergencies. Epiglottitis and severe croup usually respond to medical management in a emergency room, but if they progress, urgent intubation or rarely tracheostomy may be indicated. Severe neck infections may cause an abscess which swells into the airway compromising breathing. The most common of these is a peritonsillar abscess. These can usually be drained by needle aspiration or small incision under local anesthesia to alleviate the emergency; further surgical intervention may be needed on an elective basis. Severe trauma may cause disruption of the trachea or severe fractures of the mouth and throat area which will result in airway disruption or progressive swelling which may threaten to disrupt the airway.

The best route is always placement of an endotracheal tube either through the mouth or through the nose, but in some situations it may be necessary to take the patient to surgery and do an immediate tracheostomy or one called a cricothyrotomy, opening the trachea higher up with a tiny incision performed in the emergency room. Patients with foreign bodies in the throat or trachea often expel them after a Heimlich maneuver which consists of standing behind an individual, grasping your hands together round him just under the rib cage, and abruptly pulling in and up; this increases the intrathoracic pressure and may cause the object to be expelled from the airway. If this doesn't work, then an ENT specialist may need to remove the object with direct laryngoscopy under sedation or general anesthesia. A non-expert trying to dislodge an object may make the situation worse!

Nose fractures, while causing some obstruction and bleeding are usually not acute severe emergencies and can be managed in a less urgent manner by pain medication, sedation and very gentle cold compresses. We have already discussed epistaxis. This can be very severe and if pressure on the sides of the nose does not stem the bleeding, an emergency room physician or ENT doctor may need to place an anterior or posterior nasal packing, under sedation and local anesthesia.

Neurological emergencies include evidence of injuries to major nerves of the head and neck. While they are indeed serious, they are often not a true emergency, and need to be surgically handled by the appropriate specialist after the necessary diagnostic studies have been performed and other more emergency situations have been stabilized. We have discussed neurological emergencies in section F.

L

PEDIATRIC SURGERY

Chapter 109
CONGENITAL SURGERY
(THINGS YOU'RE BORN WITH)
AND PEDIATRIC NEOPLASMS
(TUMORS)

Pediatric Surgery is not the term
For operating on a sperm!

Many noted pediatricians have said that children are not merely little adults. They have their own specific problems and the specialty of pediatric surgery is focused on this principle. We shall talk more about this in the next chapter. In this section we will discuss the many congenital abnormalities that are now managed successfully, often when an infant is hours or days old. The whole field of pediatric surgery is one which could occupy another entire text, but I will try to mention some of the more common problems and their treatments.

Among the more frequently seen congenital abnormalities is the umbilical hernia. This is due to a defect in the closure of the abdominal wall around the umbilical cord and results in a mass covered with skin. It may be very small, about one centimeter in size, and these usually close spontaneously by age four or five; larger umbilical hernias or those that don't close by themselves, need to be repaired through a tiny arched incision around the umbilicus in a relatively uncomplicated procedure. More significant abdominal wall abnormalities are sometimes associated with genetic abnormalities, and the timing and nature of their repair is often complex, and individualized to each infant. Another abnormality is omphalocele, where a large percentage of the intra-abdominal contents is outside the abdominal wall enclosed in a saclike membrane. If too large, it may have to be returned back to the abdominal cavity very slowly over several days.

Another abnormality is called a gastroschisis, where intra-abdominal contents are hanging freely, not in a protective sac, outside the abdomen. This condition requires emergency repair in the newborn, and if the bowel cannot be returned to the peritoneal cavity, a special bag enclosing the bowel is sutured to the abdominal wall. Eventually everything fits back into place, but the infant needs careful management for several days or weeks.

Inguinal or groin hernias in children are fairly common (males more than females). Surgery is not an acute emergency unless it contains intestine or other structures which cannot be reduced, in other words, the lump cannot be made to go away. In girls this type of incarcerated hernia often contains an ovary and requires immediate repair.

In general, hernias should be repaired as soon as possible after the diagnosis has been made. Hydrocele, a collection of fluid in the inguinal area, usually goes away by itself in the first year; if not, a formal hernia and hydrocele surgery is needed. This type of pediatric surgery is performed through a tiny incision in the groin as described in Chapter 30.

Let's move on to the gastrointestinal tract. Starting from above, there can be abnormal development of the esophagus, as seen in the diagram below, and surgical correction must be done as an emergency, usually in the first few days of life (*see* Diagram 75 next page).

The repairs are delicate and require hooking the right ends back together and preventing flow of intestinal fluid into the lungs!

The pyloric stenosis means that the part of the intestine where the stomach becomes the duodenum is so narrowed by a hypertrophic or enlarged muscle, that most or all of the contents of the stomach cannot get out into the intestine.

The treatment consists of dividing the hypertrophic muscle in a surgery that has become very straight forward with minimal complications or morbidity. If the surgery and fluid resuscitation is immediately performed, the infant is usually home in two days.

Other congenital abnormalities of the infant intestinal tract may be secondary to abnormal rotation (this is a change in the position of the intestine as it matures during the fetus development in the mother's womb) or other developmental abnormalities. Sometimes the intestine doesn't get large enough in certain areas, and this causes a blockage repaired by surgically removing the segment of the intestine, usually very

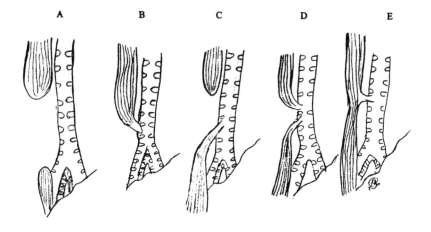

CONGENITAL ABNORMALITIES OF THE ESOPHAGUS

DIAGRAM 75

(A) ESOPHAGEAL ATRESIA WITHOUT ASSOCIATED FISTULA
(B) ESOPHAGEAL ATRESIA WITH TRACHEOESOPHAGEAL FISTULA BETWEEN PROXIMAL
SEGMENT OF ESOPHAGUS AND TRACHEA.
(C) ESOPHAGEAL ATRESIA WITH TRACHEOESOEPHAGEAL FISTULA BETWEEN DISTAL ESOPHAGUS
AND TRACHEA.
(D) ESOPHAGEAL ATRESIA WITH FISTULA BETWEEN BOTH PROXIMAL AND DISTAL ENDS OF
ESOPHAGUS AND TRACHEA..
(E) TRACHEOESOPHAGEAL FISTULA WITHOUT ESOPHAGEAL ATRESIA (H-TYPE FISTULA)

DIAGRAM OF PYLORIC STENOSIS

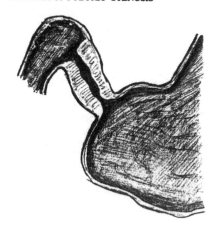

TREATMENT OF PYLORIC
STENOSIS

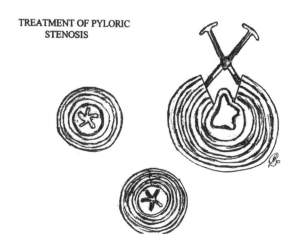

ANATOMY AND TREATMENT OF PYLORIC STENOSIS

DIAGRAM 76

localized to a small area, and the infant does well after the surgery. This is called intestinal atresia. Other abnormalities may be due to twisting of the bowel called midgut volvulus causing death of a segment of bowel, which has to be removed. Another cause of obstruction is called intussusception, which means one loop of intestine slides inside its following loop. Most of the time it can be resolved medically with air enema x-rays or fluids from above, but if the bowel is dead or will not reduce, then an open surgery is needed with removal of a small segment of intestine.

Hirschsprung's disease is a problem in children where the large intestine lacks special nerves that cause the normal peristaltic movement of the bowel. In simple words this means that part of the colon doesn't work in moving the bowels and this results in a bowel obstruction. These children have a congenital absence of the nerve plexus (collections of nerves - the ganglion cells of the myenteric plexus to be exact) and diagnosis is made by rectal biopsies. They must have this segment of colon removed surgically and some surgeons will do a temporary colostomy and wait until the infant weighs ten pounds before undertaking the definitive surgery which is called a "pull through" operation after colon resection.

Another problem is being born without a rectal opening, and of course this must be repaired immediately. There are two different types: Where the normal colon is just under the anal skin, or low in the pelvis, and where the colon is high up. The low ones can be repaired early whereas the high ones usually require a temporary colostomy and definitive surgery at about two to three months. Many of these children have associated neurological problems and must be evaluated fully before complete repair is possible. There is usually a tiny opening somewhere in the perineum and there may be abnormal connections to the bladder. It often requires complex and delicate surgery by the pediatric surgical specialist.

We won't discuss appendicitis or Meckel's diverticulitis since they have been discussed elsewhere, but the diagnosis may be more difficult in an infant or young child and the surgeon must have a high index of suspicion to make the correct diagnosis.

Let us move to the neck. The child may have a remnant left from the formation of the thyroid gland called a thyroglossal duct cyst which may get infected or form a mass which can be surgically removed. Another fluid filled cyst in the neck may come from what is called a developmental branchial cleft, a structure that is forming during the fourth week of the fetus growth and due to an abnormal development a small cyst remains which must be removed in a relatively simple surgery under general anesthesia.

A more difficult problem is the cystic hygroma, a sometimes huge mass which develops because of an abnormal development of lymph vessels in the head and neck. Complete removal may not be possible because of its massive size and possible involvement of other vital structures in the neck. For the huge hygromas, a multi-staged procedure may be the best management over several years.

There are several respiratory anomalies but most are rare and their treatment too complex to discuss here. A Bochdalek hernia, or congenital absence of the back part of the diaphragm, allows the abdominal contents to rise up into the chest causing severe, often fatal respiratory failure. Since the use of extracorporeal membrane oxygenation (long words just meaning a machine that puts oxygen in the infant's blood and keeps it alive until the lungs recover and the hernia can be repaired - sometimes several weeks!), the success rate of the surgery has risen from almost zero to 60%. Suffice it to say the surgery and pre and post operative care is very complex.

Some infants are born with jaundice, a yellow skin coloring, and certain types of jaundice resolve spontaneously. But other types are due to anatomical abnormalities of the biliary tract with names such as choledochal cyst, biliary atresia or hypoplasia. The cyst requires special drainage and the atresia requires complicated surgery connecting intestine to the liver so it can drain properly. Portal hypoplasia may require a liver transplantation if the infant survives long enough.

Congenital abnormalities with the genitalia are often related to genetic disorders which cause many different kinds of sexual developmental anomalies. These are listed under "Intersex Syndromes" and can't be discussed here. Cryptorchidism is a fancy word for undescended testicle and means that the testicle has been interrupted in its normal descent towards the scrotum. It may respond to medical treatment with chorionic gonadotropin, but if this fails, a surgical procedure is needed. Testicles which remain undescended have a much higher incidence of malignancy, produce less sperm, create psychological problems for the child and have an increased chance for other problems with the testicle later in life.

Finally, let us consider the tumors found in children. Although trauma is first in causing deaths among children, tumors are second on the list.

The most common cancer is leukemia which only involves a surgical procedure for the initial diagnostic bone marrow biopsy. It is highly responsive to chemotherapy. Brain tumors come next in frequency and may present with headache, dizziness, vomiting, facial asymmetry, lethargy, and change in behavior to name a few.

The management of central nervous system tumors in children involves a multimodality team approach including not only the pediatric neurosurgeon, but also the neurologist, oncologist radiation therapists, psychologist and support groups for the patient and the family. The diagnosis is made much as with other tumors through CAT and MRI scans, appropriate biopsies and laboratory blood studies. I will mention the most common for you, but their individual surgical management is complex and needs to be explained on an individual basis. They are: Low grade astrocytoma, often cured by surgery followed by radiation and chemotherapy; medulloblastoma, the most common childhood brain tumor - its cure rate depends on its size, extent and area of involvement, and generally poor cure rates greater than five years even with radiation and chemotherapy; high grade gliomas or glioblastoma multiforme are not curable but with optimum care the child may survive up to five years or longer with combinations of radiation and chemotherapy.

Another tumor is the craniopharyngioma which, if surgically removed, may have long term survival. One of the major problems with radiation to the brain in children is the effect on brain function, lowering the IQ by 15 to 20 points or more whereas the chemotherapy is better tolerated with many long term survivals without radiation. Cancer of the brain in children is a difficult problem for the patient, the family and the treating physicians.

Lymphoma or cancer of the lymphatic system is next on the list and again, these are diagnosed with surgical biopsies to obtain enough tissue for appropriate studies. Their primary treatment is then chemotherapy and not surgical.

The fourth most common tumor of children is neuroblastoma which is a tumor whose origin is from neural crest cells which means basic nerve tissue in the fetus. It usually presents as a mass in the abdomen and requires workup using ultrasound and CAT scan. The main treatment is complete surgical removal since radiation and chemotherapy has not been very successful in the treatment. Strangely enough, children under age one may have a spontaneous disappearance of the tumor even when there is metastatic disease, which lead scientists to believe that there must be an immunologic therapy in effect. The tumor is staged I-IV by its location; I - is tumor in one place, II -is tumor spread beyond its origin, "III" - if it crosses the midline of the body and "IV" - meaning it has spread to liver, lungs, etc. Obviously, in children over one year. the prognosis relates to the stage and resectability.

Wilms' tumor is a cancer of the kidney in children ages one to six, which usually presents as a mass in the abdomen. Researchers now feel that this tumor grows because of the absence of a special gene which prevents this type of cancer (WT1 and WT2). The diagnosis is confirmed by CAT and MRI scans followed by surgical exploration and complete removal of the tumor, even if this requires taking out part of adjacent structures. After removal of the tumor, the patients are treated with chemotherapy including actinomycin D, Vincristine. adriamycin and others and the cure rates are often in the high ninety percent range for stage I and II disease and up to eighty percent for III and IV with the addition of other chemotherapeutic agents and sometimes radiation therapy. Other cancers in children include teratomas, composed of all different types of tissue, sarcomas and liver tumors which are treated by surgical removal, if possible.

Chapter 110
WHY KIDS ARE DIFFERENT
FROM ADULTS

The infant grows to be the child, the child up to the teen,
Becoming the adult it passes through each age that's in between.
And though it's the same individual, I could tell them apart at a
glance.
The child is the one that smiles all the time, and the adult just rages
and rants.

The baby will only cry when it's wet, or hungry or hurt or cold,
The adult will cry for no other reason than it's getting a little bit old.
If we could reverse the whole process, and start out life as a little
adult,
By the time we grew down to the infant size, we'd have a much better
result.

I n the past fifty years the specialty of pediatric surgery has come of age. Children and infants are not just "little adults" and their medical and surgical care requires a whole new perspective and management. Surgery on infants and newborns was once considered highly risky because the ability to diagnose and the expertise of anesthesiologists and surgeons was not up to the job. Tremendous advances have made it possible to operate on a fetus still in the mother's uterus with excellent success and neonatal surgeries for congenital abnormalities have become routine for the well trained surgical team at the well supplied hospitals.

In general, the "principles" for pre- and post-operative care are similar for the child and the adult; the actual care itself, however, is quite different. Children can have intolerance to blood and fluid losses, rapid deterioration in conditions that an adult might tolerate much longer, and the inability to tell the physician what is wrong, where the pain is, what's different now than yesterday, etc. It many cases the infant will tolerate surgery better than an adult, heal faster and not be subject to the complications brought on by age such as arteriosclerosis and other diseases of aging, and yet we know that infants do not do well after extensive intestinal surgery and must be carefully monitored. The fluid and electrolytes of children must be expertly administered since a few cc's error can make a serious difference. The approach toward children must be somewhat different because the child is usually wary or scared of strangers and certainly doesn't want to take off his/her clothes in front of this stranger. Infants and toddlers fear separation from the parents and it is important to keep a parent with the child during the initial and follow-up examinations.

The surgeon needs to spend ample time with the parents clarifying and reassuring, since they may often be listening half to the physician and half to the child. Dehydration in children comes on rapidly and hopefully, if you are reading this and have infant children, you will learn the signs and symptoms of dry mouth, sunken eyes, lethargy, fever, little or no urine output and watch for decreased fluid intake, excessive diarrhea and high fever and general "not looking good" appearance. Infants and children do not tolerate cold and their body temperatures can drop rapidly. In surgery, the operating room for infants is always kept uncomfortably warm to prevent hypothermia (severe body cooling), since a child or infant's ability to adjust to changes in body temperature is not well developed. It should be emphasized that the pediatric surgeon is trained to handle all of these issues.

Anesthesia for children and infants is different from that of adults because of the size differences, the delicacy of the lungs and chest wall, and the different responses to anesthetic drugs. Children can go into shock from very small fluid or blood losses and the anesthesiologist must be familiar with pediatric fluid and electrolyte changes, heart changes (which can occur very rapidly) and understand the treatment of seizures and even cardiac arrest, both of which are not rare with neonatal patients but which are rapidly reversed. The surgeon and/or anesthesiologist needs to understand fluid and nutrition status, must find IV access (and tiny veins can make this a difficult problem in babies), and pain control. Pediatric surgeons have become more adept in minimally invasive surgeries using laparoscopes for hiatal hernias, splenectomy and a whole host of other procedures.

Chapter 111
CONCLUSION

I want to leave you with these words, avoiding all confusion,
That while one lives, the learning never ends, there's no conclusion.
So let me tell you, I have learned to learn by writing this book,
It's taken me back to my medical school years, to have a second look.

And I have been surprised and excited by recalling and renewing each topic,
By seeing the growth in each surgical field, and not remaining myopic.
I learn and I teach and I write with a view,
Of passing my zeal and excitement to you.

And if you have gained some few facts that you've needed,
I'll consider that my aims in this book have succeeded.

I want to emphasize that this book has taught me more than I expected. In medical school, internship and surgical residency, the young physician has a taste of most of the subspecialties and then leaves most behind to focus on an area of major interest. It has been a wonderful review for me, to poke my head into different operating rooms during the day and into journals and texts at night finding out about what the other specialties have been doing in the last twenty-five years. I have seen open heart surgeries progress from the earliest days of coronary artery bypass to doing this surgery without using extracorporeal bypass. I have seen the major advances in neurosurgery using the microscopes and the new orthopedic arthroscopic procedures and the many advances in surgery of the inner ear and the eye.

Physicians can write volumes of complexities for their own specialists. I have attempted to sift out the basic wheat from the verbiage chaff so that you too can experience some of the wonderment of your own body, and the physician's ability to overcome a whole host of abnormalities. Never look back to a so-called kinder, gentler tune somewhere in the past. It is too often a romanticized view. From a purely medical point of view, there has never been a better time to be alive. The ages past have been filled with endless suffering, painful inadequate treatments, and early death. From the peasant to the king, everyone suffered untold medical miseries with little to alleviate the discomforts. We now have comprehensive management for every aspect of health care; all we have to do is educate ourselves. And in the process of education, I think you'll find that the world continues to unfold its wonders, not the least of which is the mind of man.

GLOSSARY

I know a man who always speaks with long important words,
He may as well be talking to the clouds or to the birds.
I'm sure he's very bright and all his words are quite correct,
But I would rather use the simple terms that you expect.

However, when I write about a subject, I've agreed,
To give to you a list of words or terms that you might need.
So here's my glossary of words. I hope you'll use it often;
I know I won't stop looking up things, until I'm in a coffin!

AA - Alcoholics Anonymous: A voluntary self-help twelve step organization for alcoholics.

Abdomen: The part of the human body between the diaphragm and the pelvis containing the peritoneal cavity with all the viscera.

Abdominoplasty: Aesthetic reconstruction of the abdomen by excising excess skin and fat.

Above knee amputation: Surgical removal of the leg through the thigh and above the knee.

Abscess: A pocket of pus that forms when the body attempts to wall off an infection.

Acid phosphatase: A laboratory test which when elevated may indicate cancer of the prostate gland.

Acinus: A small sac such as in lung, liver or breast anatomy.

Acoustic neuroma: A tumor of nerve cell tissue affecting the acoustic nerve (hearing), sometimes resulting in hearing loss.

ACS - American College of Surgeons: A major organization for assuring quality and continuing education of its accepted surgeon members in the U.S.

Acupuncture: Ancient Chinese practice of medicine for curing disease, improving health and alleviating pain by insertion of needles in specific locations or meridians of the body.

Acute: Of short duration as opposed to chronic; severe, sharp pain.

Adams-DeWeese filter: A device with a "strainer" effect placed surgically around the lower vena cava to prevent blood clots from going to the lung (pulmonary emboli).

Addiction: Physiological and psychological dependence on a substance such as alcohol pills or heroin.

Adenocarcinoma: A cancer of glandular tissue.

Adenoid cystic carcinoma: A malignancy occurring in the salivary glands, lungs and breast.

Adenoids: Lymphoid tissue in the throat; pharyngeal tonsils.

Adenoma: A usually non-cancerous, benign tumor forming gland.

Adenomyosis: Benign tissue growth of glands, often in muscle.

Adenosis: Glandular appearance of tissue.

Adhesions: Scarring that causes tissue to stick together; in the abdomen it can cause partial or complete intestinal obstruction or pain.

Adjuvant chemotherapy: Anticancer drugs used to treat a tumor before it has spread to prevent or delay recurrence and used in conjunction with surgery and/or radiation therapy.

Adrenal gland: Gland above the kidney; has a medulla producing adrenaline and a cortex producing steroids.

Adriamycin: Doxorubicin; a cytotoxic chemotherapeutic drug for treating cancer.

Aganglionic megacolon: Hirschsprung's disease in children; lack of ganglion nerve structures that cause normal colonic movement (peristalsis).

AIDS - Acquired Immune Deficiency Syndrome: Caused by human immunodeficiency virus, HIV, which causes deficiency of T4 helper lymphocytes.

Air sacs: The smallest functional unit in the lungs where oxygen and carbon dioxide gas exchange occurs.

AK amputation: Above knee amputation.

Albumin: A protein in blood and other animal tissue.

Alcohol: Ethanol; intoxicating substance in liquor and wine, also used for cleansing the skin.

Alkaline phosphatase: Laboratory test which may indicate disease or blockage of the bile duct or certain bone disease.

Alopecia: Loss of hair seen with some types of chemotherapy.

Allogeneic: Referring to a graft between two genetically nonidentical individuals.

Alternative medicine: Therapy which is prescribed instead of Western Medicine, including acupuncture, chiropractic, homeopathy.

Amenorrhea: Absence of menstrual period.

American Cancer Society: Nonprofit organization for information and help with all types of cancer problems.

Ampulla of Vater: The distal end of the common bile duct where it often unites with the pancreatic duct as they enter the duodenum.

Amputation: Removal of a part.

Amylase: Enzyme produced by the pancreas to help starch convert to sugar; elevation may indicate pancreatitis.

Amyotrophic lateral sclerosis: Lou Gehrig's disease; disease of muscular weakness and atrophy.

Anal crypt: Anatomic area just inside the rectum, often site of hemorrhoids, fistulas and infections.

Analgesic: Substance that relieves pain.

Anaplastic: Usually referring to cancers; loss of normal structure.

Androgen: Hormone responsible for male characteristics.

Anemia: Condition where there is deficiency of red blood cells or hemoglobin.

Anesthesia: Loss of sensation; the field of medicine pertaining to alleviating pain; local, regional, spinal or general (going to sleep).

Aneurysm: Dilation of an artery, vein or part of the heart.

Angiogram: X-ray of blood vessels after injecting radio-opaque dye.

Angioplasty: Dilating arteries or veins with a specially designed balloon catheter after which a tube or stent may be placed.

Angiotensin: A substance which is produced from angiotensinogen by renin and which causes vasoconstriction and elevated blood pressure.

Annulus Fibrosus: Dense outer fibrous portion of an intervertebral disc.

Anomaly: A deviation from the norm.

Antacids: Substance or medication that neutralizes or diminishes acid content in the stomach.

Anterior chamber: Space in the eye between the iris and the corneas containing aqueous.

Anterior repair: In Gynecology and Urology, repairing a cystocele through a vaginal approach.

Antibiotics: A substance that stops or prevents the growth of bacteria; i.e. penicillin.

Anticoagulation: An agent that prevents or slows the clotting of blood.

Antifungal: An agent that kills fungus; i.e. fluconazole.

Anti-inflammatory drugs: Drugs which decrease the inflammatory response such as aspirin and steroids.

Antireflux: Preventing backward flow as from the bladder to ureter, or stomach to esophagus.

Antrectomy: Surgical removal of the antrum of the stomach; for treatment of a peptic ulcer removing the gastric antrum which produces the hormone gastrin.

Antrum of stomach: First part of the pylorus of the stomach where gastrin is produced.

Anus: The end of the gastrointestinal canal; end of the rectum.

Aorta: Main artery coming from the left side of the heart and progressing down to the mid-abdomen where it splits into the iliac arteries.

Aortic valve: The bicuspid or two-leafed valve between the heart and the aorta.

Aortic stenosis: A narrowing of the aortic valve usually due to rheumatic heart disease.

Appendectomy: Removal of the appendix, either through an open or laparoscopic procedure.

Appendix: A fingerlike appendage of the cecum felt to have a possible immunological significance.

Aqueous of the eye: Fluid in the anterior and posterior chambers of the eye.

Areola: The pigmented tissue around the nipple.

Argon beam coagulator: An instrument used for coagulation or stopping superficial bleeding.

Arteriogram: X-ray of a blood vessel using radio opaque contrast (dye).

Arteriole: A very small artery, small enough to attach to a capillary.

Arteriosclerosis: Age related degenerative change in an artery, hardening of the arteries.

Artery: A thick-walled muscular blood vessel carrying oxygenated blood away from the heart (except for the pulmonary artery which carries unoxygenated blood to the lungs for oxygenation).

Arthritis: Inflammation of a joint.

Arthropathy: Joint disease.

Arthroplasty: Surgical correction of a joint.

Articular: Related to a joint or joint surface.

Artificial kidney: Dialysis machine; any apparatus which takes the place of the human kidney in getting rid of waste.

Artificial heart: A man made apparatus to pump blood, assisting or in place of the human heart.

Ascites: Fluid in the peritoneal cavity.

Aspiration: Removal of fluid from the body; abnormal taking of fluid into the lungs.

Aspirin: Acetylsalicylic acid; an anti-inflammatory agent, causing decreased platelet function.

Astrocytoma: Tumor of the brain or spinal cord.

Atelectasis: Partial lack of filling of the lungs with air after surgery which can lead to pneumonia.

Atherosclerosis: Arteriosclerosis with fat type deposits on the inner layer of a vessel.

Atrial septal defect: Congenital heart defect with an opening between the right and left side of the heart through the atrium.

Atrium: One of the two upper chambers of the heart.

Atypical ductal hyperplasia: Not cancer, but abnormal changes in a cell indicating that there may be cancer in the surrounding tissue.

AUA - American Urological Association.

Audiology: Science and study of hearing.

Auditory nerve: Eighth Cranial nerve; nerve from the ear mechanisms to the brain.

Augmentation mammoplasty: Increasing the size of the breast.

Auricle: The external ear; old term for atrium of the heart.

Autopsy: Examination of a dead body to determine the cause of death and other pathology.

AV Node - Atrioventricular node: The source of the electrical stimulus that stimulates and regulates heart beat.

AVM - Arteriovenous malformation: Pathological abnormality of blood vessels which can rupture causing severe hemorrhage. In the brain this could be fatal.

Axilla: Armpit; containing nerves, arteries, veins, fatty tissue and lymph nodes.

Axillary lymph nodes: Lymph nodes in the armpit.

Axillary dissection: Surgical removal of the fatty tissue in the axilla containing lymph nodes.

Axon: The "arm" coming from a nerve cell transmitting impulses.

AZT: Retrovir, a drug used for the treatment of AIDS.

Backbone: Vertebral column.

Bacteria: A group of tiny organisms which may cause disease in humans.

Bacteriology: The study of bacteria.

Balloon pump: Intra-aortic balloon, a temporary, intermittently inflating balloon placed in the aorta and connected to an outside pump, used to assist the heart in circulating the blood.

Bariatric: Relating to the management of obesity (severely overweight).

Barnard, Dr. Christian: South African surgeon who performed the first human heart transplant in Capetown's Groote Schuur Hospital in 1967.

Bartholin's gland: A gland near the vaginal orifice which can become infected or form an abscess.

Basal cell cancer: "Rodent ulcer"; cancer of the skin which does not metastasize but can grow slowly and extensively locally.

Battle's sign: Bruising seen behind the ear suggestive of basilar (floor of) skull fracture.

BE - Barium enema: X-ray examination of the lower intestinal tract using liquid with barium.

Below knee amputation: Removal of the leg below the knee and above the ankle.

Benign: Not cancerous or malignant; a mild character of illness.

Bezoar: A mass of food or hair in the stomach or intestinal tract causing symptoms of pain or obstruction.

Bile: Green or yellow fluid secreted by the liver into the intestine which helps absorb fats.

Biliary atresia: Abnormal development of the bile ducts in the liver with resultant obstruction and jaundice.

Bilroth I: A surgical procedure after removal of part of the stomach, where the remaining stomach is connected back up to the duodenum.

Bilroth II: As above but the connection is between the stomach and the jejunum.

Biopsy: Removing tissue from a patient in order to make a diagnosis.

BK amputation: Below knee amputation.

Bladder: An organ for storing a fluid: i.e. gall bladder, urinary bladder.

Blepharoplasty: An operation to correct an abnormality of the eyelids.

Blood Clotting Factors: I=fibrinogen; II=prothrombin; III=tissue thromboplastin; IV=calcium; V=proaccelerin; factor VII=proconvertin; VIII=antihemophilic factor; IX=Christmas factor; X=Stuart-Prower factor; XI= plasma thromboplastin antecedent (PTA); XII=Hageman factor; XIII= fibrin stabilizing factor.

Blood count: Determination of blood contents including WBC, RBC and number of WBC per unit volume.

Blood types A, B, O, AB: One of the four blood groups, each of which may be Rh + or -.

Blowout fracture: Fracture of the floor of the orbit surrounding the eye, without fracture of the rim.

Bochdalek's hernia: Congenital hernia of the side and back of the diaphragm.

Body of stomach: Part of the stomach between the fundus and the antrum.

Bone graft: Transplantation of a piece of bone from one area of the body to another.

Bone marrow: The substance inside of a bone often with blood forming ability.

Bone: Connective tissue in a matrix with calcium salts making it hard.

Bony spur: An abnormal projection of bone which may or may not be symptomatic.

Bowel prep: A special cleansing of the intestine in preparation for colon surgery (i.e. GoLYTELY).

BPH - Benign prostatic hypertrophy: Noncancerous enlargement of the prostate gland.

Brain death: Absence of brain function, as in an EEG; one criterion of body death.

Brainstem: The lower portion of the brain below the cerebellum, including the medulla, and down to the upper portion of the spinal cord.

BRCA1: A gene that when altered indicates an inherited high susceptibility to developing breast cancer.

Breast: The mammary gland; the front of the thorax; a modified sweat gland.

Bronchial adenoma: A malignant lung tumor of the carcinoid type; a bronchopulmonary endocrine tumor of lung; long term survival rate over 90% with surgery.

Bronchoscopy: Examination and possible biopsy of the bronchi with a lighted tube.

Bronchus: One of two subdivisions of the trachea which continue to divide into smaller bronchi and bronchioles down to the air sacs.

Browlift: Operation to raise or elevate the eyebrows.

Bufferin: Buffered aspirin; pain killer and anti-inflammatory.

Bullous emphysema: Lung condition with increased air spaces in the air sacs; caused by smoking resulting in barrel chested appearance and respiratory embarrassment.

BUN - Blood urea nitrogen: A chemical in the blood used to measure kidney function.

Burn center: A specialized hospital unit or department for handling burn victims with all the needed support personnel and expertise.

Bypass-biliary: Mechanism for relieving an obstruction of the bile duct due to stone, cancer or scar using surgery, radiological stenting, or gastroenterological stenting with ERCP.

Bypass-vascular: Bypassing a blocked artery (or vein) with a reversed vein or synthetic artery.

CA 125: A tumor bio-marker elevated in ovarian cancer but also elevated in many non-cancerous conditions; can be followed in ovarian cancer to evaluate response to chemotherapy.

CABG - Coronary artery bypass grafting: Use of the mammary artery or vein grafts to bypass blocked or narrowed coronary arteries.

Calcium: Metallic element important for blood clotting; factor IV.

Canal of Schlemm: Sinus venosus sclerae; canal in eye through which aqueous passes to be reabsorbed; blockage can cause glaucoma.

Cancer: A malignant growth; purposeless, uncontrolled growth of abnormal cells that can destroy local tissue and may have the ability to metastasize and destroy the host.

Candida albicans: Monilia; fungus; yeast-like cells that can cause thrush, vaginal infections, and systemic infection - often secondary to broad spectrum antibiotic treatment, immuno-suppression and debility.

Carbon dioxide - CO_2: A gas produced by metabolism, excreted by the lungs.

Carcinogen: Something that can cause cancer.

Carcinoma in situ: Stage 0 cancer; cancer that has not spread beyond the basement membrane and is unable to metastasize; a very early cancer.

Cardia of stomach: The first portion of the stomach just below the esophagus.

Cardiac arrhythmias: Abnormalities in the beating of the heart usually due to some underlying heart disease.

Carotid artery: One of the main arteries supplying blood to the brain.

Carpal tunnel: Anatomical area in the wrist through which the median nerve passes; pressure in this area may cause numbness and tingling in the hand.

Cartilage: Dense connective tissue found near joints.

Cast: A rigid encasement of plastic or plaster for immobilization, as for a fracture.

CAT scan: Computerized axial tomography; an x-ray which takes thin slice pictures of the body which are reconstructed by computer.

Cataract: Opacity or loss of transparency of the lens of the eye.

Catheters: Tubes with holes; urinary catheters (Foley's) or drains.

Cautery: Electrical device for cutting or coagulating tissue.

CDP - Computerized dynamic posturography: Method of evaluating the vestibular system of the inner ear.

Cecum: First portion of the ascending colon where the appendix is attached.

Cellulitis: Inflammation of tissue cells.

Cephalic phase: Part of the physiology of acid secretion in the stomach; when you feel hungry a message passes from the brain, down the vagus nerves to the stomach to liberate acid.

Cerebellum: The part of the brain below the cerebrum responsible for control of coordination and posture.

Cerebrum: Largest, uppermost part of the brain with two hemispheres with an inner white and outer gray matter responsible for motor, sensory and thought functions.

Cervical (spine): The spine and vertebrae in the neck.

Cervical rib: An extra rib sometimes present on the cervical vertebrae which may or may not be symptomatic.

Cervicitis: Inflammation of the cervix of the uterus.

Cervix: The first portion or neck of the uterus projecting into the vagina.

Cesarean section: Delivery of a baby through an abdominal incision; Julius Caesar was supposedly born this way.

Chalazion: Inflammation of a gland in the eyelid.

Chamberlain procedure: A 6 cm. incision in the left chest for access to the chest cavity for small procedures and biopsies, eliminating the need for a large incision.

Charcot joint: Disease with joint destruction caused by loss of sensory nerves such as in leprosy, syphilis, diabetes mellitus.

Chemotherapy: Treatment of cancer (occasionally non-cancerous condition) with drugs which kill cells.

Chest wall: The bony and supportive chest outer layer encompassing the heart, lungs etc.

Chest x-ray: Radiological examination of the chest as routine or to evaluate abnormalities.

Chest tube: Thoracostomy tube; tube placed to remove air, fluid or infection from the pleural cavity.

CHF - Congestive heart failure: Heart disease usually caused by heart muscle injury from coronary artery disease or certain drugs.

Chlamydia: A bacteria-like organism that causes vaginal, lung and other infections.

Chloride: A compound containing chlorine; Cl- part of salt water solution NaCl and hydrochloric acid HCl.

Chocolate cyst: Ovarian cyst containing old blood.

Cholecystectomy: Removal of the gallbladder and cystic duct with an open or laparoscopic procedure.

Choledochal cyst: Congenital abnormality of the bile duct causing a large dilated cystic structure.

Choledocholithotomy: Removal of stones from the common bile duct.

Cholelithiasis: Gall stones; stones in the gall bladder.

Cholesteatoma: A middle ear disease caused by a chronic infection which has abnormal tissue in a cystic cavity (keratinizing squamous epithelium and cholesterol).

Cholesterol: A fattylike substance in the body which can cause gall stones and disease of arteries with eventual narrowing or closure.

Chondrosarcoma: Cancer derived from cartilage tissue.

Choroid: Part of the eye lying between the sclera and the retina.

Choroid plexus: Segment of the choroid of the eye producing aqueous fluid.

Christmas factor: Clotting factor IX.

Chromic catgut: Absorbable surgical suture once prepared from sheep intestines.

Chronic: Lasting a long time, as opposed to acute.

Cimino fistula: A surgical connection between a small artery and vein, usually in the forearm, which will cause the arm veins to dilate so they can be used for hemodialysis.

Circle of Willis: A circular arrangement of arteries in the brain connecting the right and left carotid and vertebral artery systems and, when intact, can insure continued brain blood flow if one of its supplying arteries is occluded.

Cirrhosis: Disease of the liver often caused by excess alcohol intake, but also by bacteria and viruses with development of jaundice, ascites and liver failure.

Clavicle: Collarbone.

Clear margin: Describing the normal cancer-free tissue margin of a tissue specimen.

Cleft lip: Congenital abnormality of the development of the palate and lips leaving a separation between the right and left sides of the upper lip.

Cleft palate: Congenital developmental abnormality with a varying separation of the side of the hard palate in the roof of the mouth.

Clinical medicine: The treatment of disease without surgery; Internal Medicine.

Clinical stage: A determination of the activity of a tumor by pathology, measurement and symptoms.

Closed angle glaucoma: Increase pressure in the eye secondary to inability of aqueous fluid to be reabsorbed.

Clotting factors: *See* blood clotting factors.

CO$_2$: *See* carbon dioxide.

Coagulation: Clotting of blood.

Coccyx: The last bone of the vertebral column made up of four fused bones.

Cochlea: Part of the inner ear labyrinth containing the auditory nerve endings for hearing.

Cochlear implants: Surgically implanted devices for reconstituting hearing ability after surgical or infectious destruction of the cochlea.

Codeine: An opium alkaloid used for pain control and cough sedative.

Cold cone: Gynecological procedure of biopsying the cervix.

Colectomy: Surgical removal of part or all of the colon.

Colitis: Inflammation of the colon, acute or chronic, i.e. ulcerative colitis.

Collagen: A protein of fibrous tissue needed for wound healing and strength.

Collecting system: Part of the kidney where urine is produced for excretion.

Colles' fracture: Dinner Fork Deformity; fracture of the forearm bone, radius with the hand displaced backward.

Colon: The large intestine; the bowel from the ileocecal valve to the anus.

Color blindness: Achromatopsia; inability to distinguish certain colors usually reds and greens.

Colostomy: A loop or end of colon brought to the surface of the abdomen as a stoma.

Colovesical fistula: An abnormal connection between the colon and bladder usually secondary to chronic inflammation, malignancy or trauma.

Colposcopy: Examination of the cervix and vagina with an endoscope.

Comminuted fracture: A fracture or broken bone in many pieces.

Common bile duct: Main duct composed of conjoining of the main hepatic and cystic ducts; carries bile from the liver or gall bladder to the duodenum.

Compartment of leg: A fascially encapsulated muscular segment of the lower leg.

Complementary medicine: Treatment which is in addition to Western medicine including supportive measures which do not cure cancer but control some of the symptoms and improve well being.

Compound fracture: A fracture in which the overlying skin is punctured leading down to the broken bone.

Concussion: Injury to the brain characterized by loss of consciousness, and possible cold clammy appearance and loss of excretory control.

Condylar: Relating to the articular surface between two bones.

Condyloma acuminatum: Papillomas; genital warts on the penis, vulva and perianal area.

Congenital: Condition you were born with.

Conjunctiva: Inner surface lining of the eyelids and over part of the eyeballs (palpebral and bulbar).

Conjunctival: Relating to the conjunctiva.

Conjunctivitis: Inflammation of the conjunctiva; pinkeye.

Consumption coagulopathy: Clotting disorder produced by a bleeding condition that uses up the body's supply of certain clotting factors.

Contamination: Presence of bacteria in a wound which have not colonized and grown.

Contrast dye: A radio-opaque liquid used in x-rays to enhance the ability to see a structure.

COPD - Chronic obstructive pulmonary disease.

Cornea: Outer convex covering of the eye in front of the pupil and iris.

Corneal transplant: Replacing a damaged cornea with one taken from a cadaver.

Coronary arteries: The arterial blood vessels supplying the heart.

Coronary angioplasty: Dilating a narrowed coronary artery using a special catheter with an inflatable balloon on one end, introduced through the skin, usually into the femoral artery and up to the coronary arteries; stents may also be placed to keep the artery open.

Corpus uteri: Body of the uterus.

Corpus luteum cyst: Follicular cyst formed by the expulsion of the ovum during ovulation.

Cortex of brain: Outer portion of the brain; gray matter.

Corticospinal tract: Nerve tracts from the brain through the spinal cords controlling motor function (movement).

Corticosteroids: Hormones produced by the adrenal cortex; also name used for synthetic steroids.

Cosmetic surgery: Aesthetic surgery for improving the appearance.

Coumadin: Warfarin; oral anticoagulant for prolonging the prothrombin time.

CPR - Cardiopulmonary resuscitation.

Craniectomy: Removing part of the bony cranium or skull.

Craniotomy: Opening into the skull during a surgery on the brain.

Cranium: Skull.

Creatinine: A waste product excreted in the urine and used to evaluate kidney function.

Cricothyrotomy: Incision in the neck above the level for a tracheostomy done under emergency situations.

Crohn's disease: Regional ileitis; transmural colitis; inflammatory disease of the colon and small intestine which effects all layers of the bowel.

Cryosurgery: Use of freezing temperature to destroy tissue, i.e. cancer.

Cryptorchidism: Failure of one or both testicles to descend into the scrotum.

CSF - Cerebrospinal fluid: Clear fluid surrounding portions of the brain and spinal cord.

Cure: Completely eradicating a malignancy (as compared to a five year survival or disease free interval etc.)

Curette: An instrument with a sharpened tip shaped in a loop or ring for scraping tissue for biopsy.

CVA - Cerebrovascular accident: Stroke. Brain damage secondary to impaired blood supply, tumor, trauma, etc.

CVP line: Catheter introduced into a vein for venous access and to measure central venous pressure.

Cyclosporine: An immunosuppressive agent often used in transplantations which does not inhibit antibody production.

Cystic duct: A duct from the gallbladder to the common bile duct.

Cystic hygroma: Lymphangioma; A benign congenital cystic mass caused by abnormal lymph channel development.

Cystitis: Inflammation of the bladder.

Cystocele: Protrusion of the bladder into the anterior vaginal wall due to pelvic floor weakness, occasionally after multiple pregnancies.

Cystogram: X-ray of the bladder.

Cystoscope: Light instrument for examining the bladder for tube placements, biopsy, or general evaluation.

Cystoscopy: *See* cystoscope.

Cystourethrocele: Protrusion of the bladder and urethra into the vagina wall due to pelvic floor weakness.

Cysts: Fluid filled sacs.

D&C - Dilatation and curettage.

Dacron: A synthetic fiber used for suture, grafts and patches.

DCIS - Ductal carcinoma in situ: Stage 0 cancer; cancer where the basement membrane is intact and tumor will not spread or metastasize.

De Motu Cordis: William Harvey's book describing the circulation of blood published in 1628.

Debridement: Cleansing a wound; removing dead, infected tissue and foreign bodies.

Debulking: Surgically removing a large portion of a tumor when the entire tumor cannot be removed.

Declotting: Removing the blood clots from a vessel or graft by chemical or surgical means.

Degenerative joint disease: Deterioration of a joint secondary to aging.

Dehiscence: Splitting or breaking open of the fascia with the skin still intact.

Dermoid cyst: Benign tumor, usually in the ovary, containing hair, skin, teeth.

Diabetes mellitus: Disease characterized by high blood sugar due to inadequate insulin production by the pancreas.

Dialysis: Removing waste tissue from the blood or peritoneum when the kidneys are unable to function adequately; artificially functioning as a kidney.

Diaphragm: Musculofibrous division between the thoracic and abdominal cavities; muscle aids in respiration; a rubber cap placed over the cervix as a contraceptive device.

Diaphysis: The shaft of a long bone.

Diarthrodial: Synovial joint; a freely moveable joint.

Diastole: The relaxation part of the heart action cycle when it fills with blood; as opposed to systole.

DIC - Disseminated intravascular coagulopathy: A complex bleeding problem caused by excessive hemorrhage, infection or sepsis.

Diplopia: Double vision; abnormal eye focusing causes one object to appear as two.

Direct hernia: Inguinal hernia involving the abdominal wall in the direct space, below the epigastric artery.

Disease free: No evidence of disease at the time of exam; not necessarily meaning cured. Patients with a cancer may have a disease free interval but the cancer may return at a later date.

Disk: A fibrocartilaginous "spacer" between vertebral bodies.

Diverticulitis: Inflammation in a diverticulum.

Diverticulosis: An outpouching of any structure usually in terms of the GI tract i.e., colon, esophagus (Zenker's) and small intestine (Meckel's).

Doppler study: Ultrasound study of a part of the body, especially for vascular and heart disease.

Dorsal columns: Part of the spinal cord that carries information to the brain about touch, position and vibratory sensation.

Dorsal and ventral nerve roots: Nerves exiting the spinal cord at each level joining to form the spinal nerve on each side.

Dr. Joel Berman's Comprehensive Breast Care and Surviving Breast Cancer: The best book on breast disease and one that you can't do without.

Drains: Flat rubber or plastic tubes used to drain bloody or watery fluid or infection from a wound or part of the body.

Dry eye syndrome: Sjogren's syndrome; Inadequate secretion of eyedrops by the lacrimal gland of the eye.

Ducts: Tubular structures draining fluid from an organ or gland.

Duodenum: First part of the small intestine after the stomach; site of entry of the common bile duct and the pancreatic duct.

Duplex scan: A special ultrasound study which can measure flow in blood vessels as well as general pathology.

Dupuytren's contracture: A chronic bending of a finger towards the palm requiring surgery when symptomatic or unsightly.

Dura mater: A tough outer covering of the central nervous system.

Dyspareunia: Painful sexual intercourse.

Dysuria: Painful urination.

Ectropion: Eversion or turning outward of the eyelid.

Edema: Swelling; accumulation of watery fluid in tissue.

EEG - Electroencephalogram: Instrument for recording and measuring brain electrical function and diagnosing disorders.

Ejaculation: The ejection of semen.

EKG - Electrocardiogram: An instrument for recording the electrical activity of the heart and used for diagnosis of abnormal conditions such as irregular rhythms and heart attack.

Electrolytes: Sodium Na, Potassium K, chloride CL, and carbon dioxide, CO_2 in the blood or urine.

Electrocautery: *See* cautery.

Embolization: Blockage of a blood vessel by a clot, or other substance.

Emphysema: A chronic lung condition characterized by over-aeration of the air sacs and thus, the lung, creating respiratory distress and barrel chest; usually cause by smoking.

Empyema: Pus in the chest cavity.

Endarterectomy: Removal of the diseased inner lining of an artery.

Endobronchial: Within the bronchus.

Endocrinologist: Physician who specializes in the endocrine and other secretory gland diseases of the body such as pancreas (diabetes mellitus), thyroid, parathyroid, adrenal, etc.

Endolymphatic duct: Part of the inner ear associated with vestibular function and containing endolymph.

Endometriosis: Benign ectopic occurrence of endometrial type tissue in ovaries or on peritoneal surfaces causing pain.

Endometrium: The inner layer of the uterine wall that sloughs with each menstruation.

Endonasal pituitary surgery: Neurosurgical procedure operating through the nose and into the center of the brain to remove a tumor of the pituitary gland.

Endotracheal tube: A tube placed through the mouth into the trachea during anesthesia or for emergency respiratory support in an intensive care unit.

Endovascular: Literally inside the vessel; surgery done with instruments inside a vessel such as coronary artery angioplasty, peripheral vessel angioplasty and placement of stents in   vessels.

Enterocele: Weakness of the pelvic floor with protrusion of small bowel into the wall of vagina.

ENG - Electronystagmography: A test used for measurement of vestibular system.

Enteritis: Inflammation of the small intestine.

Enterostomy: Exteriorization of the intestine through an opening in the abdominal wall.

Enterovaginal fistula: Abnormal connection between the small intestine and the vagina.

Entropion: Turning in of the eyelid.

EPA - Environmental protection agency: National agency created to standardize excellence of safety in the workplace.

Ependymoma: Glioma; brain tumor.

Epicanthus: Congenital fold of skin covering the inner canthus of the eye.

Epidemiology: The study of the causes and distribution of diseases.

Epidermis: The outer layer of skin.

Epididymitis: Inflammation of the epididymis.

Epididymis: Part of the testis consisting of tube through which sperm pass from the testis to the vas deferens.

Epidural anesthesia: A regional anesthetic causing complete anesthesia below the level of injection into the epidural space in the back; used for obstetrical delivery and some abdominal surgeries.

Epigastric hernia: Abdominal wall hernia occurring in the upper mid-abdomen.

Epiglottis: A flap of tissue behind the tongue which closes the airway when eating or drinking to prevent aspiration of this food or liquid into the lungs.

Epiglottitis: Inflammation of the epiglottitis; may be life threatening in children.

Epiphora: Overflow of tears.

Epistaxis: Nosebleed; usually from the back of the nose in adults and the front of the nose in children.

ERCP - Endoscopic retrograde cholangiopancreatography: A study of the common bile duct using a scope passed through the mouth and esophagus under heavy sedation; for removal of common bile duct stones, biopsies and placement of stents.

Erection: Hardening of the penis when its erectile tissue is filled with blood.

Esophageal atresia: Congenial incomplete development of the esophagus with many structural variations.

Esophagus: Muscular tube extending from the mouth to the stomach.

Estrogen: Any of several female sex hormones; Estradiol, estrone, estriol.

Ethmoid sinus: Air sinus near the nose.

Eustachian tube: Tubular connection between the middle ear and the pharynx, for pressure equalization.

Evisceration: Dehiscence that breaks through the skin; Complete outer wound breakdown with organs protruding to the outside of the body.

Ewing sarcoma: Malignant tumor of bone usually in young adults; reticulocytoma sarcoma.

Exophthalmus: Protrusion of the eyes seen with hyperthyroidism and other causes.

Expander prosthesis: Temporary breast prosthesis placed on the chest after extensive breast surgery and which can be inflated over several months to stretch the overlying skin. It is   later replaced by a permanent implant.

External auditory canal: Outer ear canal from the entrance to the ear drum.

External ear: The outer visible ear and canal.

Extracorporeal membrane oxygenator for infants: A machine for keeping newborn infants alive until their own lungs can take over adequately.

Extradural: Outside the dura covering the brain and spinal cord.

Extremities: Arms and legs.

Facelift: Rhytidectomy; plastic surgical procedure for getting rid of wrinkles, reshaping the face to give a younger look by excising tissue.

Facial nerve: Cranial nerve VII, motor nerve for many of facial muscles of expression.

FACS - Fellow of the American College of Surgeons.

Fallopian tubes: Tubes, one on each side of the uterus which convey the ova from the ovary to the uterus.

Fascia: Fibrous tissue between the skin and underlying body and surrounding some muscles.

Fecal material: Stool.

Felon: An infection or abscess of the tip of the finger.

Female period: Menstrual period; monthly shedding of the uterine endometrium with bloody vaginal discharge.

Femoral: Area of the body at the upper anterior thigh, related to the bone, the femur.

Femoral hernia: Hernia protruding through the femoral canal below the groin crease.

Femoral head: The head of the femur which articulates at the hip joint with the pelvis.

Femoral neck: The part of the femur just below the head and site of some fractures.

Femur: Large long bone of the upper leg/thigh.

Fetus: The unborn child in the uterus.

Fibrinogen: Blood clotting factor I; converted to fibrin in making a clot.

Fibroadenoma: A benign rubbery tumor occurring in a gland, especially the breast.

Fibrocystic disease: Benign occurrence of single or multiple cysts in the breast which may cause discomfort and are thought to be aggravated by intake of caffeine.

Fibroid uterus: Leiomyomata uteri; benign condition of the uterus with the growth of rubbery masses which may cause pain or vaginal bleeding.

Fibrous tissue: Connective tissue, also scar tissue.

Fibula: The outer bone of the lower leg.

FIGO - International Federation of Gynecology and Obstetrics.

Fissure: A slit or opening; in the anal area a painful splitting in the mucosa which may bleed.

Fistula in ano: In the anal area, a tract from inside the rectum through the side wall and exiting through the perirectal skin.

Fistula: An abnormal communication between two organs or body areas.

Five year survival: A general term often used to describe the success of cancer treatment of a specific tumor. If there is no recurrence in five years many cancers are considered cured; however, there are some cancers which can recur after ten or even twenty years.

Flank hernia: Lumbar hernia; a defect in the lateral abdominal wall, usually secondary to previous surgery.

Fluconazole: A medication for treatment of certain fungal infections.

Fluorescein dye: A green fluorescent liquid, which, when placed in the anesthetized eye, can help identify corneal abrasions.

Fluoroscopy: X-ray of the body in a continuous mode to see movement; a type of "radiological television".

Foley catheter: A rubber tube with an inflatable balloon on the end which can be placed in the bladder for measuring urine and allowing flow in obstructive conditions.

Follicle: A mass of cells usually with a central cavity.

Fontanelle: The membranous areas between the skull bones of infants.

Foreskin: Prepuce; the free fold of skin covering the end of the penis in uncircumcised males.

Fovea: A small cup-shaped depression; the fovea of the eye.

Fracture: A broken bone.

Fragmin: An anticoagulant.

Free graft: A segment of tissue which is transferred from one area of the body to another without its original attachments in place; the vessels of the donor and recipient sites are   then connected.

Frontal lobe of brain: The front of the brain usually related to function of thought.

Frontal sinus: Air sinus in the frontal bone near the nose.

Full thickness graft: Taking the entire thickness of skin for a graft.

Gall bladder: Saclike structure attached to the undersurface of the right lobe of the liver for storing bile; it is connected by the cystic duct to the common bile duct.

Gall stone: Cholelithiasis; a concretion or stone found in the gall bladder or bile duct.

Gallstone pancreatitis: Pancreatitis caused by gallstones blocking the entry of the pancreatic duct into the bile duct.

Gangrene: Death of tissue usually related to decrease of absence of blood supply or due to severe infection.

Gastrectomy: Surgical removal of the stomach.

Gastric acid: Fluid secreted by the stomach to digest food.

Gastrin: Hormone secreted by the antrum of the stomach that stimulates acid production.

Gastroenterology: The medical specialty concerned with the function and pathology of the gastrointestinal tract, including liver, pancreas and biliary tract.
General surgery: The specialty of medicine concerned with surgery of the abdomen, breasts, thyroid, cancer surgery, etc.; tremendously variable depending on the training and experience.
Genes: A basic unit of heredity; located on a chromosome; abnormalities in certain genes can cause diseases and even certain cancers.
GERD - Gastroesophageal reflux disease: Acid indigestion.
Gestation: Pregnancy.
GFR - Glomerular filtration rate: A measure of kidney function.
GI tract - Gastrointestinal tract.
Glasgow coma scale: An evaluation scale used for assessing level of brain function.
Glaucoma: An eye disease characterized by elevated intraocular pressure.
Glioma: A type of brain tumor.
Globulin: A serum protein with immunological functions.
Glomerulus: A group of coiled blood vessels in the kidney important in the making of urine.
Goiter: Enlargement of the thyroid gland.
GoLYTELY: An oral liquid used for cleansing the intestinal tract in anticipation of surgery, colonoscopy, or certain x-rays. It goes anything but lightly!
Gonioscopy: Examining the angle of the anterior chamber of the eye; i.e. to check for glaucoma.
Gonorrhea: A highly contagious disease of the genitalia spread through sexual intercourse.
Gore-Tex: A synthetic material used for vascular grafts and sutures.
Gray matter: Brain cells.
Greenfield Filter: An umbrella shaped apparatus placed through a neck or groin vein into the inferior vena cava to prevent blood clots from going to the lung from the leg veins or pelvic veins.
Groshong catheter: A centrally placed catheter for I.V. access which exits the body as a tube.
Gynecological oncology: A subspecialty of gynecology focusing on the treatment of gynecologic cancer.
Gynecology: The medical and surgical specialty of female organs, i.e. uterus, tubes, ovaries.
H&P - History and physical examination.
H2 antagonists: Substances which block the production of gastric acid in the stomach.
Hageman factor: Factor XII; a blood clotting factor.
Hamartoma: A benign growth containing multiple different tissue types.

Hammer, anvil and stirrup: The ossicles of the ear; the bones of the ear important for transmitting sound impulses to the inner ear and cochlea.

Hardening of the arteries: Atherosclerosis; disease of blood vessels often causing narrowing and obstruction.

Harrington rod: A metallic rod used for stabilization in orthopedic surgery.

Hashimoto's disease: Autoimmune thyroiditis; a benign thyroid disease causing mild hypothyroidism.

Heart valves: Two or three leafed valves in four places in the heart assuring one directional blood flow.

Heart failure: Ineffective or decreased contraction of the heart due to heart disease, causing multiple systemic problems.

Heart sounds: The normal sounds heard by auscultation or listening over the heart valves.

Heart murmur: Abnormal heart sound caused by congenital or acquired heart disease; i.e. aortic stenosis or insufficiency have characteristic sounds.

Heart transplantation: Complete removal of a failing heart and replacement with a normal heart from a "brain dead" donor.

Heimlich maneuver: Method of expelling a foreign body from the throat by standing behind the individual and pulling sharply into the epigastrium with clenched fists.

Hemangioma: A congenital malformation of blood vessels; a tumor of blood vessels.

Hematocolpos: Retained blood in the vagina; usually menstrual blood behind an imperforate hymen.

Hematology: The medical specialty dealing with all aspects of blood, blood formation and diseases.

Hematoma: An abnormal collection of blood as after trauma, surgery, etc.

Hematometrium: Blood in the uterine cavity.

Hematuria: Blood in the urine.

Hemodialysis: Dialysis.

Hemoglobin: The pigmented substance in the blood that combines with and releases oxygen.

Hemoperitoneum: Blood in the peritoneal cavity.

Hemophilia: A group of pathological conditions in which there is a coagulation problem causing increased tendency for bleeding.

Hemorrhage: Bleeding.

Hemorrhoids: Enlargement or varicosity of the veins around the anus and rectum.

Hemothorax: Blood in the chest cavity.

Heparin: An anticoagulant which elevates the PTT (partial thromboplastin time).

Hepatectomy: Surgical removal of a part or all of the liver.

Hepatitis: Inflammation of the liver due to virus, other infectious agents, or bile duct obstruction.

Hepatocellular: Relating to the cells of the liver.

Hernia: An abnormal protrusion or opening through a body cavity or structure.

Herniated disc: Protrusion of an intravertebral disc which may cause pain and nerve injury.

Hiatus hernia: Protrusion of the stomach upward through the esophageal hiatus into the chest.

Hickman catheter: An I.V. access placed in a large vein, usually the subclavian, for long term usage. It hangs out of the body.

HIDA scan: A special gall bladder x-ray to measure the function of the gall bladder and identify gallstones.

Hilum - lung, spleen, kidney: The part of an organ where the vessels and nerves enter and exit.

Hip: The joint where the femur articulates with the acetabulum of the pelvis.

Hirschsprung's disease: Congenital aganglionic megacolon.

HIV - Human immunodeficiency virus: Cause of AIDS.

Hordeolum: A purulent infection of an eyelid gland.

Horner's syndrome: Clinical findings after paralysis of the cervical sympathetic nerves of one side of the face; anhydrosis (dry skin), enophthalmos (retraction of the eyeball), ptosis   (drooping of the eye) and myosis (constriction of the pupil); sometimes seen with some tumors.

Humerus: Large bone of the upper arm.

Hydrocele: Fluid filled sac of the inguinal canal or scrotum.

Hydrocephalus: "Water on the brain"; an excess of CSF in the subarachnoid and ventricular spaces of the brain.

Hymen: A membranous perforated tissue across the entrance to the vagina; maidenhead.

Hypernephroma: A cancer of the kidney.

Hyperplasia: An increased number of cells in any given tissue, but not cancerous.

Hypertension: High blood pressure.

Hyperthyroidism: Overactivity of the thyroid gland from one of many causes.

Hypertrophic scar: Raised, unsightly, excessive scar formation; keloid.

Hypertrophic pyloric stenosis: A congenital thickening of the pyloric muscle in newborns which causes gastric outlet obstruction and requires a pyloromyotomy.

Hypomastia: Small or non-existent breasts.

Hypopharynx: Laryngeal part of the pharynx.

Hypothyroidism: Hypoactive thyroid gland, may cause low metabolic rate, weight gain, myxedema, thickened hair; old term was cretinism for hypothyroid newborns.

Hypoxemia: Low oxygen content of blood.

Hypoxia: Low oxygen content of breathed air.

Hysterectomy: Removal of the uterus.

Hysteroscopy: Examination of the inside of the uterus with a lighted hysteroscope.

Ibuprofen: Non-narcotic painkiller.

ID - Infectious disease specialty.

Ileostomy: Bringing a loop of ileum through the abdominal wall for drainage of small bowel contents; temporary or permanent depending on the disease.

Ileum: The third portion of the small intestine after the duodenum and jejunum and before the colon.

Ilioinguinal nerve: A sensory nerve running obliquely from lateral to medial across the inguinal canal and sometimes injured during inguinal hernia surgery. Cause of some postoperative   pain.

Ilium: One of the three bones of the pelvis along with the ischium and pubis.

Imuran: A medicine used to prevent immune rejection of tissue transplants.

Immunocompromised: Having decreased ability to fight off infection, tumors, etc.

Immunology: The study of the immune system, allergy, etc.

Immunotherapy: The treatment of certain diseases by boosting the immune system; gamma globulin and interferon.

Incarcerated hernia: A hernia that is stuck and cannot be reduced.

Incision: A surgical cut.

Incontinence: Loss of control of excretion such as with urine or stool.

Indirect hernia: An inguinal hernia that protrudes through the direct space in Hesselbach's triangle (lateral border of rectus sheath, inguinal ligament, inferior epigastric artery).

Infection: Growth of bacteria in a contaminated wound. Acute or chronic.

Inguinal: In the right or left lower abdomen; the groin.

Inner ear: The labyrinth including the cochlea, semicircular canals and vestibule.

Inorganic: Not formed by living organisms; neither animal or vegetable.

Insufficiency: Incompleteness of function.

Intergluteal: Between the buttocks.

Internal mammary artery: Artery inside the front of the chest, lateral to the right or left side of the sternum, occasionally used for coronary artery bypass grafting.

Intervertebral disc: *See* disk.

Intraocular pressure: The pressure inside the anterior and posterior eye chambers. *See* glaucoma.

Intubation: Placing a tube into the trachea either through the nose or mouth.

Intussusception: One loop of bowel insinuating into itself, as a invaginating sleeve.

Invasive: Going into; with tumor - invading into a surrounding area.

Iodine: Chemical element: in compounds used for antiseptic cleansing and IV dyes. Needed for normal thyroid development and function.

Iris: A colored diaphragm in the anterior part of the eye with a central hole called the pupil. Responsible for labeling of eye color; blue, brown, green, etc.

Ischemia: Lack of blood supply in a tissue.

Ischium: One of the bones making up the pelvis with the ilium and pubis.

Islet cells: Islands of Langerhans' cells in the pancreas that produce insulin and glucagon.

Isthmus of the thyroid: The tissue of the thyroid gland in front of the trachea acting as a bridge between the right and left thyroid lobes.

IV fluids: Intravenous fluids.

IVP - Intravenous pyelogram: X-ray study of kidney function and visualization of the kidney, ureters and bladder.

Jaundice: Yellow color of skin, eyes, and other tissue due to increase bilirubin usually secondary to congenital or acquired infectious or malignant liver disease, bile duct obstruction, or increased blood breakdown.

Jehovah's Witness: Religious group refusing transfusion of blood or blood products for religious reasons.

Jejunum: The second portion of the small intestine after the duodenum and before the ileum.

Keloid: Hypertrophic scar; enlarged, ugly scar.

Kenalog: Steroid injectable into tissue, as into skin to prevent keloid formation.

Keratitis: Inflammation of the cornea.

Keratome: Instrument for making extremely fine exact cuts in the cornea for refractive surgery.

Kidney cortex: The outer portion of the kidney.

Kidney medulla: The inner portion of the kidney.

Kidney pelvis: Cup-shaped cavity near the hilum of the kidney; the largest part of the collecting system and just before the ureters.

Kock pouch: Intestinal pouch used as an "artificial bladder" after removal of the bladder for cancer.

Kwell shampoo: Lindane lotion shampoo for head lice.

Kyphosis: Humpbacked; disease of the spine characterized by flexion.

Labium: Lip; of mouth, vagina, etc.

Labyrinthitis: Inflammation of the inner ear.

Lacrimal apparatus: In the eye, the structures responsible for secretion and drainage of tears.

Lamina: A thin layer, usually referring to bone.

Laminectomy: Removal of the vertebral lamina to expose the spinal cord nerve roots and for removal of an intervertebral disk.

Langer's lines: Lines indicating the best location for incisions to achieve the least obtrusive scarring.

Laparoscopy: Endoscopic examination of the peritoneal cavity.

Laryngeal tube: A special tube placed in the larynx for anesthesia without having to place an endotracheal tube.

Laryngectomy: Surgical removal of the larynx with the vocal cords.

Laryngoscopy: Direct examination of the larynx with a lighted tube.

Larynx: The organ of voice production between the pharynx and trachea.

Laser skin peel: Removal of a thin layer of epidermis and sometimes upper dermis using a laser.

Laser: Light Amplification by Stimulated Emission of Radiation: Instrument with multiple functions using a concentrated beam of energy. Types e.g. CO_2, YAG, KTP.

LASIK - Laser in-situ keratomileusis: Instrument for refractive eye surgery.

Lasix: Furosemide; a diuretic; to increase urine output.

Laser vaporization: Complete conversion of a solid into a vapor as in certain tumors and in eye surgery to remove certain structures.

Latissimus flap: Plastic surgical procedure where the latissimus muscle and overlying skin is used for breast reconstruction.

Layered closure: The closure of a surgical wound in a progressive orderly fashion to remove tension and obtain anatomical approximation of tissue.

LDS: A surgical instrument with staples used in abdominal surgery that Ligates, Divides and Staples in one action.

Leiomyomata uteri: Fibroid of the uterus; benign tumors.

Lens of eye: Transparent lens in the eye for converging or diverging light.

Lesion: Any abnormality in a tissue, i.e. tumor; an injury or wound.

LeVeen shunt: Peritoneal-venous ascites shunt; specially designed tube and valve to move intra-abdominal fluid one way into the venous system.

Lice: Pediculus; parasitic organism found in hair, clothes and in genital areas.

Linitis plastica: "Leatherbottle stomach" infiltrating stomach cancer causing a rigid thickened tubelike appearance; often advanced cancer.

Lipase: Pancreatic enzyme which helps digest fats.

Lipoma: Benign fatty tumor, often in the subcutaneous tissue of the skin.

Liposuction: Plastic surgical procedure where areas of excess fat are sucked out and remodeling of the body is accomplished.

Lithotripsy: Procedure for breaking up kidney stones by the force of sound waves.

Liver: Large gland in the right upper abdomen responsible for bile, clotting factors, and many metabolic functions on proteins and fats.

Lobectomy: Surgical removal of a lobe, as in liver, lung or thyroid.

Lobules: Small subdivision of a lobe.

Local anesthesia: Making a body part numb by using local infiltration of drugs such as marcaine or xylocaine.

Look Good, Feel Better: American Cancer Society program to help patients with cancer apply makeup, wigs, etc.

Lou Gehrig's disease: Amyotrophic lateral sclerosis.

Lucid interval: A phenomenon in head and brain injury where a comatose patient becomes alert before deteriorating further.

Lumbar hernia: Lateral abdominal wall hernia.

Lumbar: Lateral abdominal wall; flank; side of abdomen between rib cage and pelvis.

Lumpectomy: Removal of a lump; in breast surgery, removal of a tumor with free margins.

Lungs: Organs of respiration.

Lymph nodes: Round or oval small bodies of lymphoid tissue along the lymphoid channels and often the site of spread of inflammation or tumor.

Lymphatic: Pertaining to lymph nodes or lymph drainage.

Lymphoma: A malignant disease of the lymphatic system.

Macromastia: Abnormally large breasts often causing back and shoulder pain.

Malignancy: Cancer: Growth with the ability to invade and spread locally and in many cases to metastasize distantly.

Malleus, incus and stapes: *See* Hammer, anvil and stirrup; ossicles of the ear.

Mallory-Weiss tear: A tear in the mucosa of the esophagogastric area of the stomach usually caused by excessive vomiting.

Malrotation of the bowel: Congenital abnormality of the intestinal tract which may or may not produce symptoms.

Malunion: Bad joining or healing of a fracture.

Marcaine: A local anesthetic.

Mastectomy: Removal of the breast.

Mastoid air cells: Cavities in the bone behind and around the inner ear.

Mastoidectomy: Surgical removal of the mastoid air cells for chronic disease.

Mattress suture: A surgical closure technique with alternating close and far sutures to evert and approximate tissue.

McBurney's point: An approximate skin marking two thirds the way between the umbilicus and the anterior superior iliac spine, often the area of greatest tenderness for appendicitis.

Mebendazole: Vermox; drugs for treating hookworm.

Meckel's diverticulum: A sac arising from the ileum about two feet from the ileocecal valve, in 2% of people and with three potential kinds of mucosa: Gastric, pancreatic and intestinal and which may bleed or get infected and mimic appendicitis.

Median sternotomy: Opening the chest by incising the skin and bone in the middle of the sternum or breastbone.

Mediastinoscopy: Examination of the mediastinum for tumor using a special scope inserted under the manubrium.

Mediastinum: The middle part of the thoracic cavity; the space between the lungs.

Medulloblastoma: A malignant, rapidly growing brain tumor in children.

Melanocyte: A pigment producing cell in the skin.

Melanoma: A cancer arising from melanocytes; either black or red or pale occurring, in the skin or eye.

Menarche: Onset of menstruation.

Meniere's disease: Disease of the inner ear causing tinnitus, vertigo and hearing loss.

Meninges: Membranes surrounding the brain and spinal cord including dura mater, arachnoid membrane and pia mater.

Meningioma: A benign brain tumor, often symptomatic and sometimes surgically challenging for complete removal.

Meningitis: Inflammation of the meninges.

Menopause: Cessation of menstruation.

Menstruation: Evacuation of blood and endometrial lining once a month from the uterus between ages approximately thirteen to forty-five or fifty.

Mestinon: Drug for the treatment of Myasthenia gravis.

Metaphysis: The portion of bone between the epiphysis and diaphysis.

Metastasis: Spread of cancer cells from their point of origin to another part of the body and the implantation and growth of the tumor cells.

Metronidazole: Flagyl; antibiotic used for numerous infections.

Microbiology: The study of microorganisms including bacteria, fungi, viruses, etc.

Microcalcifications: Tiny specks of white calcium seen on mammograms which can indicate benign or malignant disease depending on their arrangement.

Middle ear: Part of the ear with the ossicles.

Midline incision: Abdominal incision down the middle of the abdomen.

Mitomycin: Chemotherapeutic agent.

Mitral valve: Bicuspid heart valve between the left atrium and the left ventricle of the heart.

Modified radical mastectomy: Operative procedure removing the breast, nipple and areola and some surrounding skin and the axillary lymph nodes for breast cancer.

Mons pubis: The mound of fatty tissue over the symphysis pubis of females.

Monteggia's fracture: Fracture of the proximal ulna and dislocation of the radial head.

Motility: Ability to move.

Motor nerve: Nerve to a muscle which causes contraction and movement.

MRI scan: Magnetic resonance imaging; technique of imaging the body using magnetic fields and radio-frequency and a computer to get thin slice pictures through the body structure.

Mucoepidermoid carcinoma: Type of cancer which secretes mucous.

Myasthenia gravis: A muscular weakness disorder of autoimmune etiology and occasionally related to cancer of the lung.

Myeloma: A cancer of plasma cells in the bone marrow.

Myxedema: A clinical presentation of hypothyroidism.

NA - Narcotics Anonymous: Self help twelve step group for narcotics addicts.

Naprosyn: Anti-inflammatory and analgesic, not irritating to the stomach.

Nasopharynx: The area of the pharynx above the soft palate.

Navicular: One of the bones of the wrist.

Nephrostomy: Placement of a tube in the kidney pelvis.

Nerve block: Injection of an anesthetic around a nerve to temporarily or permanently deaden it.

Nerve stimulator: An instrument used to test the function of nerves especially in surgery to locate the tiny branches of the facial nerve during parotid surgery.

Neurology: The field of medicine which studies the nervous system and its diseases.

Neurons: Basic unit of the nervous system with dendrites, nerves cells and axons.

Neurosurgery: Brain, spinal cord and peripheral nerve surgery.

Neurotransmitters: Substances in the brain and at nerve endings that stimulates or inhibits impulses.

Nicotine: Poisonous alkaloid from tobacco.

Night vision: Decreased vision as one gets older.

Nissen fundoplication: Surgical procedure for correction of reflux esophagitis and esophageal hiatus hernia disease.

NSCLC - Non small cell lung cancer: Lung cancer which has poor prognosis and is usually a systemic disease by the time of diagnosis.

Normal flora: Normal bacteria present in the intestinal tract or other areas of the body.

Nucleus pulposus: Central portion of an intervertebral disk which can prolapse - slipped disk.

Nuclear medicine: Diagnostics using radioactive material and scanning machines.

Nurolon: A synthetic suture material.

Nylon: A type of suture material.

OA - Overeaters Anonymous: Self help twelve step program for overeaters.

Obesity: Excessive fat accumulation. Excessively overweight - varies by ethnic cultures.

Obstetrics: The field of medicine dealing with pregnancy and birth.

Off pump CABG: Coronary artery bypass surgery done without placing the patient on the heart bypass machine.

Oncologist: Cancer specialist.

Oophorectomy: Surgical removal of an ovary. This can also be functionally accomplished with medications and radiation therapy.

Open angle glaucoma: Glaucoma secondary to malfunction of the absorption of aqueous fluid.

Operating microscope: Special scope which can be used in surgery for delicate procedures i.e. eye surgery, neurosurgery, microvascular surgery.

Optic nerve: Nerve from the retina to the brain.

Orchiectomy: Surgical removal of the testicle.

Organ of Corti: Sensory organ of hearing in the inner ear.

Organic: Associated with life.

Oropharynx: Portion of the pharynx below the soft palate and above the hyoid bone.

Orthopedics: The study of normal and pathological conditions of bones, joints, muscles, ligaments, etc. All aspects of the locomotion system.

Orthotopic: In a normal position.

Ossicles: Hammer, anvil and stirrup; the tiny bones of the middle ear.

Osteoarthritis: Degenerative arthritis.

Osteoblasts: Bone-forming cells.

Osteoclasts: Cells which destroy unwanted bone.

Osteocytes: Bone cells.

Osteosarcoma: A cancer of bone.

Otitis media: Middle ear infection.

Otoscope: Lighted instrument for looking into the ear canal at the eardrum.

Ovaries: The oval shaped organs, one on each side of the uterus at the end of the Fallopian tube, which produce ova.

Oversewing an ulcer: Treatment of a perforated ulcer, often use a piece of adjacent fatty omentum as a patch.

Ovum: Egg oxygenated blood: Blood which has passed through the lungs and has given off CO_2 and taken on O_2.

Pacemaker: A part of the heart in the atrium that initiates the heart beat; any artificial device that stimulates the heart to beat regularly.

Paclitaxel: A chemotherapeutic agent.

Palliation: The alleviation, but not cure of disease; cancerous or noncancerous.

Pancoast tumor: A lung cancer at the apex of the lung.

Pancreas: An upper mid-abdominal gland with endocrine (insulin and glucagon) and exocrine (enzymes) functions.

Pap smear: A smear of cells from the vagina and cervix to detect cancer.

Papanicolaou: Physician who devised the Pap test.

Papillary: Having small to microscopic papillae or fronds.

Paralysis: Inability to move.

Paraparesis: Weakness of the lower extremities.

Parathormone: Hormone produced by the parathyroid gland; increases calcium level in the blood by mobilizing it from bone.

Parathyroids: Tiny glands in the neck behind the thyroid which regulate Ca levels in the body.

Paresis: Weakness.

Paresthesia: Any abnormal sensation.

Paronychia: An infection around the fingernail.

Parotid gland: Salivary gland at each side of the face in front of the ear.

Patent ductus arteriosus: Congenital failure of the ductus arteriosus to close in the newborn causing circulation and oxygenation problems. Easily repaired by cardiac and pediatric surgeons.

Pathology: The study of disease.

PDS: A synthetic material used for sutures and grafts.

Pectoralis muscles: The large muscle on either side of the front of the chest; "The Pecs"

Pectus excavatum: Congenital maldevelopment of the front of the chest which makes it concave inward; funnel chest.

Pectus carinatum: Congenital maldevelopment of the front of the chest where it protrudes outward; pigeon or chicken breast.

Pediatrics: The study of children and their diseases.

Pedicle: A stalk by which a growth is attached.

Pelvis: The bone formed by the ilium, ischium and the pubis.

Penicillin: An antibiotic.

Penis: Male urethra.

Percutaneous: Through the skin.

Perforation: Hole or opening.

Pericardium: The sac of tissue surrounding the heart.

Perinephric abscess: A collection of pus around the kidney.

Perineum: The area between the thighs containing the external genitalia, rectum and urethra.

Periosteum: Tissue covering bone.

Peripheral vascular: Pertaining to the vascular system outside the heart.

Peristalsis: The normal movement of the intestine propelling food and liquid forward.

Peritoneum: The tissue covering the surface of the intraperitoneal organs and lining the inside of the abdominal and pelvic walls.

Peritonitis: Inflammation of the peritoneal cavity.

Permanent prosthesis: As opposed to temporary expander in breast surgery. The final implant.

Pessary: An instrument placed in the vagina to alleviate prolapse.

PET - Positron emission tomography scan: A diagnostic tool for imaging parts of the body.

Pfannenstiel's incision: Low transverse incision in the abdomen frequently used for Cesarean section and gynecological surgery.

Phalanges: Bones in the fingers or toes.

Phantom pain: Pain felt in a missing limb.

Pharynx: The part of the digestive tract above the esophagus.

Phlebitis: Inflammation of a vein.

Photophobia: Light sensitivity; dread of light.

Photoreceptor cells: A rod or cone cell in the retina.

Physical therapy: Physical treatment of injury, pain, and disease using many modalities including active, passive and ambulatory therapy.

Physiology: The study of how things function.

Pia mater: A fibrous membrane over brain tissue.

PIC line: Peripheral intravenous cannulation. An IV site.

Pilonidal: An infection in the intergluteal fold and extending to the sacral prominence usually caused by ingrown hair. Treated by wide excision and packing.

Pingueculum: A yellowish thickening of the conjunctiva sometimes seen in the elderly.

Pink eye: Acute conjunctivitis.

Pinworms: Enterobius vermicularis; a tiny white worm infection of the GI tract often in children causing anal itching. Medically treated.

Pituitary gland: Hypophysis; a small gland in the center of the brain producing many hormones such as TSH, growth hormone, ACTH, FSH, prolactin, et al.

Placebo: A harmless or inactive substance given as medicine: used in double blind studies to test the efficacy of a new drug; some get the drug, some get a placebo.

Plain catgut: Absorbable suture material made from sheep intestines.

Plasmapheresis: Process of removing blood, separating out the plasma and reinfusing the cells as treatment for certain diseases.

Platelets: Thrombocyte; disc shaped blood particle important for clot formation.

Platinum based: A type of chemotherapeutic agent.

Platysma: The superficial musculature of the neck.

Pleural effusion: Fluid in the chest cavity.

Pneumonectomy: Surgical removal of a lung.

Pneumonia: Inflammation of the lungs.

Pneumothorax: Air in the chest cavity outside the lung causing lung collapse.

Polypropylene: A synthetic suture material.

Polyp: A mass of tissue that projects outward; usually a tumor either benign or malignant.

Port-A-Cath: An intravenous access device with a tube attached to a capsule placed in a pocket made under the skin. The tube is placed in a large vein. The port is accessed by a special needle.

Portal hypertension: Increased pressure in the portal circulation from many causes, most commonly caused by cirrhosis of the liver.

Posterior repair: Surgical repair of a rectocele.

Posterior chamber: Anatomical part of the eye behind iris and pupil anteriorly and the lens and ciliary body posteriorly.

Potassium: An electrolyte chemical in the body.

Premalignant: Changes in a tissue which are felt to be indicative of possible transformation or development into malignancy.

Priapism: Painful, tender, persistent erection of the penis; a pathologic rather than sexual condition.

Primary injury: The first causative problem which may lead to many secondary problems; i.e. a heart condition may lead to hypotension, kidney failure, pneumonia, etc.

Proctitis: Inflammation of the anorectum.

Progesterone: Hormone of the corpus luteum of the ovary; used in oral contraceptives.

Prolapse: A falling out as with the uterus or rectum.

Prolene: Synthetic material used for suturing.

Prostate: A gland at the base of the bladder having a secretion discharged with the semen at the time of ejaculation.

Prostatectomy: Removal of the prostate for benign or cancerous condition.

Prosthesis: Artificial substitute for a missing part of the body, i.e. leg, knee joint, etc.

Prosthetist: Specialist in fitting and designing prosthetics.

Proteins: Compounds built of amino acids and needed for growth and repair of the body.

Prothrombin: Clotting Factor II.

PSA - Prostate specific antigen: Normal at low levels; when elevated indicative of prostate enlargement and possibly prostate cancer.

Pseudocyst: A cystic mass developing in a pathologic situation as pancreatic pseudocyst.

Psychiatry: The medical specialty concerned with the diagnosis and treatment of mental disorders.

Psychologist: A PhD or MS specialist dealing with psychological problems.

PT - Prothrombin time: Clotting factor II.

Pterygium: A degenerative condition of the conjunctiva which may partially cover the cornea.

Ptosis of breasts: Drooping of the breasts.

Ptosis of eye: Drooping of the eye.

PTT - Partial thromboplastin time: Test for blood clotting; heparin will increase the PTT.

Pubis: Pubic bone.

Pullthrough procedure: Surgical procedure for reconstructing the rectum after resection of rectal mucosa and lower colon as in Hirschsprung's disease.

Pulmonary embolism: Blood clot in the pulmonary artery circulation of the lung.

Pulmonary angiogram: X-ray of the pulmonary artery to evaluate for pulmonary embolism.

Pump team: The special technicians that run the extracorporeal circulation and oxygenation pump during open heart surgery.

Pupil of eye: The hole in the center of the iris.

Pyloric stenosis: Hypertrophic pyloric stenosis.

Pyloroplasty: A surgical procedure to widen the pyloric outlet of the stomach.

Quinton catheter: A double lumen tube inserted into a large vein and used to place a patient on a hemodialysis machine for renal failure.

Quadriplegia: Paralysis of all extremities.

Quinsy: Peritonsillar abscess.

Raccoon sign: Black eyes sign of basilar skull fracture.

Radiation therapy: Treatment of cancer with radiation.

Radical mastectomy: Surgical removal of breast, pectoral muscles and skin with an axillary lymph node dissection.

Radioisotope: A substance that emits radiation and can be used for body image studies.

Radiology: Diagnosis and sometimes treatment of disease using x-ray technology.

Radius: One of the two bones of the forearm.

RBC - Red blood cells.

Reach To Recovery: American Cancer Society program of recovering breast cancer patients talking with and helping newly diagnosed patients of same age and similar prognosis.

Rectal exam: Digital exam of the rectum.

Rectocele: Protrusion of the rectal wall into the wall of the posterior vagina.

Rectovaginal fistula: Pathological connection between the rectum and the vagina.

Recurrent laryngeal nerve: One of two nerves that supply the vocal cords.

Reduction mammoplasty: Making the breast smaller.

Referred pain: Pain from disease of an organ which is felt in another area of the body: i.e. gallbladder disease may present as left chest pain mimicking a heart attack.

Refractive corneal surgery: Surgery, usually laser or LASIK, on the cornea to correct myopia or hyperopia.

Regional enteritis: Crohn's disease; chronic recurrent granulomatous disease of the ileum and colon.
Riedel's struma: Fibrous benign thyroiditis.
Renal: Relating to the kidney.
Renal cell carcinoma: Cancer of the kidney.
Renin: Substance produced by the kidney when the renal artery is narrowed, which converts angiotensin one to two and causes elevation of blood pressure; renovascular hypertension.
Renovascular hypertension: Renin/angiotensin system caused by narrowing of the renal artery.
Replantation: Reconnecting an amputated body part.
Resectable: Surgically removable.
Resectoscope: Urological instrument for examining the bladder and surgically removing bladder or prostate disease.
Resection: Removal.
Retention suture: Large sutures placed at intervals in a wound to hold it together; usually for very sick patients with poorly healing wounds.
Retina: Light sensitive rear part of the eye with neuroreceptors for vision.
Retinoblastoma: Malignant tumor of the eye of children.
Retinopathy: Disease of the retina.
Retroperitoneum: Behind the peritoneum.
Rheumatic heart disease: Infectious heart valve disease which may lead to severe valvular disease eventually requiring surgical correction or replacement.
Rheumatoid arthritis: Probably autoimmune disease causing polyarthritis.
Rhinitis: Inflammation of the mucous membranes of the nose.
Rhinoplasty: Plastic surgery to change the size and shape of the nose.
Rhinorrhea: Drainage from the nose.
RIND - Reversible ischemic neurological deficit.
Rods and cones: Neuro visual receptors in the retina-rods for black and white, cones for color vision.
Roentgen, Wilhelm: Discoverer of the x-ray.
Roux-en-Y: A surgical procedure for making connections between intestine using a Y configuration - *see* Chapter 35.
SA - Smokers Anonymous: Self help group to stop smoking.
Sacral: Relating to the sacrum.
Salivary gland: Gland in head and neck producing saliva; the parotid, submandibular and sublingual glands.
Scabies: Skin pathology due to a mite, Sarcoptes scabiei.
Scalpel: Surgical knife.
Scar contracture: Narrowing of a scar in time.
Sclera: Part of the eye; the "white" of the eye.
Sclerosing adenosis: Benign breast disease with severe scarring and thickening.

Scoliosis: Lateral curvature of the spinal column.

Scrotum: Sac containing the testes.

Sebaceous glands: Skin glands secreting fatty, oily substance called sebum.

Sebaceous cyst: Cystic skin mass with sebum; retention cyst.

Second look procedure: Reoperating on a patient, usually the abdomen to check on the status of a cancer or infection or the intestines.

Secondary sexual characteristics: Sexual characteristics which develop because of the action of hormones on a gland or body; breasts, hair distribution, etc.

Secondary injury: Pathology which follows a primary bodily insult.

Segmentectomy -lung, breast, liver: Removal of only a part of an organ.

Sensory nerve: Nerve that reports sensation of feeling, position and touch; as opposed to motor nerve.

Sentinel node: The first node draining a particular area.

Sheath: An enveloping structure as a nerve sheath.

Sigmoid colon: The S-shaped segment between the descending colon and rectum.

Silk suture: A type of surgical suture.

Silver nitrate: An applicator stick with silver nitrate used for cautery of wounds.

Simple closure: Suturing a wound closed with individual sutures in the skin.

Simple mastectomy: Removal of the breast tissue leaving the muscles and axilla.

Sjogren's syndrome: A decrease in the secretion of saliva or tears.

Skene gland: Glands at the entrance to the female urethra.

Skin: Largest organ in the body.

Skin graft: Transfer of skin from one area of the body to another for coverage.

Skin sparing mastectomy: Mastectomy done through a very small periareolar incision for better cosmetic results.

Skull fracture: Broken bone in the skull; "depressed" if bone is pushed into the brain substance.

Small intestine: Duodenum, jejunum and ileum.

SCLC - Small cell lung cancer: A lung cancer which has often spread to other areas by the time of diagnosis and difficult to treat.

Sodium: Part of sodium chloride; salt NaCl, a body electrolyte.

Spermatic cord: The tubular structure going from the testicle to the urethra through which sperm passes during ejaculation.

Sphenoid sinus: One of the paranasal sinuses connecting with the upper nose.

Sphincter of Oddi: Muscle at the end of the common bile duct.

Sphincter: A muscle that surrounds a duct or tube.

Spinal cord: Continuation of the nervous system from the brain down the spinal canal.

Spinal stenosis: Narrowing of the spinal canal sometimes causing spinal cord or nerve root compression with symptoms.

Spinal anesthesia: Anesthesia achieved by temporarily paralysing the spinal nerves by a needle placed in the back.

Spine: The vertebral column.

Spinothalamic tract: Nerve tracts carrying sensation from the body to the brain.

Spleen: A lymphoid, vascular organ of immunological significance located in the left upper quadrant of the abdomen under the left diaphragm.

Split thickness graft: Skin graft where only a small layer of skin is taken to cover another area of the body.

Spondylolisthesis: A condition where the lumbar vertebrae may slide forward and back on one another sometimes causing nerve root compression.

Squamous cell carcinoma: Cancer arising from the squamous epithelium.

Stage 0 cancer: Cancer in situ; cancer which has not yet developed the ability to spread or metastasize.

Staging for cancer: A recognized system for grading a cancer on the basis of size, cell type, location and presence or absence of involved lymph nodes and distant metastases.

Staples: Metal clips much like paper staple which are used to close skin, connect loops of intestine and close off open ends of tissue.

Stenosis: Narrowing.

Stenting: Placing an artificial tube inside a duct or vessel to keep it open or dilated.

Stereotactic biopsy: Three dimensional x-ray guided biopsy.

Steroids: A large group of chemicals such as hormones, anti-inflammatories, etc. produced by the body or synthetically.

Stomach: The sac between the esophagus and the small intestine which produces acid and enzymes for digestion of food.

Strabismus: Heterotropia, squint; uncoordinated action of eyeball muscles.

Strangulated hernia: An incarcerated hernia where the blood supply to the incarcerated tissue has been impaired with threatened death of that tissue.

Steri-Strip: A paper wound dressing which sticks to the skin for wound edge approximation.

Sty: Hordeolum.

Subarachnoid bleed: Bleeding, usually arterial, in the subarachnoid space of the brain.

Subcutaneous tissue: The tissue directly under the outer skin layer.

Subcuticular suture: Closing the skin by placing sutures in the subcuticular tissue, like hemstitching where the suture does not show on the surface.

Subdural hematoma: Bleeding in the subdural space of the brain; usually venous.

Sublingual gland: Salivary gland under the chin.

Submandibular gland: Salivary gland under the mandible.

Suprapubic: The area above the pubic bone; the lowest midline section of the abdomen.

Suture: Material used for sewing.

Sweat gland: Gland in the skin which produces perspiration.

Swollen glands: Refers to enlarged lymph nodes.

Syme: A type of foot amputation.

Symphysis pubis: The frontal area of cartilaginous connection between the left and right pubic bones.

Synarthrodial: Articulation of two bones without a moveable joint such as the symphysis pubis.

Syngeneic: Pertaining to genetically identical individuals.

Synovium: Membrane over a joint or tendon.

Syphilis: Venereal disease caused by Treponema pallidum, affecting first the genitalia but which can become systemic.

Systemic disease: Disease process which involves not just one organ but the entire body.

Systole: The contraction phase of heart function when blood is expelled from the heart.

T&A - Tonsillectomy and adenoidectomy.

T-cell lymphocytes: Lymphocytes involved with immunity.

T3 T4 T7: Laboratory tests for evaluating thyroid function.

Temporal bone: Skull bone underlying the area of the ear and containing the inner ear.

Tendonitis: Inflammation of a tendon.

Tessio Catheter: A chronic hemodialysis access catheter.

Testicles: Male reproductive glands.

Testis: Testicles.

Tetralogy of Fallot: Complex congenital abnormality of the heart.

The pump: Extracorporeal oxygenation and circulation machine.

Thiotepa: Chemotherapeutic agent.

Thoracic: Pertaining to the chest.

Thoracic outlet syndrome: Condition where the nerves or vessels exiting the neck into the arms are compressed by bony or fibrous structures causing symptoms of numbness or pain.

Thoracoscopy: Examination and treatment of intrathoracic conditions using a lighted scope passed through the chest wall.

Thymoma: Tumor of the thymus, which may be benign or malignant, sometimes associated with Myasthenia gravis.

Thyroid: Ductless gland in the neck which secretes thyroxine and controls metabolism.

Thyroidectomy: Partial or total surgical removal of the thyroid.

Thyrotoxicosis: Extreme hyperthyroidism.

TIA - Transient ischemic attack: Transient diminished brain function usually due to decreased blood flow.

Tibia: The inner-side bone of the lower leg.

Ti-Cron: A synthetic suture material.

Tinnitus: Ringing in the ears.

TNM staging: Tumor size, lymph node status and presence or absence of metastasis for evaluating a cancer.

Tobacco: A leaf containing nicotine which when smoked can cause lung and other cancers.

Tonometry: Measurement of pressure in the eye.

Tonsils: Lymphoid tissue; the lymphoid tissue at the back of the throat.

Total knee replacement: Prosthetic knee joint for reconstructing severely diseased knee.

Total hip replacement: Prosthetic hip joint for reconstructing severely diseased hip.

TPN - Total parenteral nutrition: IV fluids given to ensure enough fluids and calories when an individual cannot take food in the GI tract for a long period of time.

Trachea: Segment of the respiratory tract between the larynx and the main bronchi.

Tracheoesophageal fistula: Pathological condition where disease, tumor or injury to the esophagus or trachea has resulted in a connection between the two organs.

Tracheostomy: Surgical procedure where a tube is place through the skin in the front of the neck into the trachea to assist with cleansing the airway and lungs, and to place a patient on long term ventilatory support.

TRAM flap: Rotation of a segment of skin and subcutaneous tissue with its own blood supply from the abdomen to the chest for breast reconstruction.

Transmyocardial laser revascularization: New method of heart revascularization in patients whose vessels are too diseased to do the standard CABG procedure by making laser openings between the heart muscle and the inside of the heart.

Trauma: Emotional state I feel in writing this glossary.

Trephination: Opening into the skull by making a trephine or small circular opening.

Trichomonas: A parasitic disease of the vagina and urethra of women and the urethra and prostate of men.

Trochanteric: One of two large bony projections off the proximal, upper end of the femur.

Truncus arteriosus: Congenital heart abnormality where there is a common arterial trunk instead of a pulmonary artery and aorta.

Tubal ligation: Tying off the Fallopian tubes to prevent possible pregnancy.

Tubes: Fallopian tubes.

TUIP - Transurethral incision of the prostate.

Tumor: Any swelling - not necessarily a neoplasm (cancer or benign growth)

TUMT - Transurethral microwave thermal therapy.

TUNA - Transurethral needle ablation of the prostate gland.

TURP - Transurethral resection of the prostate gland.

Tympanic membrane: The ear drum.

Ulna: A forearm bone (with the radius).

Ultrasound: Use of soundwaves greater than 30,000 Hertz for diagnostic studies.

Umbilical hernia: Congenital hernia at the site of the umbilicus.

Undescended testicle: Congenital lack of testicle to come down into the scrotal sac.

Ureter: Muscular tube from the kidney to the bladder.

Ureteroscope: Lighted scope used to look into the ureter by a urologist.

Urethra: Tube from the bladder to the outside; the penis in males.

Uterus: Female muscular organ in which the fertilized ovum develops into a fetus/child.

UV light: Ultraviolet light; electromagnetic rays.

Uvea: The pigmented part of the eye; iris, ciliary body and choroid.

Vagina: The female genital canal from the vulva to the uterus.

Vaginal hysterectomy: Surgical removal of the uterus through the vagina.

Vagus nerve: 10th cranial nerve with multiple functions; motor and sensory fibers to the stomach, heart, voice box, etc.

Varicocele: Abnormal dilation of the veins of the spermatic cord.

Vas deferens: Excretory duct of the testis.

Vascular: Relating to blood vessels.

VAT - Vestibular autorotation test.

VATS: Video assisted thoracoscopic surgery.

Vein: Blood vessel carrying poorly oxygenated blood to the heart (except the pulmonary vein).

Vena cava: The largest vein in the body.

Vena cavogram: X-ray of the vena cava.

Ventral: The abdominal side, belly side, undersurface, anterior side.

Ventral hernia: Abdominal wall hernia.

Ventricle of brain: One of four fluid filled cavities in the normal brain.

Ventricle: One of the four chambers in the heart.

Ventricular septal defect: Congenital deformity of the heart where the septum between the atria or ventricles is partially or completely missing.

Ventriculo-peritoneal shunt: A tube with one end surgically placed in a ventricle of the brain and the other placed in the peritoneal cavity for hydrocephalus or increased intraventricular pressure.

Versed: A strong amnesic medication used to relax patients before surgery; and during and after procedures done under heavy sedation.

Vertigo: Dizziness; sensation of spinning.

Vesicovaginal fistula: An abnormal connection between the bladder and the vagina usually secondary to infection, surgical injury or tumor.

Vestibular system: Relating to the vestibular system of the inner ear; to balance and equilibrium.

Vicodin: An oral pain pill.

VIN: Vulvar intraepithelial neoplasia.

Vitamin D: Fat soluble vitamin important for calcium and phosphorus metabolism.

Vitreous: Jellylike substance in the eyeball and behind the lens.

Vocal cords: Voicebox; membranous folds across the larynx for making sounds.

Volvulus: A twisting of the intestine occasionally causing obstruction.

Von Willebrand's disease: A bleeding disease related to factor VIII deficiency.

Vulva: External female genitalia.

Vulvectomy: Surgical removal of the vulva for cancer.

Warts: Verruca, genital warts, venereal warts; sexually transmitted genital or anal growths caused by a virus.

WBC: White blood count.

Wedge resection - liver, lung: Partial removal of an organ with a pie-shaped excision.

Whipple procedure: Pancreaticoduodenectomy: Surgical removal of the distal common bile duct, part of the pancreas, and duodenum in an attempt to cure pancreatic cancer.

White matter: In the brain, medullated nerve fibers; having myelin sheaths.

William Harvey: Physician who wrote "De Motu Cordis" first describing the circulation of blood in 1628.

Wilm's tumor: Malignant kidney tumor of children; prognosis determined by the stage and onset.

Wrist bones: Navicular (scaphoid), lunate, triquetrum, pisiform, greater multangular (trapezium), lesser multangular (trapezoid), cuneiform (capitate), hamate bones.

Xanthelasma: Yellow plaques on the eyelid.

X-ray: Discovered by Wilhelm Roentgen, electromagnetic radiation used for diagnostic procedures.

Xylocaine: A local anesthetic.

Zenker's diverticulum: Outpouching of the pharyngo-esophageal junction in the neck; if large and symptomatic must be removed surgically.

USEFUL SURGICAL REFERENCES

Ballenger, John Jacob, M.D., *Otorhinolaryngology: Head and Neck Surgery*, 1996, Williams and Wilkins, Baltimore.

Campbell's Urology, 1998, W.B. Saunders Company, Philadelphia.

Canale, S. Terry, M.D., *Campbell's Operative Orthopedics*, 1998, Mosby, St. Louis.

Chase, Robert A., M.D., *Atlas of Hand Surgery*, W.B. Saunders Company, Philadelphia.

Chutter, Timothy A.M., M.D., *Endoluminal Vascular Prostheses*, 1995, Little, Brown and Company, Boston.

Cohen, Mimis, M.D., *Mastery of Plastic and Reconstructive Surgery*, 1994, Little, Brown and Company, Boston.

Danforth's Obstetrics and Gynecology, 1994, J.B. Lippincott Company, Philadelphia.

DeVita, Vincent T, Jr., M.D., *Cancer, Principles and Practice of Oncology*, Lippincott-Raven, Philadelphia.

Gellis and Kagan's Current Pediatric Therapy, 1996, W.B. Saunders Company, Philadelphia.

Grant, J.C. Boileau, M.D., *Anatomy*, 1962, The Williams & Wilkins Co., Baltimore.

Gray, Henry, M.D., F.R.S., *Anatomy of The Human Body*, 1959, Lea & Febiger, Philadelphia.

Harvey, James C., M.D., *Cancer Surgery*, 1996, W.B. Saunders Company, Philadelphia.

Howkins, John, M.D., *Shaw's Textbook of Operative Gynecology*, 1977, Churchill Livingston, Edinburgh.

Lee, K.J., M.D., *Essential Otolaryngology*, 1998, Appleton & Lange, Stanford, Connecticut.

Linton, Robert R., M.D., *Atlas of Vascular Surgery*, W.B. Saunders Company, Philadelphia.

Lucente, Frank E., M.D., *Essentials of Otolaryngology*, 1999, Lippincott Williams & Wilkins, Philadelphia.

Little Brown Handbook Series, The Little Brown and Co., Waltham, Mass.

Netter, Frank H., M.D., *The CIBA Collection of Medical Illustrations*, CIBA.

Schwartz, Seymour I., M.D., *Surgery*, McGraw-Hill, New York.

Rutherford, Robert B., M.D., *Vascular Surgery*, 1996, W.B. Saunders & Company, Philadelphia.

Vaughan, Daniel, M.D., *General Ophthalmology*, 1992, Appleton & Lange, Norwalk, Connecticut.

Vitale, Gary C., M.D., *Laparoscopic Surgery*, 1995, J.B. Lipincott Company, Philadelphia.

Walsh-Sukys, Michele C. M.D., *Procedures in Infants and Children*, 1997, W.B. Saunders Company, Philadelphia.

White, Robert R., M.D., *Atlas of Pediatric Surgery*, McGraw Hill Book Company, New York.

Zollinger, Robert M. Jr., M.D., *Surgical Operations*, 1993, McGraw-Hill Inc., New York.

INDEX